PROMISES TO KEEP

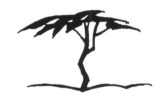

But I have promises to keep,
And miles to go before I sleep

STOPPING BY WOODS ON A SNOWY EVENING
Robert Frost

To our peerless daughters
Kim, Sophie and Rona

PROMISES TO KEEP

A British Vet in Africa

Hugh Cran

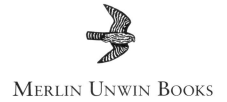

MERLIN UNWIN BOOKS

First published in Great Britain by Merlin Unwin Books, 2015

Published by:
Merlin Unwin Books
Palmers House
7 Corve Street
Ludlow
Shropshire SY8 1DB
U.K.

www.merlinunwin.co.uk

The author asserts his moral right to be identified with this work.

Designed and set in Sabon by Merlin Unwin Books

Printed and bound by Ertem Ltd STI Printing & Binding

ISBN 978-1-906122-97-3

CONTENTS

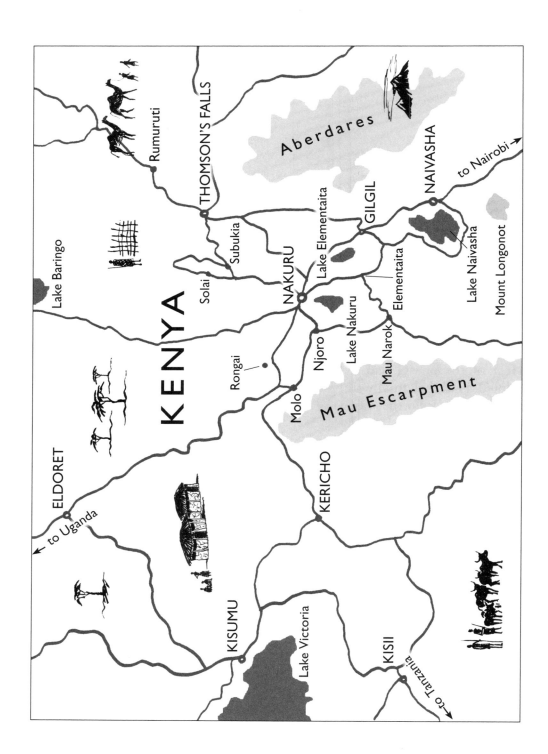

KENYA

Lake Baringo

Rumuruti

THOMSON'S FALLS

Aberdares

NAIVASHA

to Nairobi

GILGIL

Lake Elementaita

Elementaita

Lake Naivasha

Mount Longonot

Subukia

Solai

NAKURU

Lake Nakuru

Mau Narok

Njoro

Rongai

Molo

Mau Escarpment

ELDORET

to Uganda

KERICHO

KISUMU

Lake Victoria

KISII

to Tanzania

Chapter One

NIGHT GAMES

'Time to hit the sack,' I said to my Berna, my lovely and long-suffering bed-mate, 'I've got 140 cattle to pregnancy test at Beaumont-Bott's place on the other side of Eldoret at eight tomorrow morning. I'm going to have to get up at 5.30 in order get away by six.'

Eldoret was 100 miles away on the road to Uganda.

As I shuffled off to the bathroom, the phone rang. Berna lifted the receiver. 'It's the police,' she said. My heart skipped a beat. The Dixon of Dock Green type did not figure in the ranks of the Kenyan constabulary. Most of the ones I had met were narrow eyed, overweight and open palmed. Had they finally run me to earth for that time I had failed to stop at a road block on the way to Naivasha? Had the cop's hand been raised to stop me or was he just scratching his head? Naturally I had assumed the latter. 'It's the Dog Section,' said Berna. Major relief.

'Inspector Macharia here,' an authoritarian voice declared. 'One of our German Shepherds is sick.' Less relief. 'She ate all right at six, but now her stomach is swollen and she is trying to vomit and having difficulty in breathing. She doesn't look good. She's twelve years old but she's one of our best dogs.' *They always are,* I thought. I looked at my watch – 10pm.

'Right,' I replied. 'You'd better bring her to the surgery right away. This sounds serious.'

Berna came along to help me and we got to the surgery in short order. We arrived before the police. I opened the door, put on the lights and started getting things ready. 'This is probably torsion of the stomach,' I said to Berna. 'Happens in big dogs after a meal and a bit of exercise. Fatal unless treated very early.'

'So what do you have to do?'

'Probably open her up – ah, here they are.'

The police van screeched to a halt, headlights shining through the open door of the surgery. A posse of gendarmes marched in, leading a large German Shepherd bitch. She staggered slightly, stopped, salivated, lowered her head and made an ineffectual attempt to vomit. I palpated her abdomen. It was grossly distended, as tense as a drum and so hard that I feared to exert pressure lest I precipitate a terminal collapse.

I addressed the uniformed front rank. 'From what I can feel she's got a twisted stomach, which is now distended with gas. We've got to act fast, or she'll die very soon, so I want two men to stay to help. The rest can go.' A spokesman barked a command and Berna and I were left with the bloated patient and two cops.

'Right,' I said, 'first of all we have to give her fluids – i/v.'

'How much?' asked Berna.

'Well, she's about 35 kilos, so up to three litres. But we'll give her a litre and see how we go.' The policemen lifted the bitch onto the surgery table. I clipped the hair from her right foreleg below the elbow, and fed a catheter into her cephalic vein, attached it to a bottle of Hartmann's solution, held by Berna, and ran in the fluid. After fifteen minutes the litre was finished and the bitch looked no better. If anything she was worse, gasping and groaning.

'Let's give her another half litre and then try to get rid of some of the gas,' I said. I ran in the fluid.

'Right, lift her off the table and stand her on the floor. Let's see if we can pass a stomach tube.'

'A stomach tube for dogs?' asked Berna. 'I didn't know you had one.'

'I haven't, but I do have several sizes for horses. We'll try the yearling model.'

I placed a bandage roll in the bitch's mouth and asked one of the policemen to hold the mouth shut while I fed the tube through the middle of the roll. But try as I might it was impossible to pass the tube. I gave her an injection of Valium and tried again. No go. 'Right, we'll have to decompress the stomach with a large bore needle and then try again.' I rummaged in my surgical bag and located a 14 gauge cattle needle. I sterilised this, clipped an area over the bitch's right side, just behind the ribs, where the distension and tympany was at its maximum, sterilised that and pushed the needle through the skin and into the stomach. There was a rush of gas and a satisfactory deflation, before the needle became blocked with stomach contents.

'OK,' I said. 'Shall we try the stomach tube again?' This time the tube slid down and more gas was released.

'Right, a little more i/v fluid, and we're ready to open her up. Are we all ready?' Berna was. The two gendarmes looked less sure. Another litre together with i/v antibiotics, then the pre-med. The instruments were ready, the anaesthetic, ketamine, was not ideal, but I was strapped for choice. This was Africa, not Bognor or Brighton. The patient was now unconscious. We lifted her onto the table and I shaved her abdomen and clipped drapes over the incisional area.

'OK, here we go.' Very carefully I made an incision through the midline from sternum to umbilicus – carefully – as the last thing I wanted to do was to puncture a distended stomach and contaminate the abdominal cavity. As I cut, the distended stomach came into view, protruding through my incision, still distended, despite gas being removed by needle and stomach tube, as it was still rotated and still producing gas. The now visualised stomach was covered with the greater omentum, the lacy part of the mesentery which covers and protects this part of the abdominal cavity. Seeing this I knew that the stomach was rotated in a clockwise direction, as viewed from the dog's rear.

Something made me look up. One of the policemen had gone a strange grey-green colour. He was swallowing convulsively, which I knew was the horrid precursor to a burst of vomiting, the very last thing I wanted mid-operation. 'Out! Out!' I bellowed. He fled.

'And then there were three,' I said. 'On we go. Now I have to try and turn the stomach back to its correct position. But first I'd better deflate her a bit more. Berna, is she still breathing at your end?'

'Yes, looks fine to me.'

'Good, can you give me that cattle needle again. Thanks.' There was a welcome high-pitched hiss as I pushed the needle into the stomach and the mounded balloon sank until it was no longer under internal pressure. 'Great, here we go.' By pushing down on the right side of the stomach and pulling on the left, the organ slowly swivelled anti-clockwise, followed by its attendant spleen. 'Looks good,' I said, 'no sign of damage. The last thing I want to do is to resect a chunk of necrotic stomach wall. Then the outcome can be poor to hopeless. But I can feel big pieces of meat in here so we'll have to open the stomach, empty it, stitch it up and then stitch the stomach to the abdominal wall to prevent a recurrence of the problem.'

'Oh yes, and how do you do that?' asked Berna.

'You make a careful incision in the wall of the stomach, without going the whole way through, and then make another in the muscle of the nearest abdominal wall and stitch them together. They form a strong adhesion which prevents the stomach from twisting again. Simple!' Simple indeed, but it took me another hour to empty the stomach, close it up, perform the so-called incisional gastropexy and then close the abdomen. During this time I had to top up the anaesthesia. The bitch was coming round, I was pleased to see. When they don't come round, is when you worry.

My back was giving me stick. I had been bent over for what seemed like hours. 'Berna,' I asked. 'What's the time?'

'One o'clock.'

'Ye gods! And I've got to be on the road by six.' The sole remaining member of the forces of Law and Order was out on his feet, leaning against the wall, eyes half closed.

'Right, let's cut her down, give her some more antibiotic, and some more fluids and that's it. We'll put her in one of the kennels and keep her here for a few days to keep an eye on her. Nothing by mouth for the first day, then water offered on the second day and a little food, and then small meals three times daily and limited exercise.'

The bitch survived, one of the lucky ones. Many are found dead, having died within an hour or so. Others develop post-operative complications.

By the time I got to bed at 2am I felt that I was in imminent danger of developing post-operative complications myself.

But after a restorative three and a half hour's slumber I was up and by six on the road to Eldoret.

—∗—

Old B-B, as Beaumont-Bott was generally called, was an ex-submariner, with a neatly trimmed naval beard. As such he had everything shipshape and Bristol fashion when I arrived on the farm. The cows were lined up in the crush, heads to the right, backsides to the left, just as I liked them to be. Hot water was in abundance, together with soap and an array of towels. Soft fluffy ones to care for the hands, hard hairy ones for forearms and upper arms. And the other hands, namely the rustic farmhands, were drilled to perfection. B-B, wearing a nautical peaked cap, sat on a sort of wooden poop deck, directing operations and writing down my findings as I shouted them out. By 11.30 we were finished. By 12.30 I was cleaned up, had a spot of much-needed tiffin and a small glass of port and was on my way back to Nakuru. I rolled into the surgery at 2.30 to find it packed. Dogs were barking, cats were miaowing, there was even a goat bleating in the corner. By the time I had dealt with them all it was after five and I still had three farms to visit, including a cow with a prolapse.

I was home by eight, in the dark. The light dims rapidly on the equator and by seven the light has gone. The house girl had left for her well-deserved repose but Berna had the hot dinner waiting as I staggered in. 'Gad, what a day!' I gasped. 'An early night tonight I think. Can't wait to get the old head on the pillow. But the good news is that the bitch we operated on during the night is doing fine.'

'Wonderful!' said Berna.

I tucked into the hot meat pie and pastry, the house girl's speciality, followed by my favourite – rhubarb crumble. 'Ah, that's better. Thanks so much for that! Now I think I'll take a cold beer from the fridge and have a good soak in the tub. Try to unwind.'

'You do that. You deserve it.'

I lay back in the tub, sipping my beer and letting the hot water do its soothing work. I closed my eyes. I was still at Eldoret, B-B was bellowing at his workers and my arm was up a cow's rectum. Then I was behind the wheel of my Peugeot, dodging potholes. I swigged my beer, placed the bottle carefully on the floor and promptly fell asleep. But I wasn't asleep because what was that ringing noise? Then knocking. 'Hugh! Hugh! Mike Higgins is on the phone! He says that his Alsatian has been gored by a hippo and that its guts are hanging out! Can you speak to him?'

Groaning and gasping I hauled myself out of the bath, water flooding all over the floor. Wrapping a towel around my midriff I tottered to the phone. Mike lived on the shores of Lake Naivasha, 80 kilometres from Nakuru. 'Hi Mike, what's happened?'

'Hello, Hugh, I put my Alsatian bitch Sukari out into the garden so that she could have a pee and there was this ruddy great hippo on the lawn. Lifted her into the air with its enormous canines and when she came down her innards were hanging out. The hippo took off when I shone a torch into its eyes.'

'Right, you'd better get her here fast, but first soak a clean sheet in warm water and wrap it around the intestines and try to keep Sukari from standing up. Make sure you have someone holding the sheet in place until you get here.'

'Right, I'll be at the surgery in about an hour. I'll bring the askari to help.'

I put the phone down. I glanced at the clock on the wall. Nine pm. Mike should be arriving at about ten. Same as last night. Setting a pattern. I returned to the bathroom, collected my discarded raiment and put them back on. So much for the early night!

Once again Berna and I made a nocturnal trip to the surgery and prepared a tray of instruments in readiness for the arrival of bitch number two. At five minutes to ten Mike's Land Cruiser roared round the corner and screeched to a halt. Once again blinding headlights shone through the open door of the surgery.

Berna and I went out to help.

Sukari was lying on the back seat, swathed almost entirely in an enormous white sheet. Only her nose was visible. Sitting beside her was the askari (security guard), a ferocious looking individual, clad in a greatcoat which looked as though it had seen service during Napoleon's retreat from Moscow. Mike hopped out of the driver's seat and all four of us, very carefully, carried Sukari inside the surgery. As we did so an oversized raindrop fell on my forehead, followed a second later by a clap of thunder. Heavy rain began to fall.

Once inside, the first job was to weigh the patient on the scales, before undoing her shroud. This done we carried Sukari through to the operating room and laid her on the table. I undid a corner of the sheet and peeped inside. A coil of blue intestines met my gaze. I quickly closed up and gave her a pre-med injection. As I was scrubbing up I asked Mike why he had called his bitch Sukari – Swahili for sugar. He laughed. 'I just love '*Some Like It Hot*', that wonderful black and white comedy with Marilyn Monroe, Tony Curtis and Jack Lemmon. In the film her name was Sugar.' Sugar was now well sedated. I gave her a half dose of anaesthetic. Didn't want to shove her over the edge. I could top her up later as required.

We lifted her onto the operating table, laid her on her back, secured her legs and removed the sheet.

'Ye gods!' I exclaimed. A ragged open wound extended from her umbilicus to her pelvis. A mass of looped intestines hung to one side of poor Sugar. Bits of grass and dirt were stuck to the exposed vitals. Gently I lifted the intestines and laid them on a clean surgical drape. 'Berna,' I said, 'can you bring a litre of warm Hartmann's solution so that we can clean up this mess.' I picked off the debris and washed the exposed intestines until I was certain that no foreign bodies were left. Now we had to clean and shave Sugar's abdomen, without contaminating the eventrated viscera – a delicate and tedious task. I examined the intestines with care, looking at their colour, checking the pulsation of their blood vessels, searching for any punctures and leakages. All looked well. But we had to move fast. The exposure of intestines is a deeply shocking event, and can quickly lead to irreversible decline.

'Right,' I said, 'let's get this lot inside where they belong.' As I spoke there was a deafening clap of thunder, followed almost simultaneously by a blinding flash of lightning, and all the lights went out, plunging us into total darkness. But Berna was up to the crisis. Ever since we had had a night-time puncture on the Rift Valley escarpment when coming back from a right royal reception in Nairobi, she had always carried, on her person, day and night, a small powerful torch. Assisting in the replacement of a wheel in a howling gale, when you are eight months pregnant, with only a candle stub for fitful illumination is not something you wish to repeat in a hurry. Some people carry Swiss army knives, others ivory handled pistols, Berna had her Mini Maglite. She whipped it from its secret hiding place and we continued with the replacement. More warm Hartmann's solution to irrigate the abdominal cavity, then the painstaking business of stitching the muscles, the subcutaneous tissues and finally the skin. Intravenous fluids, antibiotic and we were done. As I gave the final injection the lights came back on. Sugar was waking up, and we looked at each other in relief. Mike laughed. The askari grinned.

'OK, Mike, you can either leave her here overnight, we'll check her in the morning and let you know how she is, or take her home. We've no night nurse. It's up to you.'

Mike opted to leave her. Sukari/Sugar recovered from her encounter with the hippo, finally dying many years later of old age.

—*—

I was a British vet in Africa, in Kenya's Rift Valley Province, based in the town of Nakuru, former capital of the White Highlands. After graduating from Edinburgh in 1963 I had worked for three and a half years in a large-animal practice in Aberdeenshire, in the north-east of Scotland. Tiring of the incessant rain and snow, the grey skies, cold winds and winters which seemed to extend into summer before starting all over again, my thoughts turned to sunnier climes. Nurtured on a literary diet of H. Rider Haggard and *Sanders of the River*, my overheated imagination saw me in Africa, a noble young pioneer, battling against exotic diseases in an exotic land, aided in my chosen task by a small band of faithful native followers, all clad in the colourful accoutrements of their particular tribe. Aged 26 I set forth for East Africa in December 1966 to take up a job as assistant vet to a hard-boiled Welshman. After about 14 months, a patient in the form of a hump-backed Zebu cow took objection to my ministrations and broke my right leg in several places, landing me in hospital for several months. Upon my discharge my employer announced that he was exhausted, having done the work of two men for the past six months, and that he was off to Mombasa and the coast for a spot of much-needed rest and relaxation. And that was the last I ever saw of him. He had done a moonlight flit and, in a small plane, had taken wing not to the coast but to Rhodesia, as it was then, the craft laden with saleable booty in the form of Persian carpets, game trophies and sundry exotica, but, most importantly, minus receipts of payment from the Income Tax Department to which he owed considerable sums.

He also owed me considerable sums, having paid neither my statutory health insurance nor any wages during my sojourn in hospital. Almost categorised as a Distressed British Subject and down to my last centime I wondered what to do. Help came in the shape of a group of local farmers who formed a company to keep me afloat, until able to stand on my own feet.

I ran the practice single-handed, as described in my book *And Miles To Go Before I Sleep*, working day and night and taking little time off, until in late 1978, I decided that I was also due a little rest and relaxation…

Chapter Two

A Trip to the Lake

Something flashed by my window.

Well-chilled beer in hand, I was a passenger in a Toyota Land Cruiser, and rather more than halfway to Ferguson's Gulf, on the western shores of Lake Rudolf, in Kenya's northern deserts, heading for the Fishing Lodge.

Getting away had been difficult, as usual.

It was October 1978 and things in my veterinary practice in Nakuru, in Kenya's Rift Valley Province, were brisk.

The plan was to spend the night in the town of Kitale, at the foot of Mt. Elgon, on the road to the lake. Kitale was four hours from Nakuru. In Africa a journey is measured in hours, not in miles or kilometres. The state of the road is all, whether it is dirt, rock, mud or bitumen. Kitale was 130 miles from Nakuru and the road was good. We had to leave not later than 3pm in order to get there before dark. Not easy, when the phone was ringing and clients were queuing in droves, all expecting the instant, personal touch, from the daktari.

The morning had been enlivened by a request to deal with a donkey which had fallen into a pit latrine, a cow having difficulty giving birth, a horse with biliary fever and a mysterious note from one Miss Hiroko Watanabe asking me to treat her dog for 'fukuhuom'. After much cerebral dredging I realised that she was referring to 'hookworm'!

My companions were the 'Rongai Rake', curly-headed Dick Davenport, his new wife Aileen, and stepdaughter Agnes. Dick's reputation as a lady's man had been somewhat diminished since his recent nuptials, but his enthusiasm for fishing and beer remained undimmed. Aileen was from Aberdeen, with an accent abrasive enough to rasp through pressed steel whenever she opened her mouth, which was pretty much all the time.

We were to meet at Dick's farm and to join up with other enthusiasts at the lake. The farm was 25 miles from Nakuru, so I had to leave at 2.30pm. I dealt with the last patient, an Asian-owned hound with flea bite dermatitis. The dog had been brought in by an African orderly. Asian owners rarely demeaned themselves with this undignified task. I made for my car, parked ready for a quick getaway in Club Lane, outside the surgery. As I did so, the round, cherubic features of Emilo Ferrini appeared over the swing door. Emilio had an apology of a moustache befouling his upper lip. It looked as though he had spent time with a large chocolate ice cream and had then wiped his mouth with the back of his meaty hand, leaving an unpleasant smear.

Despite his rotund appearance Emilio must have had something which attracted him to members of the opposite sex. If he had been a dog I would have put it down to pheromones. Clustered closely around him was usually a trio or more of dusky maidens.

I often wondered how he earned his daily fix of pasta and martini.

Emilio was one of Life's time-wasters. He certainly spent a lot of time wasting mine.

'Hello, Emilio,' I said. 'How can I help you?'

'Buon giorno, daktari,' Emilio replied. 'Can you have a look at my dog, Benito? He's got something wrong with one of his eyes. It looks a bit poppy. I've just come back from safari and it doesn't look too good.'

'Right, whip him in. I'm just trying to go on safari myself.'

This mild irony was lost on Emilio, who, after giving his fatuous soup strainer a fond caress, rolled through the swing door, dragging a small Heinz 57 behind him.

I looked at the patient and my heart sank.

The left eye was protruding from its socket by a good inch. The corneal surface was dry and abraded, dead and lifeless.

'Emilio, what the hell has happened here?' I expostulated as I bent to examine the desiccated orb.

'Dunno,' he replied. 'Maybe a fight wi' anoder dog. Perhap de askari hit him wi' da rungu. I've been gone for a week. Fishing at Malindi.'

He gave a smirk.

I wondered what species of fish he'd been after.

'Well, whatever, there's only one option here and that's enucleation.'

'Beg pardon?'

'Remove the eye, cut it out, it's past its prime, lost its value.'

'OK then. When?'

'Now, this very moment. I should be on my way to Rongai, so let's get on with it! Moses! Get me a tray of instruments, please, chop chop!'

Moses was my trusty Kikuyu assistant, who had worked with me since my arrival in the country 12 years before, over hill and down dale, through thick and thin. Mostly thick, it seemed to me.

Time was of the essence if I was to make it to Rongai and catch my lift with Dick to the land of the Turkana and their great Lake.

'Hey doc, you mind if I stay and watch,' asked Emilio.

'No probs, old son,' I replied.

Instruments sterilised, laid out and ready to hand, patient weighed, I prepared the intravenous anaesthetic – sodium pentobarbitone. I clipped the hair over the right foreleg in front of the elbow. Moses pressed his thumb into the angle of the elbow and the cephalic vein appeared. I swabbed the skin with spirit and slipped the needle through the skin and into the vein and trickled in the sleeping draught until Benito slumped forwards, breathing softly and slowly.

A little more and I was ready to begin.

I clipped the eyelids together with tissue forceps and gave them to Moses to hold while I made an incision, encircling the lids, peeling them back until I was able to dissect the globe from the surrounding tissues and lift it from the bony orbit. Carefully I clamped off all bleeding blood vessels and stitched the cut lids together.

'There we are Emi…Hey Moses, where's Emilio?'

'He rushed out soon after you started cutting. He looked a bit green.' Moses grinned.

'Right,' I said. 'Let's put Benito into a kennel and I'll get cleaned up. I've got to get going. When Mr Emilio returns ask him to collect his dog at about 5pm, when he should be coming round and tell him I'll be back in 6 days' time, when he can bring him back for a check-up. I've spoken to the District Veterinary Officer and if there are any emergencies while I'm away he has promised to deal with them.'

For the second time I strode purposefully towards my car, a Peugeot 504 saloon, and this time got in and drove away. In those days the mobile phone had yet to be invented, so once away no one could contact me. Free at last!

I roared down the tarmac road towards Kampi ya Simba and Dick's Kula Mawe Farm. Fortunately for me, radar speed detectors were also some way into the future and I flashed by a couple of somnolent gendarmes before they realised I was there. In my mirror I could see them gaping at my fast-disappearing rear.

I reached the farm at 4.30pm.

Dick was at ease on his verandah, sipping a pre-safari beer.

'Hi there Hugh! Good to see you! Have a snort!'

'He will not! You both get your backsides off those chairs.'

Aileen had appeared and was not in a good mood.

'So, Hugh, you've arrived at last I see. A bit late aren't we? Now we're going to be driving in the dark and getting to Kitale too late for a decent meal for poor wee Agnes.'

'Sorry Aileen, affairs of state, you know how it is.' I gave a light laugh.

'No, I don't.'

'Right, then,' interjected Dick, 'let's get on the road.'

Present day Land Cruisers are a far cry from those of 30 years ago. Moving passion wagons, dripping with every modern convenience, from wall to wall carpeting, electrically operated windows, air conditioning, to surround-sound and in-built television sets to ensure the cosseted passengers suffer no untoward discomfort. Dick's machine was spartan in the extreme. Bolt upright seats covered in an unpleasant, slippery plastic material, which was either icy cold or red hot, depending on the ambient temperature, metal flooring, windows which remained either jammed open or shut, and an all-pervasive stench of hot oil and diesel effectively prevented the occupants, no matter how exhausted they might feel, from nodding off. I sat up front beside Dick. Aileen and Agnes were in the back, which had been padded and upholstered with blankets and cushions to lessen their discomfort.

We clattered down the farm track and along the dirt road to the collection of shacks and hovels at Rongai. A few early inebriates squatting outside the ubiquitous drinking dens squinted at us as we trundled past. A crippled man scuttled on all fours across the road. A child waved. Women carrying water drawn from the nearby soupy river toiled along in the dust, eyes down, bent almost double. Goats rummaged busily in garbage, watched by a solitary, morose marabou stork, whose pendulous wattles sagged nastily beneath a hideous, red, naked neck. An avian undertaker with a cold, dead eye.

We reached the main tarmac road and turned right and up the hill, the western wall of the Rift Valley, towards Eldoret, and Kitale. Past The Jolly Farmer hotel and past the turning to Mau Summit and still upwards and upwards through cedar forest and stands of feathery bamboo, until we reached Timboroa. The nearby railway station was, at over 9000 feet, the highest in the British Empire. And the highest in Africa. I regarded it with the required reverence due to a hoary colonial relic, one of many, inanimate and animate, still extant in former British East.

Beyond Timboroa the road skirted a gloomy mere, fringed with reeds and rushes, climbed another hill covered with yet more bamboo and then descended towards the Uasin Gishu plateau. From here the Afrikaner settlers, who had struggled, with their ox wagons, up that formidable incline from Rongai in 1908, looked down upon the Promised Land, empty of people and dense with countless herds of game – zebra, kongoni, gazelle, giraffe and their attendant carnivores. The plain stretched ahead of us, now empty of game and full of homesteads and tin-roofed dwellings. Their owners were the successors to those dour bible-thumping pioneers who broke the land with ox-drawn ploughs and sowed the first crops the land had ever known. To the bearded Boers sitting on their little ponies it resembled the Transvaal as it had once been and was no more. But the wheel had turned and the Uasin Gishu plateau as it had once been was also no more and the Afrikaners had gone back whence they came, leaving the country when independence arrived. One chapter closed and another opened.

We rattled down the hill. The sun was declining to our left.

I peered through the window at the tangled crests of the Northern Tinderet Forest, wondering whether the mysterious Nandi Bear still lurked in those dark jungles. Known to the locals as the chemosit, it was much talked about, but seldom, if ever, sighted. A land-based equatorial Loch Ness Monster, albeit on a smaller scale. Was it really a bear, a giant hyena, a monster baboon, a tropical Yeti? When King Edward VII was crowned in 1901, five men of the King's African Rifles were present, one of whom was a Nandi. On being taken to the London zoo they were shown a chimpanzee. The Nandi whooped with delight, exclaiming 'There is the Nandi Bear!' Hundreds of years ago the forests of central Africa, including those of Uganda, probably connected with those of western Kenya. The nearby Kakamega Forest, a surviving remnant of the rain forest which once stretched in a continuous belt across equatorial Africa, is still home to many central African species of wildlife. So the most likely theory is that centuries ago chimps roamed the Nandi forests and this has become part of Nandi history and legend, oral and unwritten, but bearing nonetheless the smack of truth.

As the light dimmed I scanned the trees for signs of anthropoid activity, but saw nothing.

There was activity however in the back of the Toyota. Aileen was getting restive.

'Will ye just look at the time, Dick! Six thirty already and we know why, don't we? Aye! Poor wee Agnes will have to have some sustenance and soon. We'll have to stop in Eldoret for a bite before pushing on to Kitale.'

The accent was getting stronger.

'Right, we'll find somewhere.'

—*—

We rumbled down the main street, eyes peeled for a suitable eaterie. We passed Mama Juicy, the Get In Snack Bar, the Pork Palace, and the Tumbo Fill Restaurant before settling for The Black Horseman, ensnared by the neon-lit logo above the door, depicting a coal black armoured knight, seated on a rearing over-endowed stallion, transfixing a wretched lion on the sharp point of a spear, watched by a leering maiden, with breasts the size of watermelons tumbling unfettered from her decolletage.

Dick parked and stiffly we tumbled out. As we did so a ragged askari sidled up.

'Mimi ta chunga gari, bwana,' he told Dick. (I will guard the vehicle, sir.)

'OK, squire. I'll give you five bob if nothing is pinched when we come out.'

'Five bob! Ahhh! Sir! Sir! Give me ten, sir. I am a poor man, sir. What can a man do with five bob?'

'I'll give you 7.50 and not a cent more.'

'Ahh, you are a hard man, sir. Give me the money then.'

'Chunga kwanza na peza mwisho.' (Guard first and then the money.)

The Black Horseman belied its flamboyant exterior. The décor was stark, the lighting dim and grim and the furniture, such as it was, unadorned, unwashed plastic. The place was half empty. In a corner a couple of technicoloured tarts sniggered together.

A grubby, bow-tied waiter shuffled forward.

'Welcome, misters and misses, Karibu! Karibu! (Welcome! Welcome!) Please being seated while I am bringing you the menu.'

The menu suggested that a wide range of delectable, mouth-watering dishes was on offer.

We tried the waiter: 'Right, we'll have the grilled trout.'

'Sorry, we're out of trout.'

'OK, then, what about the prawn cocktail?'

'Sorry, no prawns, bwana. We are too far from the sea.' He gave a nervous chortle.

Last go.

'What about the roast lamb?'

'Ah, we are only having goat, sir. Will you have? Very nice and tender. Mmm!'

'Definitely not! Just bring a plate of chips, pesi, pesi!' (Quickly! Quickly!) 'We're in a hurry and the memsahib here is not to be trifled with!'

I glanced at Aileen. Her pinched nostrils had expanded until they resembled those speeded up plants in nature films which open with unbelievable rapidity when hit by the rising sun, or vice versa. Whatever the cause, the sight of Aileen's dilated spiracles had the waiter departing at high speed in the direction of the kitchen.

It did not bring him back at the same speed and after a lapse of 30 minutes Aileen rose and strode with purposeful tread in the direction of the kitchen. The sound of shouting was followed by the explosive entry of the wretched waiter, bearing a large plate of chips, closely followed by a triumphant Aileen.

The chips were revolting: limp, oily and slimy.

We did not tarry and after paying the askari, who examined his palm as though he had just detected the presence thereon of a malignant pustule, were soon on the road to Kitale.

Two kilometres outside the town, a police roadblock brought us to an unwelcome halt.

A battered sign, from which the original paint had all but vanished, requested the harassed traveller to STOP, as there was a police check ahead. Fifty yards further on, the feeble, flickering glow of a hurricane lamp indicated where a double set of road-wide spikes effectively barred onward progress. Here the gendarmes, invisible in their non-phosphorescent uniforms, awaited their prey. And, like most predators, their trap was well-laid. Unless one was aware that a road block lay ahead it was all too easy to come upon it unawares and more than one luckless driver found himself impaled on the spikes, surrounded by irate, but secretly pleased,

Officers of the Law. The distance between the spikes was niggardly, just wide enough to allow passage of a moderate-sized vehicle.

Dick coasted to a halt.

'Best to stop here until they wave you on,' he said. 'Creeping forward is an option, but you never know how they're going to react if you do that. And with the Old Man dying just two months ago these guys are bound to be a bit jittery. We don't want a sweaty finger slipping on the trigger, do we?'

The Old Man, Jomo Kenyatta, the Father of the Nation, had died in August and everyone was a bit on edge, watching to see how his successor, Daniel arap Moi, would cope.

A large dark figure approached.

Dick greeted it warmly.

'Evening, officer. What of the night?'

'Eh? Wat are you saying? Weh, mzungu! Wat are you carrying in here? Where are you going to?'

'To Kitale and then to Kalokol on the Lake.'

'Show me yo dliving licence.'

The proffered item was snatched from Dick's extended hand and scrutinised closely, even upside down. The policeman's torch was a faint glow, far too dim to read by.

'Toka, na fungua boot!' (Get out and open the boot!)

Dick muttered an imprecation, fortunately lost on the threatening presence at his elbow.

'Wat is all thees?' Encumbered by his gun, the policeman peered into the back of the Toyota, shoving things aside in an attempt to identify what he was looking at.

'Food, fishing rods, water, tools, spare tyre.'

'Give me samthing to keep me wam. We are cold standing here all night.'

'Beg pardon?'

'Nipa mimi chai kidogo.' (Give me a little tea – euphemism for bribe.)

'Aileen, darling!' Dick shouted, feigning ignorance. 'He wants some tea! To keep himself warm! Can you get me some tea bags, my love! Perhaps Darjeeling or Earl Grey?'

'Ach! Go! Go! Go!'

We went.

Soon we were passing Soy, stamping ground of a small relict herd of

Rothschild's giraffe. As we rumbled along, the moon rose and to the right we could see the rounded outline of the Cherangani Hills.

At Hoey's Bridge we crossed the Nzoia River. Early settler Cecil Hoey crossed the river by felling a tree across it and so it was named, until renamed Moi's Bridge, but as far as is known Mr Moi felled no trees across the river.

And so we arrived at Kitale, capital of Trans Nzoia, formerly called Quitale, a relay station on the slave route between Uganda and Bagamoyo on the coast opposite Zanzibar. The site of the slave market is now the Kitale Club and a circle of stones in the car park is said to have surrounded a ring to which slaves were chained at night.

We did not spend the night at the club but at the house of long-time Kitale resident, George Manuel, a welcome haven after the rigours of the day. George always looked as though he had just got out of bed, due to his spiky coiffure, which seemed to have a perverse will of its own, growing in several directions simultaneously, sideways, backwards and forwards.

Ham and eggs, a couple of Whitecaps and we were ready for bed. Even irritable Aileen seemed to have unbent sufficiently to be able to converse in tones which left my eardrums almost intact.

It had rained heavily during the night but the morning dawned fresh and clear and the massive bulk of Mt. Elgon – Ol Doinyo Ilgoon – the Mountain Shaped Like A Breast, unseen during our nocturnal approach to Kitale – loomed mightily over the rising land to the west. An extinct volcano rising to over 14,000 feet, divided between Kenya and Uganda, it dominates the surrounding area, which is fertile and thick with farms growing everything from apples and pears to wheat and maize.

We reloaded the Toyota and set off on the long leg to the Lake.

From now on the road would be all unsurfaced earth, dirt and rock.

As we dropped off the end of the tarmac I could see that attempts were being made to carpet the road and that earthmoving equipment had done a good job of converting what had in all probability been a fairly decent dirt road into something resembling a cross between a tank training ground and a freshly ploughed field. The nocturnal deluge had left long stretches covered in water and the rest was a choppy expanse of sloppy red mud, through which Dick drove the Land Cruiser like the captain of a cross channel steamer leaving port in stormy weather.

By the time we had covered the first few miles the Toyota was no longer jungle green, but rust red with road foundation and the windscreen was layered with a thick patina of the stuff that Maasai like to plaster on their hair. The Toyota springs were stiff and the upholstery unyielding and after Dick had hit a few potholes and I had all but brained myself on the roof as I was catapulted upwards, my thoughts towards the builders of the new road were less than charitable.

My sufferings were to a certain extent dissipated by the passing scene, which was green and pleasant. The peasantry were busy in their fields, the maize was as high as an elephant's eye and the outliers of the Cherangani Hills formed a pleasant backdrop to the rustic prospect. All sorts of sprightly birds zoomed or cruised hither and yon – herons, ibis, storks, crowned cranes, doves, hoopoes, hawks and hornbills. Now and again with a flash of red and violet a turaco rocketed from one thicket to another. To our right, seldom-seen sitatunga antelope lurked in the Saiwa Swamp. We certainly saw none.

The road itself seemed swampy enough to contain several herds of the semi-aquatic creatures. We ploughed along, swerving to avoid vehicles inconveniently embedded in the mire, grinding through stretches of Passchendaele-like bog, scrabbling frantically to avoid slithering into ditches and watercourses and, on occasion, moving sideways when the vehicle encountered a section more slippery than usual. Dick was one of those drivers who resolutely refused to engage four wheel drive unless absolutely forced to do so. He seemed to consider it unmanly and as a result we were all over the place as he struggled to keep the Toyota on the straight and narrow. Aileen voiced her disapproval from the rear in her high-pitched Aberdonian twang.

Kapenguria was drawing nigh and as it did so road conditions improved, until, by the time we passed the turn off to the town, the mud had gone.

Kapenguria was the remote one horse town in which Jomo Kenyatta and his henchmen were taken for trial for managing Mau Mau, after their arrest by the colonial authorities. According to one violently anti-British American authoress, Kapenguria then had no rail service, hotel, phones, restaurants or courthouse. It sounded most attractive to me.

Beyond Kapenguria we climbed steeply, through pine woods and onto a jutting spur of the Cheranganis. To our left the land fell sharply away into the valley of the Suam River, whose source was in the caldera of Mt. Elgon. The line of the distant river could be seen by following the green vegetation and trees growing along its banks, before it vanished behind hazy blue hills and into the Turkwell Gorge.

Almost immediately the road dropped in a vertiginous swoop down towards the hamlet of Chepareria and the valley of the Marun River and the Marich Pass. The road was rocky and rough. Mud was now a thing of the past. Stones rattled beneath the Toyota as we crashed downwards. To our right the Cheranganis soared coolly upwards to over 11,000 feet. Down in the valley we sweltered in ever-increasing heat. I drew a breath of overheated air and Chepareria was in our rear, a few dusty shacks quickly returning to torpor and lassitude after the brief excitement of our unquiet passage. We did a half circle around the mini-mountain Morobus, crossed the river and clattered ever downwards.

We were now well into the country of the Pokot, formerly called the Suk, a pejorative appellation which did not please them one bit, especially when used by their enemies, such as the Turkana. The Pokot were black, very tough and very traditional, wearing little in the way of clothing, and carrying spears and guns. A naked warrior festooned with bandoliers and carrying a rifle with studied nonchalance on his sinewy shoulder was now a common sight. In the township of Ortum they strolled to and fro among the market stalls, examining the merchandise displayed by their womenfolk, who sat, legs stretched out, before piles of vegetables, water containers, sisal ropes, twists of chewing tobacco, sandals and gourds, their necks loaded with mounds of red and blue beads.

Below Ortum the road narrowed and grew ever more rocky and rubbly, until it was a gravelly thread clinging precariously to a ledge above the right bank of the Marun. Behind us the land soared up and up to the summit of Sondhang, while to our front leapt the mighty mass of Sekerr. The brown river roared and thundered in its bed, falling over waterfalls, curving around huge boulders and rushing down rapids.

The river was progressively squeezed between the mountains until we entered the narrow defile of the Marich Pass, the final barrier before the open plains beyond.

We emerged from the pass and turned sharp left and crossed the river by a suspension bridge, the wooden timbers rumbling beneath our wheels. On the other side we stopped for a break and a bite to eat.

The air was hot, humid and still. Huge acacia trees lined the brown river. Doves cooed contentedly in the branches. The water gurgled musically under the bridge.

Pokot women were dipping gourds and plastic containers into a pool. Others were washing babies. I leaned over the side of the bridge and watched the water carriers who combined sinuous grace with strength and balance, a bit like ballet in slow motion. First the woman would squat down and with one rhythmic movement sweep the container onto her head, following this with an upward uncoiling of her body until she was erect. Then, gliding smoothly across the pebbles and sandy surface of the bank, torso swaying, head virtually motionless, she departed towards her distant homestead.

A group of children appeared and stood silently watching us eat our sandwiches. They did not beg for sweets nor ask for money, a pleasant contrast to their urban counterparts, who would by now be clawing at us, and whining for shillings. Not for the first time I thought that, the further you get away from civilisation, the more civilised do people become.

A column of ants stopped and surrounded crumbs dropped from my sandwich.

A white-bellied go-away bird flew across the river – 'gaarr, warrr! gaarr, warr! go awaay! go awaay!'

This avian omen was ignored in the interests of progression towards the distant lake and we pressed on northwards into the sandy wastes.

The road ran wide and flat through a dry and desiccated land. Grey scrub, low withered trees, empty expanses of gravel plain, shimmering hills on the distant horizon, all baking beneath a brassy sun in a brassy sky. Despite the seeming total aridity there was sparse life, gleaning sustenance from what seemed to my pampered eye to be the next best thing to total desert. A few fastidious camels were snacking on shrubs which looked as though they had died in the previous century, a flock of goats with wild, yellow eyes nibbled on a sweep of shale, a brace of dik dik peeped out from beneath a pygmy thorn tree and in the quivering distance was the solitary figure of a man, striding across the barren wilderness. There was something noble and brave about that small, dark figure, alone in the desolation, moving with seeming intent and purpose towards some goal, known only to himself. The sight of that little resolute form made me realise that here man had neither been crushed by his surroundings nor had he conquered them. Instead he had adapted his life to his environment and had assimilated what he could from what most people would regard as the worst of situations.

We rattled on.

Innumerable dry watercourses bisected the road at inconvenient intervals, necessitating constant braking and lurching into the sand and over the rocks and up the other side. Complaints about the standard of driving came our way from the upholstered rear.

The sun grew ever higher and the heat was intense. Sitting on the west side of the Toyota I was spared the direct rays but to the east poor Dick was getting the full treatment.

'Hell, Hugh, man. I'm being fried alive here. Got to have a cold Tusker before I pass out! Let's stop and open the cool box.'

I concurred readily with this sensible suggestion.

Chilled beer in hand we felt much better and even the road now didn't seem so bad. A few kilometres further on we snapped open another Tusker. After all in the present heat the beers were not going to remain cool for very much longer and we easily persuaded ourselves that a cold one now would do us much more good than a warm one later on.

Thus it was as we sped, relaxed and happy, over the endless ruts and corrugations, that something flashed by my left window and vanished, wraith-like, into the thin bush.

'What the hell was that?' I said to Dick.

'Search me,' he replied and then, 'Shit! shit! shit! Something wrong with the steering! Something very, very wrong with the steering. Bloody hell!' And from the back came loud screams as the hindquarters of the Toyota did a wild fandango.

I glanced up and about 500 yards ahead saw a camel give a wild skip as I now saw what had zipped so smartly past my window – the left rear wheel, travelling at the speed of Superman.

I clutched my beer to my bosom as Dick fought wildly to retain some semblance of control.

Luckily for us the road at this point was wide with shallow ditches – a bit like a rocky airstrip in fact, but even so I knew that with only three wheels when there should be four our forward progress was going to be severely limited.

And so it was.

With a horrid crunch of metal on rock and stone the left axle met terra firma. Out of the corner of my eye I saw a great shower of sizzling sparks leaping into the red-hot morning, together with a fountain of dust and pulverised gravel. The Toyota swung sharply to the left, but Dick, like a Great War pilot crash-landing his stricken Sopwith Camel, was up to the job. He sharply applied left rudder and steered into wind. We did a three point landing into the shallow ditch and came to a ragged stop.

My beer, I was gratified to note, was unspilt. There's nothing worse than the stench of sun-dried beer on your only pair of shorts. I took a deep swig. It was still cool. Very nice.

We waited for a few seconds for the dust to clear and then opened the doors and got out. No one spoke. I noticed a go-away bird sitting in a nearby tree, watching us.

The silence was almost palpable. A small waterfall of shattered road fell tinkling from somewhere inside the Toyota's innards onto the visible upper half of the left brake drum. It hissed gently. The lower half was ground several inches into the detritus of the ditch. The vehicle was tilted so far to the left that the right front wheel was almost off the ground.

I could feel the onset of acute marital discord as Aileen opened her mouth to say her piece.

'Right, then,' I said. 'I'll go and look for that wheel.'

I had a long way to go, following its track – almost a kilometre. The desert was flat and, apart from the jumping camel, had offered no obstacle to a runaway wheel. The wheel rim was hot and the holes for the nuts were large and ragged. I trundled it back to find Dick and Aileen engaged in bitter dispute.

'It was your job the check the vehicle. I was getting all the food ready.'

'I was up to my eyes on the farm. I couldn't do everything.'

'I knew that garage was no good. They didn't tighten the nuts did they? Did they? Now look what's happened!'

I also looked. The wheel nuts hadn't just come off. The studs to which they had once been attached, however loosely, had sheared clean off. We had a wheel, but no means whatever of re-attaching it to the vehicle. We were snookered, up the creek in fact, with no paddle or indeed any means of moving under our own steam. We had adequate provisions for the moment but this did not look like the sort of place in which a stay would offer much comfort. I looked around. Nothing but sand and splintered rock and a few spindly trees. Nothing moved. Even the go-away bird had gone.

'Where are we?' I asked Dick.

'About 20km from Lokichar, which is about 80km from Lodwar, which in turn is about 60km from the Lake.'

'So, still more than 100 miles to go before we see the flesh pots of the fabled Jade Sea, eh? And what's at Lokichar?'

'A police station, a couple of dukas and a mission.'

'Looks like someone's going to have to go for help?'

There was a silence. I looked up. Three pairs of eyes met mine.

Aileen was the first to speak. The Aberdeen accent was strident and shrill. I could imagine her on the docks, clad in oilskins and gumboots, flogging a tray of cod or haddock to a reluctant crowd.

'Yes, Hugh, you have to go. I'm a married woman and Dick's a married man and we can't send our poor wee Agnes, can we? You're single and have no family commitments and, besides, you have to atone for arriving late yesterday and making us risk our lives in the dark. Isn't that so, Dick?'

Dick nodded mutely.

'You'd better get out on that road to stop the first vehicle that comes along.'

It looked as though I might have to wait a long time, in the heat and the non-existent shade, but half an hour later I heard the distant rattle of springs and suspension stressed to their limits. Out of the shimmering, juddering haze materialised a travesty of a lorry, emblazoned with a sinister logo, Prison Break. I hesitated for a moment before raising my arm, but only for a moment.

The lorry ground to a lumpy halt, covering me in a pall of fine dust.

'Habari, bwana, naweza saidia?' (What news, sir? Can I help?)

A large, round black face with a melon-sized grin gazed down at me from the cab.

'Mzuri, asante. (the news is good, thank you – what was I saying!) Can you give me a lift as far as Lokichar? Our gari has had an accident.'

'So I see.' The grin widened until it threatened to disappear round the back of his head.

'Get up!' I walked round the front of the lorry and climbed up and into the cab. The tunny boy, sitting there, laughed and moved over and we ground away towards Lokichar.

'Karibu!' (Welcome!) he smiled.

Neither man was wearing a shirt and the heat in the cabin was intense.

The lorry was carrying cement and building materials to Lodwar and had left Kitale before we did, so somewhere along the way we had passed it on the road.

'You passed us coming through the Marich Pass,' said the driver. 'Aha! Going too fast! You wazungu have a saying I think – about the tortoise and the hare – ha! ha! – then we were the tortoise! Now you are the tortoise! And we are the hare!'

He threw back his head and gave a great guffaw, to which the tunny boy added his voice. I joined in the merriment, somewhat less enthusiastically.

'This is a very bad area,' said the driver. 'Here the Pokoti and the Turkana meet, and, my word, they are not liking each other! They are always fighting, shooting each side with guns, using spears, stealing their goats and camels and cows. Where you broke down is the very worst place of all. Not too long ago there was a big battle just over that hill you see there. Twenty people killed.'

He shivered dramatically. I felt a trifle chilly myself, despite the heat.

After forty minutes of being bounced up and down like a pea on a drum my spine felt as though it had been re-modelled by a blunt instrument. But it was all in a good cause and I knew that help would soon be at hand once I reached the mission.

The tatty township of Lokichar hove into view – a few ramshackle dukas, the police station, which looked as though paint had not been applied to its outside wall since independence, and the mission. Although it was only late morning every patch of shade seemed to hold its complement of sleepers, crashed out and unconscious, oblivious to our arrival, which, judging by the somnolence of the place, was probably the highlight of the day.

I bade the driver and his mate farewell and walked into the mission compound. I scanned the inscription over the entrance to a large, rather intimidating church –German Lutheran Evangelical Mission. Right then. Whatever you do, Do Not Mention the War.

As I was thus engaged I heard a voice at my side – 'Ja? Can I be helping you?'

I turned. A large, pale sandy-haired European had crept up on me unawares. He was wearing what looked like a pair of slept-in pyjamas and a crumpled shirt of a nondescript earthy hue. On his feet he wore a pair of yellow socks thrust into a pair of open-toed sandals, whose length and breadth was such that they could have served equally well as snowshoes in the Yukon or as a surfboard on a big curler off Hawaii. He was tall and thin and stood looking down at me, blinking and screwing up his eyes against the light. I noticed that his face was covered in freckles and that his nose was peeling.

'Yes indeed,' I said. 'My friends and I are on our way to the Fishing Lodge at Ferguson's Gulf. Our Land Cruiser has lost a wheel and we're stranded about 20 kilometres from here. Do you have a mechanic or any spares to assist us to get the wheel on?'

'Stranded? Unt in a bad place, I tink. A few veeks ago two European vimen on horses zis way rode, unt de tribesmen speared de horses, unt vun was so bad it had to be shot. So!'

'Yes, stranded, and in a Land Cruiser like that one over there.'

'Ja, we are having just such a Land Cruiser, but of spares unt mechanic, nein. But I can for you try to radio ze Fishing Lodge. Let us go to mein haus.'

I almost said 'jawohl, mein Herr,' but stopped myself just in time.

The missionary house was a stark stone structure, the floor bare concrete. I followed the missionary into a small room. A few admonitory motifs in German script hung on the walls. At least I assumed they were admonitory – German script is like that.

A bead curtain separated this room from the next.

In that room I could hear the sound of children's voices. Then the guttural voice of a woman admonishing the children. She sounded as though she had a plug of inspissated sauerkraut stuck in her throat.

'Mein vife unt kinder,' said the missionary. 'I am hafing sex children.'

Vot else did he do in his spare time? I vondered.

In the corner of the room was a table upon which stood the radio for communicating with the outside world. It was covered in a fine layer of dust and it seemed to me that this missionary did not communicate very often.

He sat down and twiddled with the knobs and a burst of static filled the room. He twiddled some more. A faint, tinny voice could be heard, as though it was calling for help from the end of a very long tunnel.

The missionary shouted into the mike.

Answer came there none.

'Zat is ze lodge,' he said 'but zey are not hearing me. I vill try again.'

Try he did, but it soon became apparent that nothing that he said could be heard by anyone, least of all by anyone at the Fishing Lodge.

The room was hot and airless. Outside, the air quivered in the noon-day heat. Spirals of dust shimmied across the bare ground, lifting debris and light rubbish into the air. I longed for a drink, preferably beer.

The missionary looked at his watch.

'You vill excuse me, ja?' he said, and vanished behind the bead curtain.

For the next half an hour I was regaled by the clashing of knives and forks, the slurping of fluids, the occasional belch, the glottal gulpings as food moved, as it does, from mouth to gullet, and finally, sighs of contentment as satiety was attained.

By this time I should have been salivating in unison to the anvil chorus of Teutonic utensils but I was so parched that I feared that my responsible glands had withered to dry acorns from dehydration.

The bead curtain parted and the missionary reappeared, brushing crumbs from the corners of his lips.

'Now I vill take you back to your vehicle. Zere iss nothing more I can do for you.'

I bowed. 'You are too kind,' I said.

Half an hour later I was back where I had started from, having accomplished nothing, but wiser in the ways of missionaries, German ones at least. This one decanted me from his Land Cruiser, executed a nifty three point turn and shot away back to Lokichar.

I could see Dick and Aileen looking on, jaws sagging.

Aileen was the first to speak.

'Now who on earth was that? That didnae stop to pass the time o'day?'

'That, Aileen, vos your Chermann missionary unt help us he cannot. He has no spares unt no mechanic.'

'Well, whatever he is, he's certainly no Good Samaritan.'

'That's for sure. The bugger didn't so much as offer me a glass of water. God, my mouth feels like the floor of a parrot's cage. I need a blimmin drink.'

I staggered over to the leaning Toyota and poured myself a much-needed beer.

'Ah, that's better,' I said. 'Now what?'

'Well, you'll just have to try again, won't you? The others, apart from the Perretts of course, will be way ahead of us by now, so they can't help.'

The Perretts from Mogotio were also coming to the Fishing Lodge. The only problem was that their view of time was decidedly elastic, and whether they would come on one day or another was a question to which even they were unlikely to be able to give a firm answer. John was married to Amanda, daughter of Jasper Evans of Rumuruti, whose own regard for the passage of the sun across the firmament was nothing if not flexible. North of Rumuruti watches were regarded as ornaments worn only by the effete.

'Right, I'll just have one more beer for the road. It might be my last!'

I gave a hoarse laugh.

Dick lay supine in the shade, eyes closed, chest rising and falling gently and rhythmically. A small pile of empty Tuskers at his side suggested that he had not been entirely idle while I was Not Mentioning the War on his behalf in Lokichar.

Dick spoke, eyes still fast shut.

'Better get on the road, Hugh. There's a lorry coming.'

I could hear nothing. Then I heard the distant crunch of tortured gears. I supposed that Dick's closer proximity to Mother Earth had allowed him to feel the distant vehicular vibration through his prone frame, a bit like a frontiersman putting his ear to the ground in order to detect the stealthy footfall of an enemy Mohawk or Mohican, padding silently in his moccasins along the trail, tomahawk in hand.

I padded unsteadily to the trail myself, tomahawk and moccasin-less, and once again raised my arm as juggernaut number two approached.

Anxiously I scanned the lorry for the omnipresent logo – Jungle Boy it was. At least it wasn't Coffin Carrier or Night Crasher. The lorry, an ancient Bedford, slewed to a stop, covering me in yet more dust. I looked up at the cab. It was crammed full of people.

A strong smell of fish assailed my nostrils.

I inquired of the driver, a jovial Jaluo, whither he was bound. 'To Kalokol on the lake, to collect fish. Get in!' No questions asked, no demand for money, no raised eyebrows. 'Great, great,' I thought. 'All the way to the lake!'

I scrambled with difficulty into the cab. Difficult because the cab was chockablock with other travellers. Most appeared to be Turkanas and Somalis. They made room for me in the middle. This was kind of them I thought, until I realised that I was sitting next to the massive differential, which seemed to fill most of the cab. And it was red hot. Fountains of perspiration sprang from my forehead. I felt faint and giddy and closed my eyes. When I reopened them we were underway, but our forward motion was painfully slow. The road degenerated into a surface like a huge washboard with corrugations stretching from horizon to horizon. The lorry shook and juddered under the strain. We all shook and juddered in synchronous rhythm. The interior of the cab was packed solid with humanity and comfort was there none. Soon I felt as though my gluteals had been worn away and that I was now sitting on the very bones of my backside. The discomfort was real and urgent.

For hour after hour we bounced, crashed and clattered across a shimmering moonscape, crawling painfully northwards towards Lodwar. The road was awful and our progress snail-like. I could see the road far,

far ahead and knew that it was going to take an excruciating age to reach that desirable point. Instead I concentrated on the twenty yards on front of the lorry, watching the potholes getting nearer, vanishing beneath the bumper only to be replaced by another crop of even deeper cavities, into which we lurched and rocked and rolled like a sailing ship breasting an Atlantic swell.

Every now and again the lorry would stop and one of the passengers would get off and without a backward glance, stride off over the blasted heath and into the baking wilderness. There was not a house or living creature in sight and yet there was no hesitation here, no nervous scanning of the horizon for landmarks. This was home and they knew where they were. Whenever a passenger alighted I hoped that his or her egress would allow a little living space for the rest of us, cooped up as we were like cattle en route to the abattoir, but on each occasion my hopes were dashed. Despite the apparent emptiness of the landscape, without exception someone would pop up from behind the nearest bush or boulder and swarm up the side of the cab and force a way into the foetid interior. No one objected. This was Africa. Everyone was in the same boat. Perhaps, I thought, suffering seemed less if it was shared.

We carried on. Although the area was basically flat, this was not a view shared by 'Jungle Boy's' engine. At the slightest hint of an incline, imperceptible to my jaundiced eye, the driver would grind the gears down to a lower level and our speed would decrease until were being overtaken by our following and attendant dust cloud, which billowed though the open windows, adding to our shared discomfort. The Somalis, swathed in muslin and cotton, covered their heads and noses. The Turkanas and I held our breaths and nostrils.

Due to the heat and the constant engagement of low gear the engine was running very hot and we had to make several stops to replenish the radiator, which voiced its discomfort with a variety of sounds ranging from falsetto squeaks to basso profundo bellows. In the sandy luggas the Turkana were digging for water. The tunny boy would jump down with a plastic container and return with a few litres and replenish the steaming beast, and then it was on over the corrugations and into and out of the potholes and through the dust wallows in the heat and the glare.

After what seemed like an age I espied a few buildings dancing in the haze at the very limit of my vision. The Holy Grail, Lodwar, seemed rather less than holy when we finally lurched along its rutted main street. Other vehicles were few, but pedestrians were many, a considerable number apparently the worse for wine, judging by their sinuous and erratic gait. Several bodies were stretched recumbent in the shade of the canopy of the acacia trees which covered the town. The driver and tunny boy made haste to join this happy horizontal and vertical band, drew into the verge, hopped off and vanished at speed into the shadowy recesses of the Casanova Inn.

I was left alone in the cab, the other occupants having descended to go about their various businesses.

The heat was intense. My mouth felt dry and sticky. A reviving beer to restore whatever was left of the inner man was vital.

I clambered out of the lorry and at once felt the sun smite my skull with brutal force. I staggered into the quaintly named Stress Remover Kitchen Den. After the blinding light in the street I could barely see where I was. The customary brace of raddled whores leered in my direction. A couple of far gone drinkers were slumped over the bar, while another lay stretched unconscious on the floor.

Afraid of missing my lift, I rapidly downed four Tuskers. My hydration was soon restored, but my sense of equilibrium had been knocked for six, as I discovered when I strode confidently forth into the afternoon sun. The acacia trees swung wildly from side to side. Approaching pedestrians bounced up and down as though on pogo sticks. The street had assumed a steep upward gradient which wasn't there before. Up this I clawed my way, tripping over pebbles now magnified to the size of footballs. In the far distance I could see the lorry, which seemed to be inflating and deflating like a horrid tethered zeppelin.

I need not have hurried over my beer. Of driver and tunny boy there was no sign.

I tackled the steps into the lorry. Raising my right foot I placed it where I assumed the step to be. It met mid-air. I tried again and almost dislocated my knee as my foot came down with a crash onto the metal rung. Finally I stumbled into the cab, whose interior temperature had risen to what felt like the mid-hundreds. I slumped back, gasping from the effort. I leaned my right elbow on the vast transmission and gave a yelp of pain. It was still almost red hot.

For what seemed like hours I waited there, head expanding and contracting, pulse pounding, occasionally glancing at the swirling scene outside the dusty windows.

Finally driver and tunny boy appeared, swaying sinuously through the clouds of dust billowing up the street. A blast of rancid beer fumes accompanied them into the cab, to which I contributed my third.

We set off on the road to the Lake. The driver almost bent the steering wheel in half as he concentrated on an approximation of a straight line down the road. The tunny boy, slack jawed and glassy eyed, gazed vacantly into the middle distance. I followed his asinine example.

The country was desolate semi-desert, rolling hills covered in yellow gravel, sand and grey withered shrubs. There was no sign of mammalian life, animal or human. The occasional carrion bird, black and menacing, soared the skies, searching for the dead or near-dead. In my present state, I felt like the latter, soon to join the former.

We rattled on, gravel and stones rattling like uncoordinated castanets against the bottom of the lorry, pinging like ricocheting bullets into the surrounding bush.

After about two hours a distant flash of blue between the hills caught my eye. The Lake at last.

The sun was setting as we rolled into Kalokol. Turkana women, legs outstretched, blue beads glinting, sat in the doorways of their wigwams, watching our passing with unblinking obsidian eyes. Turkana men, carved stools in their hands, stalked to and fro like patrolling sentries.

We came to a stop at the water's edge, where heaps of dried fish made their presence felt by an almost palpable stench, which rose into the air along with clouds of buzzing flies. The air was thick with mosquitoes and soon my arms and legs were smeared with drying blood as I crushed them against my skin.

My next task was to get to the Fishing Lodge, which was at the end of a long curving spit surrounding a large lagoon – Ferguson's Gulf. I could see the distant lights of the lodge buildings. The only means of access was by water and I did not fancy swimming. Being bisected by a crocodile or hippo did not appeal. It had to be by canoe.

But, no matter where you are in Africa, even in the remotest of areas, help may be at hand.

Along the waterfront came a Turkana fisherman, so black he was nearly invisible in the darkness. He was carrying a kerosene lamp.

'Ajok, ragone!' (Hello, my friend!) I said, using the only two words of Turkana I knew. 'Naweza saidia na taa yako?' (Can I have the use of your light, please?)

'Ndiyo, bwana.' (Yes, sir.)

So we set up the lamp on a prominent rock and by using a piece of driftwood to cover and uncover the light, flashed what I hoped was a primitive signal to the lodge. For a long time I despaired of making any sort of contact. Then, finally, there came an answering flash of light and, later, the hum of a motorised canoe. Out of the gloom it came and grounded on the shingle. I stepped in and was soon buzzing over the glassy water of the lake.

I staggered up the sand dunes to the lodge and into the open-sided bar where I could see a number of figures seated on stools, voices raised in animated conversation. For a moment my presence remained unnoticed. Then, every head turned as one.

'Hello,' said one. 'Look what the tide's washed up.'

I spotted 'Mfupi' Mackay nursing a glass of whisky. 'Mfupi' means 'short' in Swahili. Mfupi Mackay was about seven feet tall, thin and gangly.

'Hello, Mfupi,' I said. 'I've got a bit of a problem.'

'Sit down, and spill the beans,' he said. 'Have a snifter.'

'No thanks, not this time.' I explained the situation.

'Look, see that chap over there? He's a mechanic. Name's Brian Boxwood. Australian. Lives in Kitale. That's him there with his friend. Came here by road and his pickup is parked at Kalokol. Perhaps he can give you a lift back to where your vehicle is stranded. I flew in so I can't really help.'

I approached the Australian and his 'friend'. They looked up warily from their beers. The Aussie had a long sallow face and long yellow hair. The friend was a slender, effeminate half caste. The Australian was wearing shorts so short they looked like swimming trunks. He looked up. 'Howeryoudoin' mate?' He had a high-pitched voice, an alto, if one were to use a musical term. 'Meet Willie.' 'Good to meet you, Willie,' thinking exactly the opposite, and – what the dickens has happened to the stout settler of yester year, the doughty digger, the swift swimmer, the bronzed veteran? Too many sheep and too few women? Both offered me hands which felt like damp haddocks.

Once again I explained my predicament.

'Not a problem, old son,' said the Antipodean. 'Be delighted to assist. Willie, my dear, I must leave you for an errand of mercy.'

Willie looked crestfallen.

'But I return the morrow morn.'

Willie still looked crestfallen.

I had not sat down and now Brian stood up.

'OK, then, let's go. Better take an askari with us in case your vehicle can't be fixed.'

In no time I was once again beached on the torrid Kalokol shore. Brian's pickup was not large and as we rattled back to Lodwar I tried to imagine how we were all going to fit into its limited space. With three of us at the moment encased in the cab there was barely room for Brian to change gear. I glanced at my watch. 9pm.

It was 1.3 0 in the morning by the time we reached the Toyota. Dick and Aileen appeared to be at the very end of their joint tether. Agnes was asleep.

'Where in Heaven's name have you been?' skirled Aileen. 'In the time you've been gone we could all have been murdered. What have you been up to? I bet you had more than a few drinks at the lodge, eh? I can smell beer from where I'm standing! If I struck a match we'd all go up like a Roman candle! You could have driven to Khartoum and back in the time you've been gone!'

Brian had his spanners out and was examining the offending wheel. He stood up. 'No go, mate. She's buggered. You need new studs. Got to get those from down country. There's none in these parts. Maybe we can get them flown to the lodge. We'd better transfer your kag and get going before we're jumped. We'll leave the askari to mind the vehicle.' The askari looked decidedly nervous when informed of his duties. He was a Turkana and this was hostile territory.

As we were in the process of moving stuff from one vehicle to the other we heard the rumble, rumble, rumble of a vehicle approaching from the south. Lights appeared.

'I bet that's the Perrets,' said Dick. 'They're always days late!'

'Stop them! Stop them!' shrieked Aileen. 'This horrid little pickup is far too small for all of us.'

We rushed for the road, waving and shouting. The lights came closer and closer, but the vehicle, recognised as an ancient Land Rover, maintained its steady and inexorable forward motion. It neither slowed nor accelerated and, to our incredulous gaze, trundled on past at a steady 25mph. It had no rear lights and so was very soon lost to view, and only the occasional rattle and thump and crash of stressed and fractured bodywork told us that it was there at all.

'That was them all right,' said Dick. 'Must be on autopilot!'

'Or something else,' muttered Aileen.

'Probably thought we were a Pokot or Turkana raiding party,' said Brian. 'Do I look like a member of a Pokot or Turkana raiding party?' asked Aileen.

No one was brave enough to answer that question.

Transference of goods and chattels completed, we bade the anxious askari farewell and set off on what I fervently hoped was my last trip to the Lake. Aileen and Agnes sat up front in the cab with Brian while Dick and I slummed it in the back, whipped by the dust-laden slipstream and subjected to the corrugations and ruts as the vehicle bounded towards the distant waters. The journey was not a comfortable one and the innumerable dry river crossings battered us into whimpering submission.

Half way between Lodwar and the Lake we came over the brow of a hill and came across what looked like a Bedouin encampment in the middle of the road. We had caught up with the Perrets, who had stopped for what remained of the night. Not expecting traffic they had not bothered to seek a better campsite than this thorn-free spot. We motored on past.

There was a faint light in the high eastern clouds as, at 5.30am, we reached still-sleeping Kalokol.

After a much-needed sleep in my quarters at the lodge, I arose with an effort and ate a much-needed breakfast. I wandered down to the water's edge with my fishing rod and cast a spinner into the deep. A sharp tug and a silver fish leapt into the air. I reeled it in. It appeared to be mostly bones and sharp teeth and I almost lost a finger in the process of removing the hook from its mouth. I was on the point of tossing it back into the lake when I felt a hand on my arm. I looked down and found a small knot of undressed, infant Turkanas clustered expectantly at my heels. The hand was now outstretched and I put the fish into it. The owner was delighted to be the recipient of a fish which the rest of humanity would have rejected as unfit to eat. The Turkana are a tough, resilient and resourceful people, living as they do in a barren, unforgiving land. They have learned that many things regarded as inedible by more fastidious tribes are not so. As a result they have survived and flourished where most people would have perished. I cast my line again into what appeared to be a ravening shoal of translocated piranhas and was pleased to supply the gathering mob with sustenance for several days.

The sun grew hot. I felt the damp sheen of sweat bedew my forehead. I turned to return to the lodge and as I did so I staggered and almost fell. 'Must be the heat,' I thought. 'Need some fluids.'

In the lodge I had an ale with Damien Fitzwilliam-Sproat, another participant in the beer and fishing fest. Damien was a professional charmer, as more than one fair maiden had cause to regret. He always looked as though he had just stepped fully-formed from the pages of The Field. Beefy, confident and giving the distinct impression that he was moneyed, titled and had access to unlimited acres of land, he seemed to dominate any company, attracting toadying waiters and simpering women in equal numbers. A product of Durham University, he cultivated a soft upper class accent. He would stare earnestly into a girl's eyes, hold her hand and swear undying love. She fell for it every time. When I came into the bar he was staring earnestly into a tankard of beer, probably planning his next conquest, I thought. I could imagine him back in England, in his green wellies, striding across the shires behind his pair of retrievers, or aboard his hunter, surrounded by yelping foxhounds, receiving a brimming stirrup cup from a fawning ostler. Or bombing up the motorway in an open roadster, a girl snuggled up beside him.

'Hugh, old fruit, you're looking a bit flushed. You've been overdoing it again. You must learn to relax. Like me. I've made a close study of how to take it easy. Look at me. Look at you. At this rate you'll be burnt out before you're 40. Get away more often. And if an animal or two dies as a result, so what? Better an animal dies than you die from overwork.'

'Sounds great in theory, Damien. Not so easy when you're self-employed. But I have to agree with you, although it took the most almighty effort to get away, with clients pursuing me half way to Rongai! If I'd slowed up for a second I'd still be there now. Well, if you'll excuse me I think I'll have a short siesta and then a swim. I feel a bit pooped.'

'Watch out for the crocs! I've been told that they don't usually attack people, but I wouldn't bank on it!'

He laughed.

A couple of hours later saw me bobbing about in the warm, green, slippery, mildly alkaline water of the gulf, keeping a wary eye on a log drifting on the surface a couple of hundred yards away. Pelicans soared overhead, a heron stood motionless in the shallows, smaller fry pottered about on the shoreline, prodding and prying, poking and probing. Such an expenditure of energy just to stay alive. On the other hand, I mused, how else would they occupy their time?

Later that evening, I found myself occupying my own time in the company of others, holding but not downing a beer. Aileen was already three parts drunk and was telling the world all about the privations she had endured en route to the lake. Mostly my fault, it appeared. Her strident voice cut through the hubbub like a chainsaw ripping through a fallen tree. I felt very odd. I sat there, fixed, anchored to my chair, speechless, unable to move. The noise around me increased, until it reached a roaring crescendo, waxing and waning, booming and softening in rapid succession. I went hot and cold. Faces swam around me like a shoal of drifting fish. I seemed to be expanding and contracting in an alarming fashion. One moment I filled the entire room. The next I had shrunk to the size of a molecule. Then I seemed to be floating, unconnected with my surroundings, off the ground, drifting up to the ceiling.

Everything went black.

When I opened my eyes I was lying on my back in the bar, staring up at a circle of anxious faces. Even Aileen was there.

'Whaaa...,' I tried to speak.

I had another go.

'What happened?'

Dick's face hovered above me. He looked like a large pink balloon. 'You had a sort of convulsion. Your head almost touched your heels! An amazing sight! Wish I had my camera. The bottle you were holding smashed on the floor and that's where you ended up as well. Waste of good beer. Bottle was almost full.'

'Good grief! Sorry about that. Well, I'd better try and get up.'

I tried and knew at once that there was something seriously amiss with my back. A sharp pain shot up my spine. It seemed to rush up and down my vertebrae like a demented yo-yo and then settled to an area between my shoulder blades. Movement was difficult so I decided that a period of rest was in order before trying again.

I closed my eyes.

When I opened them it was to see a young and attractive lady bending in a rather alluring way over my prone body. At once I felt rather better. She bent closer and I could smell her perfume, something understated and expensive. I felt it incumbent of me to meet her halfway. I half rose and once again my back felt as though someone was stabbing it with a red-hot knife.

I sank back onto whatever I was lying on – it felt like a blanket placed on the rough concrete floor.

The young woman bent closer and her blonde hair brushed my face.

'Do not try to move,' she said in a soft, Scandinavian accent. 'You may only make things vorse. I am a Svedish nurse vorking at Kalokol and vhen I heard that you were unvell I came over to see if I could help.'

'Many thanks,' I replied. 'I feel a whole lot better already for seeing you.'

She smiled. 'I will give you a pain killer and after a while we vill try to get you to bed.'

With practised movements she filled a syringe from an amber-coloured vial and slid the contents into my upper arm.

Her potion was a powerful one, and within a very few minutes I could barely keep my eyes open. A mattress materialised and upon this I was carried to my quarters.

I passed the night in what they call fitful slumber.

Morning brought little improvement to my discomfort, and walking was little more than an undignified, geriatric shuffle. Then I recalled having seen polio victims propelling themselves with singular speed and remarkable agility around the streets of Nakuru, using a stout pole. This ability I was determined to emulate.

Poles at Ferguson's Gulf seemed to be in short supply. A Turkana orderly was dispatched to scour the foreshore to see what the tide had washed up. He returned with a sun-bleached, wind-polished, nicely rounded wooden length. It looked like the mast of some small fishing craft. Probably lost in the lake with all hands. Sunk by the fierce harmattan-like winds which nightly howl across the Lake from Mt. Kulal on the eastern shore. Still, it's an ill wind, etc..

Poling was not without its difficulties, especially on soft sand. It was not a comfortable means of getting around and initially I tended to sag and sink to the ground when crossing the dunes which surrounded the lodge. However, with practice, I mastered the method and became quite an adept at the esoteric art of body poling.

A couple of days passed. I began to wonder how I would get back to Nakuru. Even if Dick's Toyota was repaired, my return in it was not to be considered. The corrugations would very soon render me hemiplegic.

Help was in the offing, however. The lodge manager, who rejoiced in the memorable name of Nutter, belied his appellation by requesting an incoming flying guest to convey Toyota spare parts in and my body parts out. The latter he would do after he had completed thrashing the Lake for Nile perch.

The fisherman was Lofty Reynolds, a rough-hewn farmer, whose rugged features had been rendered even more so by numerous bruising encounters on the rugby field, which had left him looking like an uncompleted masterpiece by the sculptor Rodin.

At the end of the designated period of piscine slaughter I was levered into his plane and we set off on the flight back to Nakuru. What had taken the best part of three days on the way up now took only three hours on the way down.

We landed at Nakuru Airstrip and taxied to the Club House, an establishment noted more for alcoholic indulgence than for things aeronautical. Seated at the bar was Byron Comis, Greek pilot and agricultural contractor. It was peculiarly gratifying to note how so many Greeks still held the English poet Lord Byron in high regard. The patriotic British thorax still, despite so many recent rebuffs and reversals, had occasion to expand with pride.

Byron gladly acceded to my request that he drive me to the War Memorial Hospital for assessment. Swiftly downing a pint of the Kenyan equivalent of ouzo, he slid off his stool and ushered me towards his battered Mercedes, whose exterior was seriously disfigured by bubbles of blistered paintwork and areas where there was no paintwork at all. With painful difficulty I inched onto the left front seat, the stuffing of which was protruding in several places as though some maniac had just attacked it with a sharp instrument. Of seat belt there was no sign and the back of the seat seemed to be jammed in an almost horizontal position. Comis cranked the gears and set off at a great pace, swerving round potholes and leaping over irregularities in the road surface as though it was a matter of life and death to get to the hospital in the shortest time possible. The journey was not a comfortable one and my back was not improved by the experience.

The matron of the hospital was no longer the formidable Scottish spinster, Miss Brown of myth and legend, but Mrs Victoria Fanshawe, a widowed lady of impressive bulk and stature, a woman of mature years and the possessor, not of an earthy Lowland Scot's burr, but of an aristocratic you-stay-in-your-place-my-man tone of voice. She liked to have the distinctions of rank well preserved.

The lady was present when Comis roared and rattled his way into the hospital car park, belching dense clouds of rank blue and purple exhaust fumes into the sterilised surroundings. I eased myself out of the Merc, thanked him for his help and, in gentle slow mo, perambulated slowly towards the matron's sanctum.

Knocking on her door was not necessary. It burst open as I approached, closely followed by Matron Fanshawe, snorting and heaving like a disturbed buffalo, nostrils dilated as though searching for prey.

'Who was that? Who was that? Coming in here, making that ghastly racket, befouling the air and disturbing the patients with his disgusting car. I want to know his name so I can ban the brute from ever coming here again.'

I knew the lady but slightly, but she knew me. That was her business and vocation.

'Who was that?'

Her massive abdomen pulsed with indignation. She seemed to be more concerned with venting her personal spleen than with what I was doing on the premises.

'That, Mrs Fanshawe,' I said, 'was a Good Samaritan,' and said no more.

She gave a harrumph and a grunt, and finally, after staring fixedly over my shoulder, as though willing Comis to return and face his punishment, turned to me.

'Well, Mr Cran, and what are you doing here?' The implication was that it had better be something serious – or else. Anything less than a coronary thrombosis or terminal injuries, would be an appalling waste of her valuable time.

I explained.

'Mmm, well, strictly speaking, you should have been referred by a physician, but in this case I'll make a very rare exception. I'll call the resident doctor, Mr D'Souza, and ask him to have a look at you. Come into my office and wait.'

She gave an upper class whinny and departed.

Mr Felix D'Souza was a Surgeon – with a capital S – and did not hesitate to let you know it, implying that he was doing you the most almighty favour merely by casting his lordly eye upon you. Hence the Mister D'Souza and not Doctor D'Souza. The pecking order seemed to run deep within the medical fraternity.

He was a Goan, of mixed Indian and Portuguese ancestry. Like many Goans he did not regard himself as strictly Indian, leaning more towards his European genes and his descent from the seed sown by Vasco da Gama and his conquistadores in the receptive wombs of the Indian maidens of the Malabar Coast.

After about an hour the man himself appeared. Tall, lean, bespectacled and of studious mien, he was not one with whom to bandy flippant quips and irresponsible jokes, especially those concerning the medical profession. Doctors, in his eyes, were gods descended from Mt. Olympus to graciously tend to the needs of undeserving mortals. To subject them to music hall comedy was disrespect of the lowest order.

'Well, Mr Cran, and what appears to be the matter?' was his initial remark – a stock medical opening which always seemed to me to cast certain responsibilities concerning the diagnosis upon the shoulders of the suffering patient.

I told him what had happened.

D'Souza said nothing, appearing to be wrapped in conjecture and differential diagnosis.

Probably thinking about his next golf tournament, I thought. D'Souza was an inveterate golfer.

He seemed to come to with a start.

'Right,' he said. 'We'd better get an X-ray done. We'll wheel you down to the X-ray department and take a few pictures.'

After the usual fiddling around in the semi-darkness, an acceptable X-ray was produced and presented to the good doctor for his professional assessment. He looked startled, pursed his lips, and almost whistled.

'Well, no wonder your back's painful. Your second, fourth and sixth thoracic vertebrae are broken. The vertebrae have collapsed, been crushed into half their original height.'

At this moment the bulky anterior of Matron Fanshawe protruded round the doorway, followed a few seconds later by her equally bulky posterior. I closed my eyes and shuddered. She took this to be a manifestation of ongoing discomfort.

'Right, Mr Cran. I couldn't help hearing Mr D'Souza here say that you've got a broken back. Into bed with you!'

'Yes,' interjected D'Souza, before Ma Fanshawe stole his thunder, 'until we know what caused that convulsion, we must keep you under close observation.'

I was incarcerated in a single room. D'Souza prodded, poked, palpated, auscultated, peered into my ears, shone bright lights into my eyes, tapped my skull and stared intently down my throat, in an effort to discover why I had had the convulsion. He was unable to come to any diagnosis.

Meanwhile, apart from a degree of sharp stiffness in my back, I felt in fine fettle, and I decided that alcoholic beverages were indicated. So I put out the word and was much embarrassed by the response. For the remaining six nights I spent at the hospital my lonely room was lonely no longer and reverberated to the clash of beer mugs, to the tinkle of tooth glasses and to the sound of song and laughter. Matron Fanshawe did not dwell on site, departing each evening to the comforts of hearth and home.

But it was not long before what was afoot reached her upper class ears.

For the first few nights all went well. Then Dick's father was admitted with a condition yet to be diagnosed. 'Par for the course!' I thought. Rumour had it that he was suffering from a heart condition, but it might just as easily have been dyspepsia. An insatiable omnivore, his feeding habits were random and voracious. He was housed in a room at the end of the corridor. An irritable blighter at the best of times, when the nightly parties got underway he complained in no uncertain terms to the night nurse, who made a note in the duty book. This came to the attention of Ma Fanshawe, who entered my boudoir the following morning, unannounced, patrician features empurpled with righteous indignation. Her authority had been flouted and she had come seeking vengeance.

'Mr Cran, it has come to my attention that you have been hosting nightly orgies in your room. Alcohol has been drunk. There has been noise, shouting, laughter, the peace of the hospital has been disturbed. I have even heard talk of women!'

'Just a few friends in to raise my flagging spirits, Matron. You wouldn't like me to get depressed, cooped up in here, all on my own, now would you?'

The matron snorted with such violence that the expiratory effort involved knocked her backwards against my modest locker and there was a clash of bottles from within – pleasantly musical I thought, and redolent of good times and good company.

Mrs Fanshawe thought otherwise.

'Right, Mr Cran! That's it! This locker and its contents will be removed forthwith. Any more nonsense from you and out you go. I don't care if you are recovered or not. There are other patients in here, including Mr Davenport, whose condition I have to consider, even if you don't. He is in a delicate state. He could easily die!'

'Fat chance!' I thought. 'The old brute's as strong as an ox.'

'Very well, Matron. I will do my best to keep my visitors under control. I am allowed visitors, aren't I?'

'Yes, but this is your last chance! One more incident and you are out!'

Mr D'Souza was still no nearer a diagnosis. Finally, he decided to refer me to Nairobi Hospital for further examination. A friend, Edmund Hemsted, offered to fly me there the following day in his light aircraft.

When news of my imminent departure leaked out, an inordinate number of friends, laden with fresh alcoholic donations, made their way that evening to my room. Even Dick was there.

I recounted my doom-laden encounter with the Matron. They roared with laughter.

'OK. OK.' I said. 'It's all very well for you lot, but I've got to face her in the morning, so for God's sake tone it down! It's like being in the bull ring and meeting the bull with both hands tied behind your back.'

They gave another roar and broke open the Tusker and Whitecap.

Next morning I was up well before dawn, desperate to get away. Edmund had promised to come early to fly me to Nairobi. As far as I was concerned it could not be early enough.

Just as I was beginning to give up hope, he popped his head round the door.

'Come on! Let's go!' he hissed. 'You're in big trouble! The matron is hopping mad. Old man Davenport got the night nurse to phone her last night when your party was at its height and she's after your head. She wants to eat you alive! I met one of the nurses as I came in and she told me the old bag's frothing blood!'

We scuttled out of the room and tiptoed down the corridor. It was empty. We reached the exit – almost there! I breathed a sigh of relief, turned the corner and ran straight into the Matron.

Shock and horror on my side, fury mixed with leering satisfaction on the other.

'Leaving us, are you, Mr Cran?' she barked.

'Yes indeed, Matron. Got to get to Nairobi to get my problems sorted out.' I laughed lightly. I could see that Matron Fanshawe was seething. Her aristocratic nostrils dilated and contracted like the blowholes of a killer whale. Her shapeless bosom rose and fell like a strong Pacific swell. Her abdominal mass quivered and shook like a vast living blancmange. For some reason I was reminded of a colossal deep-sea jellyfish, pulsating with controlled venom, whose very touch meant instant and painful death. I stared, mesmerised, a quivering calf for the slaughter.

When she spoke, her tone was icy.

'You've been nothing but a damned nuisance since you arrived. I'm glad to see the back of you. Old Mr Davenport might very easily have died from stress due to your selfish lack of consideration.'

I thought this was trifle harsh. He probably just wanted a beer and was livid because he couldn't have one.

'I'm very sorry to hear that, Matron,' I replied, 'and I apologise unreservedly. How is the old gentleman, and what was his problem?'

She hesitated.

'He's rather better now, but no thanks to you, I have to say! He had major constipation but he passed a massive stool in the night.'

Rage-induced intestinal propulsion, I thought. He's got us to thank for that.

Supressing a smile, I inclined my head. Should I tell her the joke about the constipated mathematician? I thought not, and passed on my way.

Once in Nairobi I presented D'Souza's referral note to the Nairobi Hospital and was admitted. A battery of tests was carried out – an EEG to check if my brain was normal and whether I had aberrant epilepsy, an ECG to ascertain if my heart was functioning correctly, tests on blood, tests on urine, liver function tests, my blood glucose was examined – the list was endless and exhaustive. But nothing significant was discovered.

There was speculation about toxins, idiopathic epilepsy, vitamin deficiencies and imbalances, mineral deficiencies, meningitis, brain tumours, brain haemorrhage, skull fractures, the effects of alcohol, diabetes, and malaria. The list was endless and terrifying.

Before I went on the ill-fated safari to Lake Rudolf I had been dealing with an outbreak of abortions in cattle, which had been diagnosed as due to the bacterium Brucella Abortus.

'I wonder,' I thought, 'if it might be that?'

It was. My blood was positive to Brucella Abortus. Not only that, it was also positive to Brucella Melitensis, which causes abortions in sheep and goats and is responsible for Malta Fever in people – a disease which frequently terminates in death. The symptoms in both include an undulating fever, muscle and joint inflammation, depression, nervous prostration and general non-specific malaise.

Antibody levels of more than 1 in 20 are considered to be positive. Mine rose to previously unknown stratospheric heights. These results engendered much medical excitement. Doctors came to look and wonder. Consultants came to stare and speculate. They theorised that the organism had been lurking in my vertebrae after I had been infected by the cattle I had been treating. The combination of stress, dehydration, the hammering on the endless corrugations to and from and to the lake, plus the heat, had triggered the convulsion and the collapse of my vertebrae. It sounded plausible. As for the Malta Fever, I could have contracted this when I had been to an old sheep or goat pen, whose floor was covered with dry faecal pellets. From these I might have inhaled the infection. All surmise, but it seemed to fit.

After the diagnosis came the treatment – a diabolical combination of various antibiotics, unpleasant yet effective. For a while I wondered if it was really worth it, as I rushed for the umpteenth time for the toilet, bent double, bowels bubbling, groaning with discomfort as yet another spasm gripped my suffering entrails. But my back healed perfectly and gave me no trouble from then on.

Edmund flew me back to Nakuru, where a host of impatient clients awaited my return, wondering why my fishing trip to Lake Rudolf had taken so long.

Chapter Three

NIPPED IN THE BUD

With my spine more or less connected, I had no time to ponder on the depressing possibility of ending my days as a truncated dwarf. There was work to be done. The New Year festivities were over, the healing sojourn at the coast was a fading memory and I was back in the Highlands. These had formerly been called White, but now they had a distinctly Piebald tinge. Tattered remnants of settlerdom still survived, clinging like shipwrecked survivors in isolated enclaves to their privileged past. As former white strongholds were eroded by the creeping tide of rising population, by encroaching smallholders and by the destruction of the environment, these colonial throwbacks gravitated to areas where others of similar persuasion had laid down fresh, if ephemeral, roots. One such area was Naivasha, where numbers of post-colonial relics had established themselves in circular laager-like hill stations. Here they lived in secluded splendour with their dogs and servants and horses, playing bridge and golf and tennis, attending polo tournaments, directing garden boys on how best to prune the roses and mow acres of lawn, supervising the polishing of the family silver and the bwana's riding boots and generally living a life of high feudalism. Due to their almost mediaeval devotion to their animals – horses, dogs (generally the larger the better), cows and, by extension, to wildlife, they were excellent clients, forever summoning me forth to deal with their problems, serious and trivial. Some were high-handed and demanding, others easy-going and relaxed. But I knew that barons and baronesses, mediaeval and modern, were generally flush with ducats and doubloons and so regarded them with that respect due to those who provided me with a substantial percentage of my bread and butter. And the vast majority paid their bills without demur, a most important consideration from my point of view in a country where the avoidance of the settling of debts was almost a national pastime.

Colonel Roger Chadwick-Smee and his good lady, Suzanne, lived on their small farm at Kongoni, Naivasha, where they kept a few Jersey cows and stabled a small string of hunters. They also had a mixed pack of dogs, including two dachshunds and a German Shepherd, called Monty. The Colonel had served under Montgomery in North Africa and Italy and revered the name of his late commander. Although I did not know it at the time, Monty was every bit as short tempered as the Allied General.

The Colonel was on the phone.

'That you, Cran?' he barked one evening as I was half way through the evening repast, served with characteristic off-hand aplomb by my long-serving cook and bottle-washer, Njoroge.

'Yes, indeed,' I mumbled through a half masticated mound of glutinous potato.

'What's the matter? You got adenoids or something?'

'No, Colonel,' I replied. 'Just trying to consume my lunch.' Which indeed it was.

'Well, that's all right then. Now look here. I want you to come out tomorrow morning, first thing, and vaccinate our dogs and then Suzanne wants you to rasp all of our horses' teeth.'

Kongoni was over 100 kilometres from Nakuru, and the road from Naivasha town to the Colonel's homestead was all dirt and dire in the extreme, a corrugated nightmare of deep volcanic dust, hidden boulders and camouflaged pits, deep enough to conceal a machine gun platoon.

Before I had time to reply to the Colonel's request, the phone went dead.

'Damn,' I muttered. I tried to return the call, but without success. I endeavoured to contact the operator, an exercise akin to a latter-day attempt to raise the dead. But it was patent that the Age of Miracles was past. My efforts were met by the silence of the long deceased. I already had work booked in for the following morning, but I knew that if I did not attend to the Colonel's needs I would never hear the end of it. But first I had a bitch to spay, a dozen bullocks to dehorn and several cows to pregnancy test.

By the time I had completed these mundane tasks, the morning was far advanced. Summoning my assistant, the faithful Moses, I set forth with all possible speed for the farm of the distant Colonel. But not as fast as others on the road. Jungle Boy, Japanese Warrier, Coffin Carrier and The Last Dinosaur, together with Gorilla Unit, grossly overloaded matatus (minibus taxis,) swept past me, gears whining, bodywork rattling, horns blaring, closely followed by the dreaded Eldama Express, a long-distance bus which, for reasons unknown, bore the mystic logo, Black Market. The bus was packed, the roof a mountain of luggage – beds, bicycles, water containers, mattresses, chairs, plastic baths, and crates of chickens, whose dislodged feathers streamed out behind like jet contrails.

To my right Lake Elementaita lay blue and limpid, backed by purple hills, its soda shores fringed by a pink edging of chattering flamingos. Flights of pelicans circled effortlessly on the thermals rising from the surrounding ochre plain. Not for the first time, as yet another matatu came howling towards me on the wrong side of the road, the words of Bishop Heber's much maligned hymn came once again to mind – 'though every prospect pleases and only man is vile.'

I drove up a steep escarpment and into the outstandingly decrepit township of Gilgil. A furnace-hot wind blew dust and dirt and plastic rubbish across the filthy main street, which was lined on both sides by prime examples of modern African architecture. Grey breeze block buildings, shabby shops, piles of second-hand clothes and shoes, dingy bars, butcheries with whole carcasses hanging like criminals from gibbets in their unrefrigerated windows, ambiguous lodgings, screeching off-key loudspeakers blaring earsplitting messages to a totally indifferent public, pedestrians wandering with free abandon across the street with utter disregard to personal safety, cyclists weaving to left and right, goats and sheep and cattle grazing on piles of festering debris, it was the sort of place which prompted no stimulus to linger. But it was impossible to escape at speed from this gruesome conurbation. That bane of the motorist in Africa, humps, transected the road at distances nicely calculated to allow him to accelerate to a satisfying velocity before forcing him to come to an abrupt halt, grinding down to low gear and easing his protesting vehicle over the approaching obstacle. These humps were rarely marked with paint to alert the unwary to their presence. Others seemed to have been deliberately sited so they were covered by the shade of an adjacent tree, rendering them practically invisible, until one's car hit them with a crash that almost tore its wheels from their moorings. None of these humps had smooth forward slopes. All seemed to project upwards at 45 degrees, so that before one reached the summit, forward visibility had all but vanished. Some were small and irritating, others were huge and alarming, and potentially life-threatening. On the Solai road three enormous humps had been constructed. One morning, as I was carefully approaching the last of these monstrosities I saw a small saloon car, driven by a European nun, coming at speed towards me – and the shadowed hump. Too late I flashed my lights at the ecclesiastical carriage. It hit the hump with force sufficient to lift all four wheels off the ground and as it passed me in mid-air I saw the nun's lips moving with what I was certain was not the language approved by the Pope for use in church. By the time I had reached the noisome outer limits of Gilgil I had reached the outer limits of my stock of expletives. Was I alone in regarding these barriers to progress as a personal attack on my access to the freedom of the road? I noticed that African drivers often took the humps without even slowing down, often accompanied by a tympanic clang as exhaust or sump came into violent contact with the ground. They seemed to regard the obstructions as little more than a minor inconvenience to be overcome as quickly as possible. On the other hand they probably weren't driving their own vehicles and it's amazing how fast you can go on a rough road when you're driving a car or lorry belonging to someone else.

Beyond Gilgil the land was glorious open road through bush and leleshwa plain, zebra grazing unconcerned as I passed by, warthogs rushing for cover, tails erect, baboons sitting on rocks, indifferently watching the passing traffic, but alert to anything edible cast into the verge by environmentally-unfriendly drivers. Of these there were many, hurling empty beer cans out of car windows, tossing milk cartons into the slipstream, flinging banana skins into the face of oncoming traffic, punting plastic bags filled with unmentionable garbage onto the tarmac, there to burst and void their revolting contents across the highway. Whenever this happened the baboons would scamper across to investigate. Anything edible would be borne to the side of the road to be sampled at leisure. Tetrapacks of milk would be sucked dry, half eaten maize cobs would be picked clean, beer cans would be emptied of their last drops.

The background to this desecration was the lovely triangle of the extinct volcano Longonot, grey and sombre in some lights, dark blue and purple in others, brooding over Lake Naivasha below.

The road to the Colonel's farm was every bit as bad as I expected it to be and after a few miles Moses and I were covered from head to toe with the volcanic dust which jetted into the Peugeot through every possible opening. It entered through the windows, through the floor, through the air vents. A possible solution was to close the front windows, partially open the rear windows and turn on the blower. This we did and the end result was less dust but near suffocation from the heat within the hermetically sealed cab. So, hot and sweaty, covered in a brindled patina composed of an amalgam of perspiration and a congealed sample of road material, we arrived at the HQ of Colonel Chadwick-Smee.

Our arrival was not greeted with unalloyed rapture. The Colonel, a tall, lean, angular individual whose upper lip was besmirched by the tattered remains of a military moustache, was marching up and down his verandah, shaking his watch and holding it to a large leathery ear.

As I levered myself out of the Peugeot an over-flying fish eagle threw back its snowy head and gave a loud yelping cry. Was it a warning? A mocking call of derision? I looked up and into the flinty eyes of Chadwick-Smee. He did not look friendly.

'Call this morning, do you Cran? Gad, if you'd been under my command, I'd have had you on a charge! I'd have had you on jankers! White-washing the kerbstones. Running round the parade ground in the sun with a 50lb haversack on your back! Where have you been, sir? I've been sitting on my arse all morning waiting on your pleasure.'

'Sorry, Colonel,' I said. 'Your phone appears to be out of order. I've been trying to contact you ever since you phoned last night.'

'Really? Seems all right to me.' He gave a snort of disbelief. As he did so his lady wife, Suzanne, appeared. Small and pugnacious, with a narrow pointed face, she was another no-nonsense, dictatorial type, forever expressing unsolicited opinions and supremely confident that she would never be contradicted. And on the whole, due to the all-powerful combination of class and money, she seldom was.

I looked around at the groves of flat-topped acacias, at the grey hills sloping down to the lake, at the fishing canoes far out on the blue water, their occupants tiny cut-out figures, listened to the softly repeated notes of an unseen bird, and thought once more of Bishop Heber.

'Right,' I said. 'Shall we vaccinate Monty and friends?'

'Yes,' replied the Colonel's lady. 'Jumaaaa!' she shrilled, lifting her head like a baying jackal. Almost at once a tall, tarbooshed African, wearing a red embroidered waistcoat, materialised, like a genie popping from his bottle. Was that the Chadwick-Smee's coat-of-arms on his waistcoat? Now that really *was* arrogance.

'Jambo, Juma,' I said.

'Jambo, daktari,' he replied. His ebony features remained impassive, but I thought I caught a gleam of ironic sympathy in his large, luminous eyes.

'Juma,' said the mensahib, 'can you lete the mbwas?' (Can you bring the dogs?) I shuddered in sympathy with Juma at this verbal mangling of his native tongue. Juma remained impassive. 'Ndiyo, memsahib,' he replied. (Yes, madam.)

He vanished, to return minutes later dragging a patently reluctant Monty behind him. Monty was large, mobile and keen to display rows of sharp, white teeth. Juma held him firmly by the head while I injected rabies vaccine into a hind leg and a cocktail of viral vaccines under the skin of his neck. Juma released him and Monty jumped away and lay down under a nearby bush.

'Right, Juma, now bring me Fifi. I will hold her while the doctor injects her. You're far too rough with the poor darling.' Fifi was a dachshund bitch. Juma did as instructed. 'Come along Fifi, pettikins. Mummy will hold you while the bad man injects you.' The bad man did as he was told. This left Mimi, the final dachshund bitch. The Colonel's wife clasped Mimi to her withered bosom. I manoeuvred for position, trying to get the needle into the bitch, which, snuggled deep into the folds of her owner's pectoral anatomy, presented a target so small that I was in serious danger of skewering her mistress's shrivelled mammillae. Screwing my courage to the sticking-place, wherever that was, I made a sudden thrust and got the first injection into the little beast, without her being aware that anything untoward had happened. One more to go. I filled the syringe. The vaccine was a rather lovely rose colour, a bit like the wine in which I had over-indulged a few nights previously. I held it up to the light and gave it a little shake to disperse the bubbles. What was it that Keats had said – 'beaded bubbles winking at the brim' – yes, that had been a good thrash! One of the best. 'Come along! Come along! Mimi's getting impatient!' snapped the Colonel's lady. 'So would I if I were stuck down there!' I thought.

'Right. Hold tight!'

Once again I was right on target. But this time Mimi realised that her person had been violated and she voiced her displeasure with a discordant yelp. Or was it Suzanne? The noise had a galvanising effect on Monty and before I was aware of what was happening there was a sudden, snarling rush and he was lunching off my left leg. He sank his fangs into the flesh on the inner side of my knee and gave it a good worrying. I wasn't having this and said so in plain unvarnished, politically incorrect, Anglo-Saxon English.

'Oh!' said Suzanne. 'Oh!' And then, 'Come away, Monty, you bad boy. Naughty doggie!'

Monty did come away but the uproar brought the Colonel to the scene. He staggered down the verandah steps, a brimming beaker enveloped by a gnarled fist.

'What the devil's going on? Frightful racket. Can't you deal with the dogs without disturbing the whole neighbourhood?'

'It's Monty, dear. He's given Mr Cran a bit of a nip on the leg.'

I looked down the mentioned leg and saw what looked like a chunk of fresh steak sticking out at the bend of my knee, together with a not inconsiderable effusion of blood.

Chadwick-Smee approached and stared at my leg and at the welling pool of gore forming around my boot. 'Pah!' he said. 'That's nothing to write home about. When I was fighting Rommel in North Africa chaps were losing limbs on a daily basis. We just slapped on a bandage and they carried on as though nothing had happened. You couldn't afford to pussy foot around when you had the cream of the Afrika Korps breathing down your neck.' I looked around, half expecting to see Erwin, goggled and leather-jacketed, binoculars hanging round his neck, looking pleased and squinting in my direction.

The lady of the manor reappeared. She looked at the blood as though I had just vomited on her polished parquet floor. 'What a mess! And your language, Mr Cran! Was that really necessary?'

'Sorry about that. Spoken in the heat of the moment. The baser man rising to the surface.' I gave a light laugh. Mrs Chadwick-Smee did not laugh. Her narrow mouth wrinkled with distaste. 'Really? Well, I hope my herbaceous border doesn't suffer. Too much protein and my precious shrubs just die.'

'Blast your shrubs!' I thought. 'What about my precious leg?'

'Well, we'd better get on with the horses, hadn't we?' she said. 'But can you get rid of all that blood first. Horses don't like the smell of blood. Panics them. Juma! Can you lete ndoo ya maji.' (Can you bring a bucket of water.)

Juma brought the water and, while I was swabbing away the blood, he told me in sotto voce Swahili that only the day before Monty had attacked the Colonel and had knocked him to the ground and were it not for Juma's intervention might have done him some serious mischief. And the week before he had attacked and debagged a passing cyclist. I raised my eyebrows. Thanks, Colonel.

I cleaned away the blood and brought to view an impressive wound with a mass of what looked like personal muscle tissue protruding from somewhere inside my leg.

'This is going to require stitching.' I said.

'Can't you do it yourself?' Mrs Chadwick-Smee asked. I didn't reply to that. 'Well, cover it up with a bandage. Vets always have bandages in their cars.'

I bandaged my offending leg and hobbled to the stables where a group of hunters and attendant syces awaited my attention. The latter were suitably impressed by my bloodstained limb and gallant limp, and gave me the deferential respect normally only accorded to war-wounded and campaign veterans. For the next hour, under the weasel eye of the Colonel's wife, I rasped and chiselled away at a never-ending succession of molars and incisors until I was satisfied they passed muster. By that time my leg was rather stiff. As were my hands and arms from manipulating the heavy rasp. But their ache and my rising endorphin levels lessened the throb emanating from my leg. The benefits of counter irritation. A bit like a horse having a twitch applied to its nose. Another pain to deflect the original pain.

As I was reflecting thus on the conferred wonders of physiology, the Colonel came to the car window. 'Look, old chap, take yourself to a doctor and I'll settle the bill. Shouldn't be much. A mere flesh wound, what!' He gave a dismissive laugh.

Two hours later I proffered my leg to Dr D'Souza for his consideration. By the time he had finished I had fifteen neat stitches adorning my inner knee.

Colonel Chadwick-Smee never did pay the bill.

Chapter Four

DICK THE DOG

Richard Ingram Crawford was the proprietor of the Blue Cross Kennels, at Lanet on the outskirts of Nakuru.

Here he dwelt in insalubrious squalor, sharing his house with a pack of unprepossessing canines of mixed parentage, several cats and a small flock of chickens, who laid their eggs in suitably-sited nest boxes in various corners of the house.

Dick was a bachelor, and it was apparent that he suffered from a severe form of gamaphobia (a morbid fear of marriage). His single status was reflected in his lifestyle. Piles of mouldy unread copies of the *Daily Express*, airmailed from Britain, lay heaped upon the dining table. The sagging sofa was occupied by a huge, grossly overweight Great Dane cross bitch. Ancient cobwebs hung from every corner, filled with the victims of years of arachnid endeavour. Desiccated flies, withered bluebottles, even the husks of long-dead lizards, bore mute testimony to years of non-dusting endeavour by Dick's chief major domo, the well-larded Paulo, who oiled his way about the premises with proprietorial ease. Paulo had not allowed the grass to grow beneath his feet while in Dick's employ. While Dick clothed himself in moth-eaten pullovers, hideous nylon shirts of a bygone era, and antique shorts of dubious vintage, Paulo presented himself to the world in sharp suits, wide ties and patent leather shoes. Dick's socks were full of holes. Paulo's were the very latest in fashion. Paulo was regarded with awe, and not a little fear, by the rest of Dick's entourage, a motley bunch of ne'er-do-wells, work-shy layabouts and intellectually challenged wheelbarrow pushers, who shuffled about the precincts in slow slow motion. They always appeared to be engaged in positive action, but closer scrutiny revealed that this was a subtle smokescreen, the result of long and patient practice, designed to fool Dick into thinking that their monthly wages were a well-deserved recompense for four weeks of sweated toil.

Dick had been born in Chile in 1928, went to school in Argentina, graduated in economics at Cambridge and then worked for ten years for Shell Oil in East and West Pakistan, an experience which put him off curry for life.

'When I first went to Pakistan,' Dick told me, in his fruity voice, 'I shat through the eye of a needle for seven years. After that I was fine.'

'Once, when spending a night in a hotel in Karachi, I looked down at the street below, from my window. A vendor squatting on the pavement was showing and selling something to passers-by. He made some strange waving motions with his hand, what looked like a black, undulating Persian carpet rose into the air and from below this he would give something to the person, who would then hand him something in return. Then the black carpet would descend and the process would be repeated with someone else. I was totally mystified and intrigued. Finally I could stand it no longer and went down to the street to find out what was going on. The black carpet was thousands of flies gathered upon a tray of sweetmeats. Whenever a buyer wanted a particular item the vendor would wave away the flies, which rose protesting into the air, the transaction would be concluded, and the flies would descend once more. Is it any wonder that I had the galloping trots during most of my time in Pakistan?'

As a result of his lengthy sojourns in South America and Pakistan Dick was fluent in Spanish and Urdu. He was a great favourite with the Asian merchants in Nakuru with whom he was able to converse in their mother tongue, accompanied the while by appropriate head wobbles and soprano intonations.

Dick's 'kitchen' was a soot-encrusted cell, half filled by an enormous, blackened, wood-fired stove. The walls were thick with grease, to which were added the particulate exhalations of a huge kerosene-powered refrigerator. Beneath a wooden table littered with scraps of food and unwashed dishes, cats skulked waiting for the inevitable remains, both pre and post prandial, while in hidden corners hens sat silently incubating their eggs. The occasional rat or mouse might be observed, venturing forth to participate in the feast.

Within this noisome crypt Dick's mpishi (cook) prepared his meals. Having survived ten years of daily dysentery in Pakistan, Dick was probably immune to the heaving mass of enteric bacilli which accompanied every dish. The cook would march in, clear a space amid the mounting piles of unread newspapers, sweep aside the cats, terriers and hens which had leapt upon the table to participate in the banquet, and advise Dick that his meal was ready for consumption.

Dick's character was naturally introspective and taciturn, but when he was in his cups he ripened into a teller of tales of the first order.

'When I was in Pakistan, West Pakistan that is, I was a member of the Yacht Club, which was sited on the banks of the Indus. Very nice it was too, with turbaned, white-gloved waiters, fans, punkah wallahs, members only of course. The Secretary was a starchy old buffer, ex-Indian Army, mustachioed and stiff-backed, a great stickler for the rules. We used to go picnicking on the sand banks and generally living the life of Riley. One day, while we were at tiffin, a bearer came rushing in and, after the appropriate obsequious formalities, spoke to the Commodore, as the Secretary was rather regally called. 'Sahib, sahib. Body is stuck on pontoon! What to do, sahib?' The Commodore tugged at his soup strainer and stared at the bearer. 'Is he a memba?' 'No sahib!' 'Then push him off!'

Dick had devised a number of strategies to allow him to indulge his aversion to the local cuisine without giving offence to clients and hosts, who were forever pressing him to join them in a bewildering variety of palate-scorching dishes, seasoned with chillis, cardamom and tumeric.

'Oh, Mr and Mrs Khan,' he would say, with feigned regret. 'I am most terribly sorry, but today is the Feast of the Sanctification of the Blessed St. Theophilus, when I must fast for 24 hours, abstaining from all food and drink, be it flesh, fowl, water or wine.'

'Mr Crawford, Mr Crawford, sir,' they would reply, hands clasped. 'We are most fully and completely understanding. We are having same situation ourselves on Saints Days.'

At which point Dick would retire to his appointed room, open his tin of sandwiches and unscrew his flask of gin, square his elbows and indulge in a private feast in unchillied privacy.

Dick's fondness for privacy in Pakistan extended to travelling by rail. As is well known, the trains in the Sub-continent are notoriously overcrowded, with every space occupied by a body, or more. People cram themselves into the compartments, into the corridors, they squeeze into the toilets, they hang from the doors, they balance precariously on the buffers between the coaches and swarm onto the roof with their baggage and belongings. Dick was having none of this. He would send a servant ahead to identify an empty first class compartment. Dick would dash inside and lock the door and pull down the window blinds. Passengers would begin to arrive in larger and larger numbers, searching desperately for seating. Finding Dick's compartment locked they would knock on the door, demanding entry. Dick would reply in Urdu in a high-pitched female treble.

'Please! Please! I am in purdah! I am in seclusion! My husband told me not to open door! He said that I must always travel alone, lest I be profaned by the proximity of men or unveiled harlots! Go away and leave me alone!'

And, after some disgruntled mutterings, they did, leaving Dick to stretch out in luxurious comfort in the six person compartment, together with his sandwiches and gin and to sing, sotto voce, a favourite ballad:

'I love a lassie
A great big fat Madrassi,
She's as black as the tadpoles in the well.'

Harry Lauder would have turned in his grave.

Now Dick was in Kenya, running his kennels, which had boarding space for 150 dogs and 30 cats.

With so many resident dogs and cats I was in high demand to treat and vaccinate the inmates. These demands frequently occurred at night as Dick had the peculiar habit of inspecting his canine and feline tenants during the hours of darkness. This, he claimed, was due to the fact that the animals were fed in the evening and only by checking them post-dejeuner could he determine whether they were eating or not. Fair enough, except that invariably when he phoned I had barely had time to scent my own dejeuner, far less taste it, and, by the time I had dealt with Dick's problems, my dejeuner was likely to be yet another congealed mess coagulating on the table, where Njoroge had left it.

Night visits to the kennels found Dick making his rounds, clad in tattered shorts and a knee-length sweater, which had more holes in it than material. These, Dick patiently explained, were caused by the dogs which loved him, jumping up and rending the garment with their claws. 'What,' he would say, ' is the point of buying a new one? It would last no time before becoming just like this one. Bloody waste of money.' So the upgrading of his kennel attire was not on Dick's agenda.

Dick was a fervent believer in economy. As I followed him round the kennels, he would switch his torch on and off in a mesmeric, rhythmic fashion, a bit like a distressed mariner signalling for assistance. By so doing, he claimed to save on batteries. As I stumbled behind him in the inky darkness, rats the size of young rabbits scrambling over my feet, I cursed Dick's misplaced parsimony.

But Dick was devoted to his dogs. His whole life revolved around them. He even captained a football team in Nakuru called 'Dick's Dogs'. He took no holidays and expected no one else to take any either. If I had the temerity to take a couple of days off Dick would expostulate in the strongest possible terms.

'So! Taking another holiday are you? And what's going to happen if something falls sick, eh? Remember what happened the last time you went away? OK, then, off you go.'

And off I would go, feeling a first-rate cad for leaving Dick in the lurch.

And, if something did go wrong, as it occasionally did, I would never hear the end of it. Years later, Dick would bring it up.

'I saw old Mrs Marlow the other day. She hasn't spoken to me since Squeaky was taken ill in the kennels, eight years ago. You were away, climbing some bloody mountain. I took her to a local vet, but she died. I remember every ghastly detail but you were away, enjoying yourself. I never take time off, but I suppose *you* have to.'

In other words, you abandoned me, and, as a result, poor Squeaky died. I never take time off. I'm always on duty. But, I suppose if you must go, you must. It's just like all these bloody public holidays. I've got to pay my workers for sitting around scratching themselves while I carry on, on my own.

But, in reality, Dick was grateful for what I did for him.

One day Brownie, Dick's favourite dog, a cinnamon-coloured mongrel, strayed into Lake Nakuru Park, whose boundary was only a mile from the kennels.

A game ranger saw the dog, raised his rifle and fired. At the sound Brownie leapt away, the bullet missed his head and chest, but struck his right foreleg, shattering it.

While the acrid smell of cordite still hung heavy in the ranger's nostrils and as he contemplated the results of his handiwork, I was busy pregnancy-testing cattle on Glanjoro Farm, the property of Cen Hill, on the outskirts of Nakuru. Task completed, ordure removed, I returned to the surgery, there to find pencil-thin Linda Vaughan-Ryall, Dick's lady assistant, waiting for me.

'Hello, Hugh,' she said in her deep, gravelly voice as I got out of the car, 'sorry to trouble you. I've brought in Dick's Brownie. Both are in one hell of a state. Brownie's leg's been smashed by a bullet and Dick's in terminal decline, raging and shouting and almost frothing at the mouth. Brownie strayed into the park and got shot. His leg's a right old mess.'

'Right, let's have him in.'

My right-hand man, Moses, and Dick's driver, Rono, carried Brownie into the surgery. Rono was a Kipsigis from Kedowa, a village on the road to Kericho. Tall, friendly, easy-going and intensely loyal to Dick, his head was surmounted by a great mass of frizzy grey hair, combed from back to front.

Brownie's leg was, as Linda had just said, a right old mess. The bullet had smashed through the radius and ulna, breaking them into several pieces. Sharp spicules of shattered bone protruded from a gaping wound. The muscles overlying the bone were ripped and torn. Severed veins hung from the mangled meat like purple lianas suspended from a forest canopy. I could see grit and bits of vegetation embedded in the pulped flesh. Surprisingly, Brownie did not appear to be overly upset by this massive damage to his leg, certainly, if report was correct, on nothing like the scale affecting his master.

'Well, Linda,' I said, 'this doesn't look good. I can't tell if this leg's salvageable until we get Brownie anaesthetised. If it's not we'll have to amputate.'

'OK,' rasped Linda. I looked up – did she always talk like that, like dragging sheet metal over concrete? – 'Do whatever you can do and let's hope for the best. I'll tell Dick. He's ranting and roaring about the Game Department. You know what he's like.'

'Yes, his fuse is pretty short. If we'd chucked him at the Germans in the last war things would have been over much sooner than they were.'

Linda gave a hoarse bray and departed.

Moses and stout office messenger Bernard prepared the instruments, plenty of them, so that, if necessary, I would have enough to perform an amputation. Amputations can be pretty bloody affairs and there's nothing more annoying than running out of haemostats when confronted by fountains of spouting arteries, especially when you have told your assistant for the thousandth time that you would always prefer to have ten times too many instruments on the operating table than one too few at the moment of crisis. No matter how often I said this, my words always seemed to fall on deaf ears, and as I reached for the critical forceps, or ligature, to stem some massive crimson geyser, it was to discover none at hand. Why I was never deported for the words spoken on such occasions I shall never know.

I filled a syringe with the computed dose of anaesthetic, sodium pentobarbitone, clipped Brownie's left foreleg below the elbow, and asked Moses to press his thumb into the crook of the dog's leg, in order to raise the cephalic vein. I had to get this right, first time. With the right leg looking like the remains of a hyena's breakfast, I had no second cephalic vein to fall back on. 'Get this right, Cran,' I thought, 'or Brownie's buggered. May be buggered anyway!'

The needle found the vein and Brownie slumped into temporary oblivion.

I examined the shattered bones. The central section was little more than a casserole of fragmented mush. But the top and bottom thirds still remained, although split and cracked. The best option would have been to use an external fixator, which I did not have. So it would have to be an intramedullary pin. Insertion was not difficult. Clamp it into the hand-held chuck, push it up the marrow cavity of the upper fragment, push it through and then reverse the pin into the lower shaft until it embedded in the cortical bone. Finally, with a hacksaw, I cut through the spare length of pin protruding from the upper fragment.

But so much skin and tissue had been torn away by the bullet that the wound could not be closed. Everything looked, and was, very unstable, subject to rotation and twisting and there was a section in the middle totally devoid of bone, supported only by the stainless steel pin. I left all the bony fragments *in situ* in the hope that they would form some sort of osteogenic nucleus to bridge what looked like an unbridgeable gap.

Linda came in and scrutinised my handiwork.

'Ye gods! What's this? The bionic dog?' she laughed. She sounded like a parrot with laryngitis.

A little later Dick appeared in person, still almost incoherent with rage, eyes popping, stamping his feet and still fulminating against the Game Department.

'Calm down, Dick,' I said.

'Calm down? Calm down?' Dick shouted, 'when my poor dog has just been riddled by some unfeeling blackguard who, just because he's poxed up in khaki fatigues and has a gun, thinks he can open up on anything that moves. Poor Brownie! Look at his poor leg!'

'Right, Dick,' I said, 'now you must keep him in a kennel, keep him confined, no exercise for a few weeks. I've pinned the leg, but as you can see there's a big chunk of bone missing, so movement must be kept to an absolute minimum.'

Dick was appalled by the prospect of confining Brownie to a kennel but finally agreed.

Weeks passed. The wound slowly healed. The pin remained visible. Months went by and slowly Brownie began to use the leg, tentatively at first and then with more confidence. He always limped and the pin was always visible, but he had a viable leg and for this Dick was grateful.

Others who were also grateful, but for different reasons, included members of Dick's kennel team.

In order to feed the canine and feline inmates, Dick encouraged local farmers to bring him meat, usually from cattle or sheep which had died. This, after a cursory inspection and a query to ensure that the animal had not died from anthrax or poisoning, was taken by wheelbarrow to a large vat within the kennel compound, where it was cooked. Alternatively it was lugged to a cold store of impressive dimensions, whose all-pervasive stench reminded visitors of the transitory nature of its working parts.

The cooking area was adjacent to a high wooden fence, part of the kennel perimeter.

Linda would pay the meat bringers, having first weighed their offerings, which were either fresh and dripping or rank and also dripping. Normally that was the end of the matter. But for some time Linda had had the impression that the amount of meat coming in had increased by a considerable amount. And, what was more, the volumes brought in seemed to be similar. No sooner had she paid for a mass of meat than ten minutes later someone else would come cycling in with a lump of carrion balanced on the crossbar.

A few days later Linda opened the cold store and was puzzled to discover that the amount of meat stacked inside was less than it had been before the inrush of new supplies. How could this be? Had it been stolen? Where had it gone?

She quizzed the staff, to be met with expressions of blank incomprehension and wide-eyed incredulity. Someone knew something but no one would talk.

Dick exploded when informed.

'Right!' he shouted, 'that's it! That's it! Someone's pinching the meat and I intend to find out who it is. The police are bloody useless. There's no point in getting them. It'll have to be the witch doctor!'

One morning I drove to the kennels to vaccinate some dogs and was confronted by a scene straight out of *'King Solomon's Mines'*.

Under a large acacia tree ten Africans, eight men and two women, stood in a rigid motionless line. There was none of the laughter and the movement and the foghorn conversation which accompanies Africans, off or on duty, day and night.

To one side I could see Dick sitting in a camp chair. He looked like the main character in a 1920s sepia version of *Sanders of the River*, Sanders himself in fact, presiding over a native court, a strong, still, magisterial figure, even frightening, stern, but impartial and just.

In front of the silent line capered a grotesque figure, clad in monkey skins, whose furry tails whirled around it in a wild fandango. It jingled with ankle bells and rattles, face bedaubed with grey and white paint, animal bones clashed around its neck, and its head was covered with a spiky busby.

The witch doctor had arrived.

I stopped the car and stood to watch.

Behind the bizarre figure, stamping and cavorting before the stationary figures of Dick's petrified employees, stood a smoking brazier. The smoke billowed and blew, gusting over the participants in this fantastic drama. Dust rose. Dick sat immobile, chin in hand, a modern Caesar, cast in stone.

The witch doctor scuttled along the line of suspects. He rummaged in a skin bag, tossed some powder into the air and brought out a long thin bone with a black feather bound to one end. The men and women looked grey. Most were sweating profusely. Three were swallowing convulsively. Two were trembling.

The witch doctor crouched low, bone in his right hand. Slowly, looking like a stage version of Richard III, he hobbled along the line, staring up at each person in turn, twirling the bone in his fingers, muttering and moaning.

One man looked as though he was about to collapse. The women whimpered, gasping and hyperventilating.

The witch doctor turned to the brazier and picked up a shovel, which, I had failed to see, was lying on the ground. He filled the shovel with a pile of red-hot coals and returned to the terrified row of suspects. The air above the shovel trembled and quivered. The witchdoctor stopped before each gasping prisoner and stared through narrowed eyes. 'Your name?' he whispered in a low hiss. When the victim, quaking with terror, had answered, he was told, in a sibilant snarl which seemed to rise from the very depths of the sorcerer's bowels, to 'spit onto the coals!'

Four men and one woman succeeded in raising sufficient spittle to expectorate onto the shovel. With a sharp hiss a thin snake of steam and ash rose into the superheated air. Try as they might the other five failed to perform as requested. It was as if their salivary glands had atrophied and shrunk to nothingness from sheer silent terror.

The witch doctor spoke to the five who had successfully spat.

'You five can go. You others…,' he turned, eyes rolling in his head, only the whites showing… 'shall remain.' They looked as though they would rather not, but, rooted to the spot, they seemed incapable of movement.

The four free men and woman took to their heels. They did not look back.

The witch doctor groped in his bag.

'What now?' I thought.

He produced a loaf of sliced bread, opened it and folded each slice into four and gave a folded slice to each suspect. The lone woman appeared to be bereft of her faculties.

The bread looked dry and stale.

'Now eat and swallow!' he ordered in a low, grating voice.

I watched, fascinated, as the jaws began to move. I glanced at Dick. He was leaning forward in his chair, intent on the outcome.

Throats bunched convulsively, jaw muscles bulged, eyes watered and tongues flickered over parched lips as the unhappy wretches struggled to swallow the bread.

First one man, then another, followed by the woman, managed to get their pharynxes over the bread, before it vanished, with painful and glutinous propulsion, into the owner's upper oesophagus. It was like watching an egg-eating snake tackling an ostrich egg.

The final two were in serious difficulties as they fought to surmount the cannon ball like masses which stubbornly refuse to shift from oral cavity to oesophageal tube. Wild-eyed, they chewed and chewed. The witch doctor capered and giggled with manic intensity. Dick sat on, a majestic Olympian figure. At last, after a tremendous struggle, one man succeeded, like a python swallowing a buffalo, in getting himself over the solidified mass obstructing his maw. Balloon like, his gullet distended as the obstipated mass moved in the direction of his waiting stomach.

For the last victim, a desperate, pock marked youth, all hope had gone. His jaws champed, his teeth grated, his neck muscles bulged, a bloody foam flecked his swollen lips. It was hopeless. Nothing short of surgery was capable of transposing the Saharan mass.

The witch doctor hopped across to where Dick sat in his camp chair.

'This ees tha guilty mann.'

'Thank you very much,' said Dick. 'Please ask him how he did it.'

The unhappy youth prised the inspissated gobbet from between his lacerated gums and muttered to his tormentor who, after a few minutes, returned to Dick.

'Ya, he is a very cleva boy! You pay for meat, he takes it to be cooked. But it is not cooked. It is thrown over the fence to a fliend, who takes it to you. You pay again! Again he takes it to be cooked and once again over the wall it goes! Another fliend takes it to you and again you pay! You pay for same meat three times! This has happened many times. So you think much meat is coming but not so – little meat and much money. This boy is tooo cleva!'

Simple psychology and the effect of fear were the witch doctor's tools of trade – basic but effective. I was impressed.

Dick sacked the youth on the spot and paid the witch doctor for his services.

'So, the solution of the one mystery and the termination of another waster's employment. But, mark my words, there will be more mysteries to be solved and more wasters to be sacked. La luta continua! The struggle continues!'

Indeed it did.

Chapter Five

SHOWTIME

Once a year, at the end of June, or at the beginning of July, the annual Nakuru Show was held. About two weeks before the event, I would receive a formal request/summons to act as Official Veterinary Surgeon, to deal with any problems affecting the livestock and competing horses. I regarded these invitations with a mixture of satisfaction and dread. The Nakuru Show was not a relaxed, rural, social get-together, but a frantic, grossly overcrowded bunfight, attended by tens of thousands of visitors, paying and non-paying, presided over by His Excellency the President Himself, screened on television and covered in detail by the local press.

During the rest of the year the showground remained empty, a waste of weeds and deserted buildings. A couple of weeks before the show, frenetic activity indicated that time was short and even as the first visitors were queuing up, paint was being slapped onto crumbling woodwork and nails were being hammered into stands and placards. If the weather was wet the place was a sea of mud. If it was dry it was a dust bowl. There seemed to be no happy middle ground.

Getting into the showground was difficult. Getting out was a nightmare, especially on days when the President arrived by helicopter to make his official visit. Nervous and aggressive police exercised their authority by harassing drivers and pedestrians alike. When the President sat godlike on his throne in the Presidential Box, jet fighters screamed overhead, bands played and parachutists floated down into the arena. Sometimes they dropped into the arena. Sometimes they missed it altogether, as when one luckless parachutist drifted gently over the town and into Lake Nakuru Park, several kilometres away. He survived the drop. His subsequent fate was unknown. Rumour had it that his next posting was to an isolated fort on the Ethiopian border.

Hundreds of sleek, pampered cattle, sheep, goats and pigs were exhibited and were judged by experts from overseas. Scores of horses took part in the show jumping competitions. Their riders fell into two distinct camps – European and African. The former were mostly women, generally well-heeled, top drawer, dominant, confidant, sitting proudly aboard their glossy mounts, and when not, striding about in thigh- and buttock-hugging jodhpurs, slapping their boots with their riding crops and generally sweeping the peasantry before them. The latter were either upgraded syces or members of the Stock Theft Unit – later renamed the Anti-stock Theft Unit in a belated attempt to convince the public that their real role was catching stock thieves and not actually doing the thieving themselves. The syces and Stock Theft Unit rode small, wiry horses, their saddlery was dull and scuffed, their boots and riding gear baggy and colourless, their helmets unadorned by silk or ribbon. But they were good riders and did well.

In charge of the European ground crew was Marian Swift, otherwise known as Ayatollah Swifti. The Ayatollah was elderly and large, pleasant but firm. She stood no nonsense and spoke her mind.

On the other side the troops were commanded by Inspector Kiptanui, a sharp, ambitious policeman, keen to demonstrate the skill of his men to the watching public. So, in addition to competing in the show jumping competitions, they enacted gymnastic displays, thundering the length of the arena, swinging themselves from one side of their mounts to the other, standing on the horses' backs, and doing handstands at full gallop as a variation on the athletic theme. The audience loved it.

The Inspector was gratified. He decided to expand his team's repertoire, and to regale the people with pig sticking exercises. The riders, armed with long, sharp lances, rather like mediaeval knights jousting at a tournament, galloped at top speed before the open-mouthed mob, aiming at small squares of wood, embedded in the ground. This was a tremendous success. A hit had the crowd on its feet. 'It would be much better with real, live pigs,' thought the Inspector. 'Maybe warthogs. The audience would go wild.' He put his view to the show committee. The members were alarmed, envisaging pigs running amok amid the audience, hotly pursued by men on horseback. Blood would be shed. A latter-day gladiatorial Roman Games was not on their agenda, much though it might appeal to some people. The Inspector was not to be deterred. What about a mass display then, a sort of controlled Charge of the Light Brigade? Reluctantly the committee agreed.

The team practised their equestrian exercises at their home base near the town of Gilgil, before unleashing it onto an unsuspecting public. Complicated crisscrossing movements were involved, culminating in a mass triumphal stampede towards the Presidential dais. It did seem to me a bit like something which had once happened a long time ago in the Coliseum. The sort of thing which would have had Nero giving the thumbs-up sign. Still, I thought, they must know what they are doing.

After dealing with a small mob of clients in the surgery I made my way to the showground. Today was Friday, the day when the President was due to grace the citizenry with his presence. The streets were crammed with traffic. The weather was hot and dry, dust rose into the air. Pedestrians weaved between the creeping vehicles, bellowing hawkers lined the roads, policemen confused drivers with conflicting arm movements, matatus forced their inconsiderate way into every opening, their interiors packed with an amoeba-like mass of scarcely-breathing humanity, faces squashed against windows, rumps projecting from doors, feebly moving arms sticking out of any available opening. I crept with agonizing slowness towards the favoured gate which allowed those with business within to enter relatively unmolested.

Once inside I drove to the enclosure where the private equine entries lurked in pampered seclusion, away from the bedlam which enveloped the rest of the showground. A small wooden structure formed the headquarters of the Ayatollah. She sat at a camp table, surrounded by a stern politburo of female lackeys, while the jodhpured magnificos strutted disdainfully to and fro on the dusty grass.

'Hello, Marian,' I said, 'what's happening? I thought the show jumping was just about to start.'

'Yes, it was, but the Camp Commandant has had it put forward so that the President can see the Stock Unit's display.'

'Right, so that explains the general air of displeasure out there?'

'Yes indeed.'

I strolled out to see what was happening.

In front of the gated entrance to the arena milled a mob of uniformed riders, apparently jostling for position in what was to be the Event of the Day. Behind them were assembled the members of the various bands, due to make their entry once the equine events were over. I noticed with concern that all of the riders were carrying sharp pig sticking spears. Too late to reason why, I thought. Finally in rodeo-like fashion the riders entered the arena, spears held aloft. Half of them galloped clockwise around the perimeter, the other half anti-clockwise, until they met, following which the combined mass thundered towards the Presidential Box, where they reined in their mounts and dipped their weapons in salute. Graciously he responded with a languid wave of a cambric kerchief. Next followed a complex series of manoeuvres, circling, weaving, zigzagging, trotting, cantering, galloping. I was impressed. It was exciting and held the crowd enthralled. The speed of the horses grew breakneck, until the mob of mounts and riders seemed to mesh into a serpentine river in full spate. The two lines separated and, lowering their spears, charged at each other so that each horse passed between another two at full speed. Perfect timing. Wonderful! They turned again for a final charge, and the riders spurred their mounts for all they were worth. Closer and closer they rushed. The horses' nostrils flared. Foam flecked their necks. Their flanks were black with sweat. This is what it must have been like at Balaclava! All that was wanted was the odd cannonball screaming overhead. A sudden trumpet blare shrieked above the thunder of hooves. Some idiot in the massed bands had decided that this was an opportune time to tune his instrument. Whatever his reason it had disastrous results as horses at full bore swerved in panic. It was too late for the riders to raise their lethal weapons. One horse was transfixed through the chest, and collapsed on the spot, the rider thrown several yards through the air in an ungraceful parabola, to land with a mighty thud on his back, winded and concussed. His horse, blood cascading in torrents from both nostrils, thrashed violently on its side for several minutes before dying, surrounded by pools of rising gore. Two other horses were also speared, less severely, receiving stabbing wounds to neck and chest. And one rider had his calf all but pinned through his boot to his horse as an opposition lance thrust home.

And all the while the great Kenyan public was kept up-to-date with the situation as the television cameras kept rolling. I glanced up at the Presidential Box. All occupants were on their feet, staring in horror at the mayhem before them.

As soon as I saw what was happening I rushed into the arena. I dodged a couple of policemen who tried to stop me.

'Mimi ni daktari!' I shouted.

There was an element of danger out there. Horses were milling around in great clouds of dense red dust, horses were bucking and kicking, some loomed up riderless, reins flapping, stirrups swinging wildly, a lance resembling something that Henry VIII might have carried in the lists appeared through the murk, but the atmosphere was so dense I could not see who was holding it. Slowly the dust settled.

An ambulance crew was carting off the concussed rider. I checked his horse – it lay in grotesque rigor mortis, hot, dead and steaming, eyes wide and staring, nostrils dilated and in front of them a great mound of pulsating, clotting, still rising, mound of gore. I turned to find the two wounded animals.

They were held by their riders, to one side of the general mêlée.

One had an angulated wound in the neck, the other a thrust into the brisket. Neither horse seemed perturbed and stood quietly while I examined and probed. Their riders were more upset than the horses. A little blood trickled from the wounds. I assured their riders that both animals would be fine and that I would give them antibiotic and tetanus antitoxin once the horses had been stabled.

I walked back through the excited crowds to the European enclave. People were chattering and laughing. There is nothing like a disaster, especially one involving blood – someone else's blood – to stimulate the average African to throw back his head and whoop with merriment. This was a show to remember, that was certain. It would be talked about for years. Whether the Inspector was an idiot or not, he had made his mark and would, for a while at least, go down in local history – a Local Hero.

In the domain of the Ayatollah there was no doubt what the opinion was.

'Bloody silly thing to do, if you ask me,' said Phoebe Butterworth, kneading her haunches as though they were dough ready to enter the oven. 'Could easily have killed someone.'

'That would have pleased the crowd!' chortled big-bosomed Amelia Atkinson, snapping her XL sports bra over a massive shoulder.

'How did ze Old Man take it?' inquired Ursula Oidtmann Dietrich von Stumberg, glacier-blue-eyed, sitting at attention, not quite clicking her heels but obviously wishing she could.

'Looked a wee bit stunned to me,' said Suzy McNab, in a broad Lowland accent.

'Yes,' said Rosalinda Whitaker-Jones. 'Half stood up and then sat down rather abruptly. Next thing he was gone, together with his entourage. Anyway, the coast, my dears, is now free for *us* to perform – at long last. After that primitive nonsense it's time to introduce some class and breeding into the proceedings!' She gave a tinkling, queenly laugh. 'Syce! Lete farasi yangu! (Groom, fetch me my horse!) I think I'm first.'

Her horse was trotted up, held by a wizened syce wearing ancient corduroy breeches. He had a face like a withered prune left on a shelf in the sun for a couple of years after its sell-by-date. The fair Rosalinda's flawless complexion looked as though it had been nurtured in ass's milk. She raised a slender left leg and inserted her booted foot into the stirrup, but gave the other to her ancient ostler. He seized her glossy foot and heaved mightily, a bit like a competitor at a Highland Games trying to toss the caber. Rosalinda rose with practised ease into her polished saddle. The syce breathed heavily. Rosalinda cantered off without a backward glance.

A bell clanged.

I could see Rosalinda enter the ring and approach the first jump. Her horse cleared it with ease. And the next and the next. Rosalinda was obviously an expert and returned with a clear round.

She cantered gracefully back, a small smile of patrician complacency on her handsome features.

'Your turn, Amelia,' she laughed. Amelia was aboard a beast which looked as though it had spent the better part of its life hauling coal through the back streets of London. It had great tufts of hair obscuring its lower legs, a head with a colossal Roman nose and a back as broad as the billiard table in the Men's Bar. Amelia's personal seat was such that nothing less would have sufficed to have borne the spread of her massive backside. She lumbered into the arena and charged the first fence. Miraculously she cleared it – just. Her mount seemed to go over sideways. She looked like a motorcyclist on the wall of death. There was a gasp from the audience. With a bit of luck there might be another disaster. The horse stumbled almost to its knees and then recovered, looking a bit like a camel staggering out of a pub. Amelia almost lost her hat, but hung on grimly.

She hit the top pole of the next jump with a great clang. It shook but didn't fall. She cleared the next jump by two feet and scraped over the next one. And so it went on, until she too returned with a clear round, trotting back into the enclosure, panting and gasping and peering through a mixed lather of sweat and saddle soap. Rosalinda's sunny features darkened ever so slightly.

Phoebe, Ursula and Suzy entered in succession, failed to make the grade and returned, chastened and downcast, leaving in their wake the wreckage of dislodged jump poles, scattered like strewn matchsticks across the turf.

Rosalinda cheered up considerably.

The survivors of the simulated Charge of the Light Brigade came next and their small rangy horses took the jumps almost at their leisure. More dismay among the etiolated aristos.

The Ayatollah asked for the jumps to be raised.

Rosalinda re-entered, tense and pale.

The jumps looked enormous. But Rosalinda had guts and went for the jumps with everything she had – or rather with everything her horse had. Her horse was an Arab and jumped like a stag. It performed magnificently and once again Rosalinda returned with that small maddening smirk with which to taunt the others. Amelia was less fortunate and pole after pole crashed to the ground. She returned, puffing and wheezing, lolling in the saddle, head bent, hat askew.

The Light Brigade entered and lost all their riders bar Sergeant Langat Kiprono, whose mount looked like a donkey on steroids. He seemed to regard his minor achievements as part of the day's work. No visible sign of emotion flickered across his thin, dark features.

So it was to be a jump-off between the white female blueblood and the black male non-com. I could feel a light but unmistakable crackle of racial tension sweep through the crowd.

The Ayatollah spoke. 'Raise the jumps by another notch.'

It was done. The crowd was silent.

Kiprono went first. His pony was dwarfed by the huge jumps. I could not see how it was possible for it to clear any of them. But it did. All of them. A sigh went through the crowd. Then they bayed their approval. It sounded like the roar that greets a matador after he has successfully killed an excessively dangerous bull. Or when a gladiator skewers his opponent on his trident. Very slightly worrying.

Now for Rosalinda.

The Arab showed no sign of tiring. Neither did Rosalinda. Both were of the nobility and behaved as such. Retreat or anything less than the best was unthinkable. Like Waterloo it was a damned close run thing but they won through and returned, breathing faster then usual, but otherwise unfazed.

The Ayatollah sat, chin in hand, a female version of Rodin's Thinker.

'Mmm. Should we run them against the clock or shall we raise the jumps yet again?'

'Raise zem, unt if zey both go clear zen run zem against ze clock,' said Ursula.

'Right,' said the Ayatollah. 'That's what we'll do.'

There was a great cheer when Kiprono again went clear. Silence when Rosalinda did the same. There was muttering and I could hear the word mzungu (European) uttered in less than friendly tones.

Once again Kiprono entered the arena, but this time at high speed. Time now was the thing. He shot from jump to jump, slithering over them, scraping over the poles, turning his pony at such an angle that it looked at one moment as though it might fall onto its side. He rushed into the last jump, took it from the side and rapped the top pole. It rocked, toppled and fell. There was a great aaagghh! from the crowd. But the time was fast, very fast – two minutes, 25 seconds.

As he rode out of the arena Kiprono glanced at Rosalinda coming in. 'Beat that if you can!' he seemed to say.

The bell rang for Rosalinda to begin. She had to be careful as well as fast. Faster than Kiprono and to beat him no poles knocked off. She seemed to be slower but the Arab had a deceptively smooth gait. Very economical with never a moment's hesitation as it approached the jumps. It seemed to flow round the course. I checked my watch. A fraction slower than Kiprono but Rosalinda could not afford to make any mistakes. A little faster now. Over the second last jump, a double. Touched the top pole. A gasp from the crowd. It rocked but did not fall. Into the last jump now. Two minutes, eighteen seconds. Careful now! Careful! Over and clear, – and the time? Two minutes, 23 seconds and Rosalinda was the clear winner.

There was a reluctant scattering of applause, but it was evident that the result was not a popular one. A mzungu, and a woman at that, had beaten their native son. Already people were leaving the stands. And the Presidential Box was empty.

I glanced at Rosalinda's horse as she rode out of the arena. There was a tiny fleck of blood at one nostril. The horse looked tired. Not surprising, I thought. But before I had time to examine the Arab a stentorian announcement came over the loudspeaker – 'Would Dr Clan prease go to Gicheha Farm. Would Dr Clan prease go to Gicheha Farm.' This was the farm of the late president Jomo Kenyatta and as such any delay was not to be entertained.

'Right! OK! OK!' I thought. 'Keep your blimmin hair on! I'm coming!'

'I'll see you later, Rosalinda,' I shouted. Now, how to get out of here!

Easier said than done. The place was packed with a seething mass of humanity, a goodly percentage of which appeared to be rather the worse for wine, including women and children. As is often the case this brought out the worst in many of them as they lurched in front of my car, making obscene gestures and banging on the side of the vehicle. The Guardians of Law and Order appeared to be no better, grinning in a threatening manner as I did my best to avoid members of the mob. From ghetto blasters and loudspeakers, raucous Congolese music raged at me from all points of the compass. Smart-suited evangelical fanatics, operating in pairs, perched on wooden stands, microphones in hand, one roaring his message of doom and destruction in Swahili while his mate yelled the English equivalent, harangued an indifferent audience. Hawkers flourished everything from second-hand ski-boots to coconuts and baseball caps. Herds of lacquered whores minced through the dust, leering at potential customers and lurching over the uneven ground. At the exit a large-buttocked policewoman vainly endeavoured to control the chaotic traffic jam, totally ignored by one and all, including myself.

Once out of the gates I sped with all possible dispatch to the ex-presidential farm, which was now, I was relieved to see, unguarded by members of the dread red-bereted General Service Unit. They were probably in full carouse at the showground, together with colleagues from the traffic unit, leaving the roads hassle-free for a blessed few days.

On the farm I met the normally ebullient manager, the circular, moon-faced Kamau, who led me to the patient, a large Friesian cow. Mr Kamau was less than cheery today.

'Jambo, daktari. So, you have come to see our cow.'

'Yes, I said. 'She looks very ill indeed.'

The cow was standing in the centre of a dirt boma, head down. Blood was dripping from her nostrils. She took a step forwards and as she did so she coughed, staggered and almost fell. As she coughed a stream of bright red blood poured from her nose and sank and disappeared into the soft dust at her feet.

'Mr Kamau, I'm afraid your cow is on its way out. Dead on her feet, in fact. I've seen this before and in every case it's been due to abscesses in the lungs. Probably a sequel to a foreign body in the stomach penetrating the diaphragm. Treatment is useless and in this case it's too late even to get her to a butcher.'

'She started to cough and bleed from her nose about three weeks ago. A local daktari came and gave her an injection of antibiotic and she

71

seemed to get better but now she's much worse.'

'Yes. That's the usual scenario. They may seem to improve but they always die, sooner or later. I never treat them. It's a complete waste of time and money.'

We heard a hoarse bellow and turned towards the cow. As we watched, she took a couple of steps backwards, coughed convulsively and collapsed, more blood cascading onto the dirt floor of the boma. Within a few seconds she was dead.

'Right, let's do a PM and confirm what I suspect.'

'OK, daktari. I'll get some water.'

I went back to my car, my trusty Peugeot 504, and fetched a sharp knife from the boot. I knew better that to rely upon local weaponry, whose edges were usually dull and blunt, often lacking handles and frequently made of soft, useless metal.

Most of the farm staff were at the show so I had to make do with a woman wandering by, and a deaf and dumb labourer, to hold the carcaseswhile I delved within.

'Mr Kamau, can you bring a panga or an axe so that we can open the chest?'

Pangas are littered all over Africa and used for a wide variety of benign and malign uses. Within a few minutes I had the chest opened. It was just as I had expected. The lungs were full of large abscesses, but the most striking thing was within the rumen, the cow's main stomach, which contained a monstrous clot of blood, comprising many litres of the cow's vital supply. As blood from the lungs passed up the windpipe she had swallowed most of it. Only a very small amount reached the outside world in the form of blood emanating from the nostrils. The greatest amount of blood lost ended up in the cow's own stomach.

'Right, Mr Kamau, there you are. She has bled to death and nothing that you or I could have done would have saved her. Let's have a look in the stomach and see if there is a foreign body in there.'

I rooted around for a while searching for a wire or nail but could find nothing. If there had been one it must have long since been dissolved by the stomach juices.

Time to return to showground madness.

'Goodbye, Mr Kamau.'

'Asante, daktari! Kwa heri!'

Re-entry into the showground was an even more chaotic experience than getting out, due to the fact that the number of people under the influence of toxic stimulants seemed to have doubled or trebled, until I was under the impression that I was moving through waves of drug-fuelled addicts and that I was the only one still in possession of his faculties.

Catatonic booming from loudspeakers racked up to maximum volume made the dust-laden air quiver and tremble in protest. The sun was beginning to dip below the trees which lined the perimeter walls. Grotesque shadows from moving figures expanded and contracted as they crossed and re-crossed the lowering shafts of reddish light.

As I approached the equine enclosure the aged Ayatollah came staggering out, puffing and blowing, waving her arms.

Something was up. I coasted to a stop.

'Thank God you're here, Hugh,' she gasped, leaning against the car like a sack of old potatoes. 'Rosalinda's horse, Jupiter, is in a bad way. Ever since you left he's been pouring blood from both nostrils. A fool of a vet from the veterinary department has been here to look at him and he just stood there bleating and wringing his hands and doing nothing. You'd better get there as soon as possible.'

'Right, thanks, Marian.'

I finally reached the opposite side of the arena, where the stables were sited. Outside one I could see a small knot of rubber-necking passers-by, craning over the upper half of the stable door. I pushed my way through, opened the door and stepped inside.

The place looked like an abattoir. There was blood all over the whitewashed walls, and great clots of gore lay thickly on the straw-covered floor. If there had been a ceiling it would have been on there as well, but there was no ceiling – only beams and thatch.

Rosalinda was there, together with her syce and another African, a shabby, shambling figure with grizzled hair. I recognised Wallace Wamagata, a long-time member of the veterinary department. Rosalinda turned as I entered. She looked drawn and haggard.

'God, Hugh, what's wrong with him?'

Her grey horse stood, head bowed, in the centre of the stable. A steady drip, drip of bright red blood stained the yellow straw.

As I approached he took a step forwards and staggered slightly. An ominous sign.

I knew Wallace slightly. 'Hello, Wallace,' I said. 'This looks bad.'

'No, no,' he replied. 'Lots of horses bleed from the nose like this after exercise. I've read all about it. It's called epistaxis. Nothing to worry about.'

I looked about me, at the blood bespattered walls, at the clotted mounds congealing on the floor, and thought otherwise.

Rumour had it that after 30 years in the veterinary department Wallace's sum knowledge of animal ailments could be succinctly inscribed on the back of a postage stamp.

As I moved around Jupiter I laid a hand on his back. It was cold and clammy. Temperature was subnormal and his heart rate fast and weak. As I moved my stethoscope over his chest he gave a convulsive cough and a gobbet of clotted gore shot from his nose and hit the wall with a glutinous smack, before sliding messily to the floor.

I listened to his lung sounds, and they did not inspire confidence – an unpleasant symphony of bubbling, wheezing and crackling.

I turned to Rosalinda.

'He's got Post Exertional Pulmonary Haemorrhage. It occurs sometimes after strenuous exercise in horses. Usually it's mild and of little consequence, but this looks serious. A major blood vessel must have ruptured.'

'What's this epistaxis thing that Dr Wamagata mentioned?'

'Epistaxis just means bleeding from the nose. A description of symptoms, nothing more. What you see, in other words.'

'What I see looks bloody awful.'

Silently I concurred. With a major blood vessel bleeding from the lungs, death was the inevitable and depressing outcome. I knew that drugs would make no impression on this condition and that surgery, heroic or otherwise, was not an option.

'Sorry, Rosalinda, but I don't think he's going to make it.'

She gave a convulsive sob. This was her best horse. It always seemed to be the way. The dross survived while the best died young.

'Poor Jupiter. Is it better to put him down?'

Before I had time to answer, Jupiter staggered again, this time right across the stable until he hit the opposite wall with a crash. He lurched back, fell forward onto his knees, recovered and reared up. We – Rosalinda, the syce, Wamagata and I – made a concerted rush for the stable door, to avoid Jupiter's flailing hooves. In what looked like excruciating slow motion he rose on his hind legs, eyes glaring, nostrils flared, until he stood upright, like a grotesque caricature of a circus horse, before falling backwards against the stable door. The others had escaped. I was not so lucky and one hoof struck me a glancing blow on the forehead. I could feel the hot blood coursing down the left side of my face.

Jupiter was dead. He lay in a horrid heap against the door. Upside down. A tangled mass of stiffening legs, blood seeping from his nostrils. Wallace, Rosalinda and the syce stood in a silent group outside the door. The door was jammed tight shut by Jupiter's rigid corpse. With difficulty I clambered out and into a gathering crowd of ghouls and voyeurs.

I sought out Rosalinda. 'So sorry, Rosalinda. Your best horse, I believe.'

'Yes, win some, lose some. I won the competition but lost my horse. He was a hero.' A tear trickled down her alabaster cheek.

'He was that.' I squeezed her arm.

On my way home I was stopped by a traffic policeman. He was large, pot-bellied and drunk.

He waved me into the verge and asked me to switch off the engine.

'Sweetch off yo engine. I want to examine yo ca. Geeve me yo dereving licence.' He snatched it from me and paraded around the car, waving it in the air. He looked at the insurance and road licence stickers which I knew were in order. He looked at the tyres, he checked the lights, he examined the wipers, he ordered me to switch on the indicators. He was looking for something and was determined to find it.

He looked at my driving licence again.

'Theese dereving licence eet is ees is defaced. Look at eet!' I looked at it. It looked all right to me. There was a smear of mud across one page, but apart from that it was in pristine condition. I normally kept my licence in a cubby hole in front of the gear stick. About a month previously I had driven through a rather liquid mud wallow and in the process a fountain of what looked like caramel chocolate pudding had erupted through the gear stick housing. When it had subsided my licence was left limply floating on the surface of a little pool of the stuff. Hence the smear, which, rather picturesquely, I thought, distinguished my licence from everyone else's.

'You weel go to cot on Monday! You have defaced govoment property and I am going to chage you. Get out of thee ca!'

I knew that what he really wanted was a bribe, the euphemistically named 'tea', or 'chai' and that he was dragging things out in the hope that I would cave in.

I got out of the Peugeot and turned to face my tormentor. As I did so he gave a hiss of alarm.

'What has happened to yo face? Eet is covaed in blood!'

I had forgotten about the gash caused by poor Jupiter when he had met his Maker, and which had resulted in such an interesting effusion of blood down the left side of my face and which I had yet to wash off. It had not been noticed by the cop in his state of inebriation when he had come at me from the right hand side of my right hand drive car. Now the blood had clotted and was congealing and hardening into a disgusting carapace. I must have resembled the victim of a homicidal attack.

I gave an indifferent shrug as if to suggest that blood on my face was nothing out of the usual. 'Oh – that. A kick from a horse at the Show.'

'A horse! In yo face!' He paused and then thrust my driving licence at me. 'You go! Go! Go!'

Back at home as I waited for my ever-so-slightly inebriated cook, Njoroge, to dish up yet another culinary masterpiece, I poured myself a whisky and thought, 'What a perfectly bloody day!' Everything had died in a welter of blood and gore and it was high time I cleaned off my own blood and wiped that odd look off Njoroge's face as well.

Chapter Six

FRENCH DRESSING

'Allo! Allo! Iz zat ze docteur?' 'Ah oui,' I almost said. 'Yes, it is.'

'Luc leBoeuf 'ere. Can you come zis week to castrate for me four 'orses? Zey are a little bit wild, but I zink we can manage. And you must stay for lunch.'

Luc was French. To say that he was eccentric would be a gross understatement. Some would have said that he was barking, especially so when the moon was full. He lived on a ranch not far from the collection of foetid shacks which constituted the township of Bumuguti, to which global location he had been banished by his wealthy parents in order to get him permanently out of their hair. The ranch ran at a considerable loss, but the parents paid Luc handsomely to enable him to stay there. He was, in effect, a member of a dying breed, a remittance man. They also paid for a psychiatric nurse, female by gender, to live on the ranch and deal with his more violent mood swings. Her name was Simone and she was well paid. She had to be.

'Right,' I said. 'Would Thursday morning be OK? In the morning?'

'Ah oui,' said Luc. 'Bien sûr.'

The ranch was 80 miles from Nakuru and the road was not good. So by the time I arrived it was mid-morning and the sun was high in the sky – not the ideal time to castrate colts.

A few hundred yards from the ranch buildings I saw a group of horses in a field. Assuming that these were my patients I stopped the car and walked across the dry wiry grass to examine them at closer quarters.

I did not like what I saw. The animals were large, very large, with tangled manes and endowed with massive gonads and were far from tranquil. As I approached they rolled their eyes, threw up their heads and stampeded out of sight into the bush. Great!

On the phone Luc had informed me that the horses were 'a *little* bit wild.' I had taken him at his word. I should have known better. These animals, I could see, were rampant monsters. If I had known that I going to be dealing with wild horses I would have brought along my darting equipment and treated them as such.

Too late now.

As I drove up to the farmhouse Luc appeared at the door. He was a tall individual, in his mid-forties, with a wild shock of dark hair sprouting like a mass of tangled weeds from his large bulbous head. Behind him I could see Simone, pale and plump and emanating an air of frightening efficiency.

'Allo, docteur!' said Luc. 'So, you 'ave come.'

Over a cup of coffee on the wooden verandah, with weaver birds chirruping in what passed for a garden and nesting swallows zooming over our heads bearing breakfast to their open-mouthed young encamped in their saucer-shaped hammocks cemented to the eaves, we discussed our, rather *my*, plan of attack.

The horses were all large, mature and totally untouched by human hand. They were mobile time-bombs, ready to explode into violent action at the slightest provocation. Giving these horses an injection *en plein air*, so to speak, was not to be contemplated. Even if one were able to approach close enough to give them an injection the result would be a volcanic muscular eruption and I had no wish to be in the firing line of snapping teeth and lashing hooves. I proposed using Immobilon as the anaesthetic. This drug, originally developed to chemically immobilise elephant and rhino, had the advantage of being able to be given by intramuscular injection. And there was a convenient antidote, Revivon, which, if given by intravenous injection, would have the animal back on its feet within a few minutes. It had the disadvantage of being rather dangerous to the user if he, or she, were to be the recipient of the injection rather then the animal. A derivative of morphine, it was 10,000 times as strong. The merest prick would, in the absence of immediate medical intervention, have one knocking at the pearly gates and bowing to St. Peter in very short order. A modicum of care was advisable.

As we spoke we were joined by two men. One was tall and thin and carrying a video camera, the other was dark and squat and clutching a notebook. 'Ah docteur,' said Luc, 'let me introduce you to mes copains from France. Zey are 'ere en vacances but they wish to film you in action and to record ze show! You do not mind?'

'No indeed!' ('Great! As though the job's not got enough complications! Now I've got a couple of Gallic paparazzi breathing garlic fumes down my neck!') 'Right let's go and get on with it, shall we?'

'Ah oui, oui!! Allons y!'

We located the horses in their field, in one corner of which was a rough cattle crush, whose weathered timbers, half eaten by termites and almost diaphanous with age, I feared to lean against, lest I bring the whole structure tumbling to the ground. By this time a posse of ranch workers had been assembled to drive the reluctant horses into the crush. Slender Somalis, tall Turkanas, black, wiry Pokot and loose-wristed Samburu, with whoops and yells and wild leapings herded the nervous nags towards the V-shaped rear of the crush. This tribal cacophony whipped the agitated mustangs into a state of high anxiety until they were lathered with sweat and blowing gobbets of fear-induced foam from their nostrils.

The French connection was delighted and filmed and scribbled for all they were worth. I was not so happy, wondering whether all this ethnic vociferation would affect the ability of the anaesthetic to do its job. Finally the stallions were within the crush and I prayed that they would stay within it.

The foremost horse was grey, a large, coarse beast with matted mane and an impressive Roman nose. At one time he might have been white but now he was a dirty cement colour, due to a light epidermal powdering with a mixture of dried mud and dust. I estimated his weight – about 500 kilos I thought – and filled the syringe with the requisite volume of Immobilon. As I approached the crush he bared a set of huge yellow teeth, laid back his ears and did his best to rip off my arm. I jerked back just in time. 'Hey, Luc,' I said, 'just how old is this horse? His teeth look very mature to me.' But Luc was in a close huddle with his confreres – probably discussing whether they could sell an exclusive to Paris Match. I tried again. I asked one of the native whoopers – a youthful Samburu clad in rather foppish red drapery which fluttered picturesquely in the breeze, to approach the horse from the other side of the crush, in order to divert his attention from my needle. As the horse made what I thought was a legitimate lunge for the lad's flamboyant wardrobe I whacked the syringe into the side of his neck, and stood back to observe the effect. It was not long in coming. After two minutes he began to stumble. Then, to my dismay, he gave a convulsive leap forwards, crashed through the front of the crush, which collapsed in splinters around him, and staggered off sideways into the bush and vanished.

'Ooh, la, la!' exclaimed Luc. The two hacks looked at each other. I was so taken aback by the turn of events that I had nothing to say.

We could hear a lot of smashing and crashing in the nearby bush as our patient destroyed the local vegetation. For a minute all was quiet. Then the noise started up again and seemed to be getting louder, and louder, until, with a splintering of branches and a falling of small trees, the grey emerged from the thicket, wild-eyed, dishevelled and panting, and collapsed at our feet.

The two French visitors burst into a round of applause. I almost clapped as well, but remembered just in time to maintain due British aplomb, striving to give the impression that I had planned this brief equine foray into the bush for their personal diversion.

I grabbed my instruments and set to, swabbing two enormous gonads, prior to their removal. Such was their size that only the bold, sweeping incision so favoured by the professorial writers of veterinary textbooks, would suffice for their removal. Behind me I could hear the whirr of the Gallic camera, coupled with what sounded like convulsive swallowing. I clamped the huge spermatic cords, and their accompanying, blue, bulging blood vessels, with my emasculator and, with the thickest catgut in my possession, ligated the lot. I knew that bleeding here would be unstoppable and that this horse would never, ever, be persuaded to re-enter the crush.

'Oh, docteur,' piped up Luc, as I was tying off the second bulbous mass of arteries and veins. 'I 'ave just checked. Zis 'orse. He 'as 14 years of age.'

'Whaaat?' I exclaimed. 'No blimmin wonder he's got testicles like coconuts! He should have been done about a decade ago!'

North of Bumuguti the inhabitants, both white and black, took little note of the passage of the sun across the firmament, nor of which day of the week it was. Some were barely aware of which month it was. No rushing pell-mell to the office here. No anxious scrutiny of ticking timepieces. No vital deadlines to catch. But to miss out a whole decade seemed like rank carelessness to me.

I gave the horse his intravenous injection of antidote and in a few minutes he was nowhere to be seen, having taken his leave without a backward glance.

The other three horses were models of decorum compared to their grey companion and as I tied the last ligature my salivary juices began to flow freely as I looked forward to a groaning board bearing the best that French cuisine could offer. I knew that items guaranteed to stimulate even the most anti-French of individuals into culinary excitement were regularly flown in to satisfy Luc and Simone and their guests, who included from time to time such doubtful luminaries as venal right-wing demagogue Gaston Renard whose main occupation on arrival appeared to be the indiscriminate slaughter of the local game.

I straightened up and as I did so a worker approached Luc. I could hear him say something about a dead bull.

'Sorry, docteur, but my best bull, he 'as died in ze night. He is at ze far end of ze ranch. Can you do ze post-mortem?'

'Certainement oui,' I replied, visions of pâté de fois gras, crêpes suzette flambé and beakers of bubbling champagne fast fading before visions of the exposed innards of dead bulls.

'Right, let's go in my Toyota,' said Luc. 'Zere was a shower in zat part of ze ranch last night and it's all black cotton zoil, zo you nevaire know how bad ze road will be. We can have lunch when we return.'

Fat chance, I thought.

I grabbed my post-mortem knife, microscope slides, a few plastic bags and scrambled into the Toyota as Luc came roaring round the corner. The two hacks, I noticed, did not offer to accompany us. In the mirror I saw them strolling gently in the direction of the house, heads together – probably discussing magazine deadlines and wine vintages, I thought.

Luc drove like a man possessed. False teeth clattering like demonic castanets, he seemed to be oblivious of gears and their uses and he had the rev counter needle permanently in the orange zone and hovering within a millimetre of the red. Engine screaming we leapt over ruts and howled along a dirt track at the speed of light. Luc was having one of his periodic mood swings and the disruption to his lunch seemed to have been the trigger. Whatever it was, it was not a restful ride. From time to time he glared in my direction as though I had no right to be there. In the distance a lone gazelle decided that this was a good time to cross the track. Luc saw it, gave a Neanderthal grunt and went for it, closing the gap with frightening speed, eyes popping, dentures bared in a grotesque rictus. Killer instinct aroused, it was patently obvious that he meant business.

This was too much.

'Hey! What the hell are you doing?' I bellowed.

It was enough to put Luc off his stride. He swerved, almost turned us over and tore on along the track, nose twitching, eyebrows clenched, forehead furrowed, wrenching the wheel from side to side, bouncing the Toyota over the ruts and crashing over potholes with oblivious abandon. The gazelle skittered across the plain, white tail scut twitching. 'Hell,' I thought, 'I'm out here alone with this maniac. I've obviously displeased him. Just hope we don't break down. On the other hand we're more likely to crash before we do that.'

As I clung grimly to my seatbeltless seat I noticed with a mite of concern that the track ahead was damp and that in the distance I could see pools of water, glinting in the sun. I remembered that this was the dreaded black cotton zone, where no one in his right mind would venture when it was wet. I glanced at my shock-headed companion and knew the answer to my unvoiced thoughts. Within a minute I could hear the racket as the sticky stuff was thrown up underneath the vehicle, clinging to the wheel arches, adhering to the chassis, slowing us down. It seemed to drive Luc into a fresh frenzy. He gave vent to a fearful Gallic oath, crashed the gears into four wheel drive and surged forwards, swinging wildly from side to side, muttering words like 'merde' and 'sacré bleu' under his breath – at least, that's what in my overheated state they sounded like.

We skidded round a wide corner and ahead of us lay what looked like a mile of treacle pudding. Luc did not hesitate and went for it like a man possessed, which by now I was sure he was. Several times I was almost brained as my head hit the roof when the Toyota leapt like a demented dodgem into the air, returning to Mother Earth with an almighty crash. With gobbets of goo and clumps of sticky mud flying in all directions we reached the end of this horizontal obstacle course, but at the far end there was an open gate and a right angle bend.

I felt that nemesis was near. The passage was narrow and as we got nearer the less likely it seemed to me that we would emerge unscathed. Fifty yards from the gate Luc went into a broadside skid. I braced myself for impact. Then we hit dry land. Someone had laid a layer of impermeable murram soil on either side of the gate, presumably to fortify its supports. That layer saved our joint bacon. Luc straightened up and we shot through the narrow gate with millimetres to spare on either side, turned the corner and at once re-entered the black cotton. Momentum had been lost in the turn however, and it was all too obvious that travel by Toyota was almost at an end. A few hundred yards ahead I could see the carcass of the bull, lying near the track. But Luc was slowing. That turn had been his swan song and the wheels were slipping, losing their grip, digging into the mire. We began to skid towards the side of the road, into the ditch. Luc was wrestling with the wheel, gunning the throttle. It was hopeless and we came to an ignominious halt, axle-deep in mud. Luc beat the wheel with his fists, raging in gutter patois. 'Merde! Merde! Zis bloody heap of Jap crap! Zose shitty slitty-eyed bastards. If zis car had been made in France we would not be stuck like zis! We must try to push.' By *we*, I knew that he meant *me* and I got out and immediately almost fell down. The surface was as smooth and slippery as the side of an iceberg. I clawed my way round the vehicle carrying several pounds of glutinous mud on each foot. I leant my weight on the back of the Toyota while Luc burnt out the clutch and sprayed me with more mud in futile efforts to extricate himself. It was useless. I was stranded miles from anywhere with a psychotic and possibly violent Frenchman.

The sun was hot and the mud was steaming and from the mud rose clouds of biting flies. Soon we were both slapping and waving our arms and vocalising our dismay in words unfit for polite society.

'Well,' I said to Luc. 'I've come to post mortem the bull so that's what I'm going to do.' Luc remained in the Toyota with the windows closed against the flies.

Carrying my knife and plastic bags I left the road and walked through the light bush to where the carcass lay. As I approached a couple of jackals slipped away and disappeared. A vulture hopped clumsily across the wiry grass, while another rose with difficulty into the air. I smelt a smell and knew before I reached the carcass that others had arrived before me. I pushed my way through a patch of thicket and saw at once that I was here on a fool's errand. The carcass was empty, eviscerated by scavengers, probably hyenas, in the night. There was nothing left for me to examine. The bull had been opened from the rear, the innards had been dragged out and eaten and now bluebottles in their thousands were hard at work, laying their eggs and rising into the air in evident irritation at my presence.

I walked back to the Toyota, whose windows were now opaque with French steam. Luc wound down his window down.

'Zut alors, docteur, zat was quick. What iz your diagnosis?'

By the time I had given him a terse report on my finding Luc was in full cry again.

'Zat bloody herdsman! I will kill ze lazy bugger with my bare 'ands when I see him! Zis animal must have died days ago. Not during ze night like 'e said. Now we are stuck 'ere in zis stinking mud, being bitten to death by flies and missing our lunch as well. Now we will just 'ave to wait for help. Zey will come when we do not return after an hour or so.' His voice rose to a final falsetto crescendo.

I thought of the two hacks, by now well into our share of the feast.

Luc wound up his window and disappeared into his personal sauna. Outside, the heat and the rising humidity were driving the swarms of insects to a renewed frenzy of attack, whining and pinging and biting and driving me mad. I walked up and down, shaking the mud from my boots, waving my arms, flapping my hands, slapping my legs.

'Hell,' I thought, 'if I'm walking then I might as well be walking in the right direction.'

I tapped on Luc's grey window, moisture streaming down its glass. It opened an inch. 'Luc, I'm going to walk back – OK? Don't suffocate in there!'

Luc waved a languid hand and flopped back. The window closed.

It took over an hour and a half of sweated labour, slogging my way through the glutinous mud, swatting a dense cirrus of flies and no-see- 'ums, to reach the ranch headquarters and on the way I passed a tractor going to Luc's rescue.

As I expected, the festive table had long since ceased to groan and apart from a few tired sandwiches and a quarter bottle of dead wine with a moribund fly desperately doing breast stroke on its frothy surface, there was nothing left for the workers. From the verandah I could hear French voices – Simone and one of her compatriots. They sounded merry and at peace with the world. Luc and I were obviously far from their thoughts. I entered, leaving a trail of black-cotton mud across the polished wood. They looked up from their drinks.

'Allo, docteur,' slurred the swarthy dwarf, ''ow was your post mortem? You look hot and muddy! 'ave a drink.' He waved his wine and gave a throaty laugh. Simone regarded me slowly with a glassy stare and then suddenly burst into hysterical giggling. The tall one was asleep, head back, mouth open.

'No thanks, I must be going.'

'As you must,' and they poured themselves another drink.

I walked to my Peugeot 504 – everything was French today – got in and turned the key. As I did so Luc's clutchless Toyota, with himself at the wheel, was towed clanking into the yard.

Luc was in irascible mood. 'Ah, zo you are leaving us, after willfully deserting me in ze bush, eh? Trying to get away before I was rescued, no?'

'Certainly not. You were in no danger, on your own ranch and a tractor was on its way to help you. What good could I have done waiting out there? I do have other work to do.'

I was wearing a hat which had seen better days. For some reason it seemed to drive Luc into fresh frenzy. He drew nigh, and before I could stop him he had seized the brim of my headgear with both hands and yanked it downwards. Under such violence the crown was ripped untimely from the brim, leaving the latter lodged ludicrously upon my shoulders.

'Que je deteste les chapeaux comme ça!' he snarled.

Time for Simone to swing into action, I thought. But, in her present state, there was not much chance of that.

I slipped the car gently into gear and drove away.

Chapter Seven

A WALK IN THE PARK

In the south-west corner of Lake Nakuru Park were three horses, running wild, pathetic remnants of the hundreds which once roamed free in the glades and forests between the limpid lake and the Mau Escarpment to the west. They derived from the estate of the late Black Prettejohn, a rough-and-ready colonial character who had run his property in the manner of a mediaeval baron crossed with a Texas rancher, dispensing rough justice in one hand to his black employees and basic management to his herds and flocks in the other. He bred horses, Arabs and Somali ponies in large numbers, and they ran freely in the untouched wilderness which formed the major part of his land. Mostly grey in colour with long tangled manes, they were a fine sight as they galloped across the rough pastureland and through the open glades. When old man Prettejohn died the farm was broken up and sold to the new African farmers. They did not want horses on their land and either drove them off or employed gangs of Maasai to spear and kill them. A small percentage of the horses had been rounded up by well-meaning individuals and sent to other farms for safe keeping. I had darted and gelded several of the colts and stallions. But the majority had met a nasty, brutish end.

So when Ian Slack, the manager of the Kenya Horse Stud at Elementaita heard that three horses were still surviving in the park he contacted the warden, one Mr Mburugu, and requested permission to remove them. This was readily granted in the form of an official letter addressed to Ian. After all, horses were not indigenous to Kenya so their removal would be doing him and the park a modest favour.

One evening, as I was lifting a morsel of rhubarb crumble, made by major domo Njoroge's less than fair hands, towards my hungry lips, the phone rang. Not for the first time I wondered how it was that the majority of evening calls always seemed to coincide with this most basic of acts, just when I was trying to reconstitute the inner man.

'Ian Slack here,' the voice said. 'Sorry to trouble you at this late hour. You remember those horses in the park I was telling you about? Well, I've just been given permission to remove them. The only problem is that they're to all intents and purposes completely wild. So, I need you to come and dart them. Then we can halter and hobble them and walk them to Elementaita. It's not so very far.'

'Right,' I replied. 'Give me a few days and we'll make a plan. Oh and do you mind if Judy Drews comes along as well? She's very keen to help.'

'No problem. We may need all the help we can get.' Prophetic words.

Judy was married to Lofty, who in his spare time was a notable rally driver and navigator, participating in all the local and international rallies in East Africa and beyond. Lofty was of Teutonic extraction, whose elderly father lived in Tanzania, formerly German East Afrika. Lofty's real name was Harald Willy. Sensibly he stuck to Lofty. He was tall, with a very non-Germanic sense of humour. Ribald mention of the Fatherland and the War, Hitler and the shape of German heads were quite in order in the Drews household. Lofty was the manager of the local branch of D.T. Dobie, a motor firm specialising in Japanese cars.

Judy was a vivacious brunette, with a passion for horses and dogs. She even had stables in her suburban Nakuru garden. Her dogs did not regard me with much favour, despite my having snatched them from the Jaws of Death on more than one occasion. One, the ungrateful Minnie, was able to recognise my car long before I had even reached the gate of the Drews' house and would set up the most dismal, incessant barking from the moment I arrived until the moment I left.

A few days after Ian's call we – Ian, Judy, myself and six syces – found ourselves crammed into a 4WD Toyota Land Cruiser, entering the park at its south-west corner. There was no perimeter fence here to delineate the boundary, merely a dirt track. I had brought my Cap Chur pistol and rifle, together with a supply of projectile syringes and Immobilon and its essential antidote, Revivon. Ian had his letter.

The weather was fine, dry and sunny; the date was 13 March 1980. Birds sang in the bushes. A group of waterbuck grazed unconcernedly in the distance. Crickets rasped unceasingly in their underground bunkers. An eagle turned in lazy circles far above our heads. The long brown grass sighed softly in the wind. Ian turned the steering wheel and bumped slowly into the park. The ground was uneven and pitted with the deep holes excavated by aardvarks and a warthog suddenly erupted from one of these holes, closely followed by four piglets, all with tails held stiffly erect, and rushed towards distant trees. A long-tailed widow bird fluttered above a grassy thicket. In the back of the pickup the six syces clung to the sides of the rocking vehicle. One was wearing a T shirt with the logo 'Danger – Explosive Gases – Keep Clear' on his back. Another, a brawny blue-black Turkana from the far north-west, had an ivory plug inserted in a hole in his lower lip, which sagged slightly, exposing his splendid glistening teeth. A third had the arrogant aquiline features of the Somali nomad, narrow eyed and sneering, spare of flesh and long of limb, wiry hair shining with oil.

We entered a wide clearing and at once sighted the horses. We looked at them through binoculars – two stallions and a mare.

Time for action.

Ian stopped the Toyota. The syces got out and I climbed into their places. I had already prepared my weapons but was undecided whether to use the rifle or the pistol. If we could get close enough I favoured the pistol. I was less likely to miss the target and the impact on the animal was not so great.

Ian approached the group slowly. One of the stallions and the mare lifted their heads and trotted off. The other stallion, a bold grey, continued to graze, until we were within a hundred yards.

Ian stopped. 'Let's go for him,' I said. I checked the pistol to ensure that there was a projectile syringe in the barrel, and slipped off the safety catch.

Ian crept forwards. At fifty yards the stallion decided that it was time to depart. Ian accelerated with a rush over the rough ground with all the speed he could muster. The horse twisted and turned but Ian was hard on his tail. I aimed at the grey stallion's substantial rump over the bonnet of the Toyota and pulled the trigger. There was a whack and he shot away and out of the clearing with the barbed syringe with its red feathered end hanging from his backside.

Ian slowed the Toyota and we followed the darted stallion at a more sedate speed. After a few minutes we found him in a patch of bush to the east of the clearing. He was staggering drunkenly from side to side.

Then he began to goose-step in slow motion like an inebriated member of the Prussian Guard. Finally he collapsed in a heap. The syces, who had been waiting on the edge of the clearing, appeared, and rushed to the scene with ropes, head collar and hobbles. Soon we had the stallion haltered and hobbled. I removed the syringe, nicking the skin with a scalpel blade to facilitate its exit. Then I slipped a dose of Revivon into the jugular and awaited developments. Two minutes later the handsome head came up and he struggled to his feet. The syces steadied him and held him firm, two on either side and one at his head. He made no effort to escape. Instead he stood quietly, snorting softly though dilated nostrils, skin damp with sweat.

'Right, let's return to the clearing and see if we can find the other two,' I said.

'Good idea,' said Judy.

'Mohamed, can you go and see if you can find the other two horses and drive them into the clearing?' 'Ndiyo, effendi.' He loped off and vanished.

Judy and I squeezed into the left seat of the pickup.

'Funny,' said Ian, 'never known that bloke to break into a run before. He usually struts around like a turkey cock. Somalis seem to think they're a cut above everyone else. Cocky buggers.'

'Johnny Nimmo of Naivasha led a company of them against the Italians in the last war up in the Northern Frontier District,' I said. 'He told me that he always led them from the rear as otherwise they were likely to shoot him in the back!'

'Charming,' said Judy.

We re-entered the clearing but saw no horses and no Somali syce.

'Let's go back and pick up a couple of the syces and see if with their help we can find those horses,' said Ian. 'They can't be that far away.'

As the captured stallion seemed to be quiet and amenable to being held by two men we asked the other three to jump into the back of the pickup. We drove back to the clearing and drove slowly across it, rocking and swaying over the tussocks and molehills and swerving to avoid holes and dips.

'Hey, look,' said Judy. She pointed towards the western side of the clearing. 'There's the syce, but who are those four men with him?'

'Search me,' said Ian. 'Let's go and see.'

'They look like park rangers to me,' said the eagle-eyed Judy.

'They don't look too friendly,' I said. I could see the Somali syce lurking behind them, a wolfish grin distorting his vulpine features.

Two of the men were armed with rifles. As we approached they raised their rifles. 'Simama! Simama! Stop! Stop!' they screamed. 'Wat are you doing here, in the Park? Get out of the vehicle! Now! You blaady facking wazungu!' (white people) 'We will shoot yo tyres!' They aimed their rifles at the wheels.

'Shit,' I said. 'They look deranged to me. Are they on drugs?'

'Get out! Get out! You blaady bastard kaburus!' (South Africans)

Ian stopped the Toyota. The four men encircled the vehicle, glowering and glaring at us. The two armed men were especially aggressive, pointing their rifles at us and baring their teeth, spittle flecking their lips.

'If looks could kill...' muttered Judy.

'Wapi farasi? (Where is the horse?) We know you have darted a horse. We are going to shoot it! Get out!'

They struck the side of the Toyota with the butts of their rifles.

We held our breath, not knowing what to expect next.

Ian produced his letter from the warden. 'Look. I've got a letter of permission from your boss to capture these horses...' Before he could finish his sentence the shorter of the two armed rangers snatched the letter out of his hand and thrust it into his pocket and pranced away.

'Thees letter means nathing to us! Who is thees peson who signed it? Hah! He is a bladdy nobody!'

The other armed man, the taller of the two, was wearing a beret with an elephant badge on it. Suddenly he went berserk. 'Wapi bunduki? Wapi bunduki?' (Where is the gun? Where is the gun?) he shouted.

I had my Cap Chur rifle between my knees with a loaded syringe up the spout. Suddenly he reached through the open window and grabbed it by the barrel. The gun was not cocked but knowing the potency of the enclosed Immobilon I deemed that discretion was the better part of valour and let him take it. He paraded around brandishing it in the air. Now he had two guns. Great!

'Look, mate,' I said, 'the dawa in that rifle will kill you if you pull the trigger. Do you want to be permanently anaesthetised? Give it back to me, there's a good chap.' The wrong words. They goaded him to a fresh outburst of vocal virulence.

'Who are you calling 'mate'? I am not your mate, muzungu! I am not a 'chap'!'

He began to walk away with it, when one of the unarmed rangers, an older man, looked at me. With a start I recognised him. He had brought a dog to my surgery a few months previously. I beckoned to him and showed him my firearm certificate.

He turned and approached his rabid colleague, who was stamping up and down with both rifles, his and mine, raised aloft. There was a heated argument, with lots of drop-dead looks cast in my direction. Finally, with great reluctance, he approached, the yellowed whites of his eyes rolling, a gust of beery breath, mixed with fermenting mealies, preceding him like a toxic cloud, and shoved the rifle at me, the muzzle pointing at my head.

'Weh, muzungu! Shika!' (You, white man! Take it!)

'Asante!' (Thanks) I said. 'You are too kind.' This witticism was lost on the wind.

'Right,' said Ian, 'let's go and attend to the stallion and get him and us out of here,' and started the engine. Another wrong move. It goaded the two musket-carrying maniacs into another eruption of anti-mzungu madness. The taller of the two even cocked his rifle.

'Perhaps,' murmured Judy, 'it's time to leave. If we try to get the stallion now someone is going to get hurt. We'll just have to go to Park Headquarters and report all of this and hope they don't open fire on us or the horse.'

As we turned to leave I saw Mohamed reappear, a malevolent smirk on his ferrety facade. What was his disreputable role in the whole affair? Was he getting back at Ian over some minor slight, a perceived affront to his touchy Somali honour? What had he to gain apart from personal satisfaction? Certainly not money.

'No way am I employing that treacherous swine again. He's out, out!' said Ian as we rattled along the rutted road to Elementaita and Nakuru. 'An inside job if I ever saw one. He must have been in contact with those rangers ever since we arranged to capture the horses. How did he know when we were going? Someone else *must* have informed him. Who? Did he pay them? We will never know. No one will speak. They never do.'

'What about the stallion and the two syces?' asked Judy. 'What will those brutes do?'

'I don't know,' said Ian. 'Who can understand the mind of man in Africa?'

Finally we reached Park Headquarters in Nakuru. Of the Game Warden there was no sign. There was a clerk behind a desk, head nodding over a copy of the *Daily Nation*. When he had roused himself from his torpor we told him what had happened.

'That is so bad,' he said. 'And you have an official letter?'

'Yes, but one of your uncontrolled rangers has now got it.'

'Ah, that is too bad, isn't it?' He grinned.

'Yes indeed. Can you phone the Elementaita game post?'

By some latter-day miracle he got through to be told that two syces were under arrest there for poaching and illegal entry into the park. They had been marched across the park under armed guard by four rangers.

'What has happened to the horse?' we asked. Ah, that had been released back into the wild!

'Well, you'd better release the syces back into the wild as well, or someone's head will be on the block!' we raged. More disjointed conversation.

'OK. We have agreed to let them go with a caution, but can you make a donation to our community fund?'

Bile in our mouths, we turned away and left.

Chapter Eight

ITALIAN DESSERT

Maria and Marco Magaletti lived on a small property at Lanet, on the outskirts of Nakuru, where they had a small farm, on which they had stables catering for a modest string of horses, paddocks for a few cows, and housing for geese and turkeys. They also had a couple of irascible ostriches, which wandered around looking for someone to attack. They themselves were quartered in a splendid Italianate villa, which was appropriate, being Italians themselves.

Until I met the Magalettis I had laboured under the impression that all Italians were chubby opera singers, jolly Neapolitan ice cream salesmen, friendly amateur soldiers who surrendered in their thousands to a couple of British Tommies rather than run the risk of being shot at, that sort of thing. Of course, if I had given the matter some thought, I would have realised that Italians were not like that at all. After all, Nero was an Italian, as was Caligula, and the Borgias and Mussolini. And then there was the Mafia.

The Magalettis used to farm near Lumbwa, now renamed Kipkelion. In Swahili 'mbwa' means 'dog', an appellation which did not please local sensitivities and at Independence the name was promptly changed to one with more politically correct overtones. The canine cognomen apparently arose during the early pacification of the country when the Nandi, who did not regard the invading Brits with much favour, sacrificed a dog on the railway line being built from Mombasa to Lake Victoria, as a token of their displeasure. They showed their displeasure in other ways, such as spearing missionaries and beheading messengers, but in the end succumbed to the juggernaut of imperial colonialism.

The Magalettis were born complainers. Nothing seemed to please them.

The signora was small and hunched, with dehydrated hair dyed the colour of old horse urine, squinty eyes and with the rasping sort of voice I had heard fishwives on Aberdeen quayside use to advertise a recent catch of cod to prospective buyers.

The signor was of about the same stature, with a large fleshy nose and a mane of flowing white hair. He looked like General George Custer after the Sioux had got at him. But it was obvious that his role was a subservient one. He did not wear the trousers, and padded along behind his wife like an old labrador following his mistress.

They loved to moan about everything and everyone and no one was immune to their vitriol. They were the sort of clients vets would rather do without, in that in addition to their constant dissatisfaction with all and sundry, they never stuck with one vet for long. As soon as something happened which displeased them, which was often, they would contact another vet, at the same time voicing their grievances about the previous incumbent.

When they lived at Lumbwa they occasionally used a German government vet based at Kericho, to do pregnancy tests on their cows.

'Zat Cherman vet, he is useless! When he has his arm up ze cow, he falls asleep! Zere he stands with us waiting for him to say whether ze cow is or is not pregnant and zere is no answer! Why? Because he is asleep! We are paying him to do a job, not to sleep on ze job! We will not be using him again!'

Whether the German had been out enjoying whatever meagre nightlife Kericho had to offer or whether he was exhausted from a surfeit of work did not affect the Magaletti's decision. The German had to go.

One night I was called to Lumbwa to attend to a mare which had been seen by yet another vet, the local African District Veterinary Officer. The horse had had mild abdominal colic. He had treated it and she appeared initially to have recovered, but now the animal was ill, very ill, and was straining to pass dung. My heart sank with a thump towards my socks when I heard this ominous report.

'Dr Cran, she is straining and passing very leetle dung and sweating and not eating for three days now and losing weight. Can you come and see her?'

There being no suggestion that I delay my coming till the morrow morn I had to ask in four letter words why I had not been contacted before the sun had fallen below the yardarm. To that I had no answer bar that the Magalettis were acting to form.

The Magaletti's farm was a mere 65 miles from Nakuru. What was that on a dark, moonless night on a crumbling death trap pitted with potholes and travelled by unlit, unroadworthy vehicles manned by drivers hopped up to their eyebrows on lethal concoctions of drink and drugs? I clamped my jaws around one of Njoroge's charred offerings and set forth into the night. Half an hour later it started to rain so I switched on the wipers. To my consternation nothing happened. I switched them off and tried again. Nothing. 'A fuse must have gone,' I thought. 'Do I have any spare fuses and if so where are they?' I drew into the verge and made a fruitless search. I opened the bonnet and scanned the engine by the light of a torch. I twitched a few wires and tapped the windscreen. Lorries and buses roared past, sending up fountains of muddy water. The rained sheeted down. I returned to my driver's seat, and set off again. In my right hand I now held a towel and with this, by reaching out of my window, was able to clear a small porthole of visibility on the windscreen sufficient to allow me to see where I was going. In very short order the right side of my manly torso was drenched as the rain, driven by an icy wind, poured into the car. As time passed and as the rain kept up its infernal deluge, other parts of my anatomy were similarly soaked. I turned on the heater, to little effect apart from steaming up the inside of the windows, adding to further loss of visibility. I pelted on, right arm tiring and drooping as it performed overtime clearing away the mud and water on the windscreen. The towel was a sopping wet rag, heavy with water. Overtaking other vehicles on the road was a nightmare as I was unable to see through about 90% of the windscreen. How I failed to have an accident and why I did not drive off the road I will never know. According to time-honoured local custom the road had no markings, its broken verges abutted onto ditches whose hidden depths I did not care to imagine and with the rain and the darkness the car seemed to be magnetised to the innumerable potholes into which it crashed with spine-jarring regularity.

At the Rongai junction I knew that there was a police checkpoint, with a double barrier of 6-inch spikes set across the road through which, provided the gendarmes were in accommodating mode, one had to thread one's narrow way. If they were not vehicle-friendly then one was liable to be subjected to an interrogation the outcome of which depended, not on the roadworthiness of one's vehicle but on the rapacity of the man in uniform. How I was going to pass the narrow gate, virtually blindfolded, far less avoid running down a member of the forces of law and order, invariably clad in midnight black, I hesitated to imagine. But I also knew that the cops did not like getting wet and often drew the spikes aside in inclement weather while they sheltered snug and lubricated in the nearest tavern. Not always, of course, and I had seen more than one luckless motorist impale his vehicle on spikes lying unseen in dense mist or heavy rain, while gleeful gendarmes rushed whooping to the scene.

I was in luck. The roadblock was unmanned and the spikes had been pulled aside. The rain thundered down. Through my porthole I could see no sign of the police.

Once through, as though by divine signal, the rain began to ease. Finally it stopped. I was soaked to the skin. I stopped the car, got out and took off my shirt, wrung it out and laid it on the back seat to dry, got back in and, shirtless, drove on, heater turned fully up. Forty five minutes later I reached the Magaletti ménage.

I drove to the stables. As I turned off the engine the gnome-like figure of Mrs Magaletti appeared, hair like an unkempt haystack. Behind her skulked Mr Magaletti, a furtive pickpocket-like figure. 'Where have you been?' she skirled. 'We have been waiting for you for hours! Did I not tell you clearly that my horse is very sick? I am most displeased!' (So am I, you old bitch!) She stared at me. 'And why are you only half dressed?' I decided not to answer that one. Let her think what she wants.

The horse, a bay mare, stood forlornly in her stable, head lowered. A syce held her bridle. I checked her conjunctivae – a horrid brick red. Heart rate – 70 beats per minute. Over 80 and she was on the line. With my stethoscope I listened to her abdomen – deathly silence. I asked for a bucket of warm water. When it came I soaped my unshirted left arm and inserted it into the mare's rectum. At once I came across a massive hole, a rent through the rectal wall going right into the abdominal cavity. The mare was doomed. She could not possibly survive. She was dead on her feet.

'I am sorry,' I said. 'She has a rectal tear. Someone has put a hand through the wall of the rectum. She cannot recover. She should be put down – now.'

They looked at me. They were thinking, I could see, that I had put *my* hand through the rectum.

I spoke to the syce – 'When the daktari came – did he do a rectal examination?' 'Ndiyo, bwana. And there was blood on his arm when he took his arm out.'

The Magalettis refused to have the mare destroyed. She died two days later.

When they first moved to Lanet they brought with them from Lumbwa a pony gelding with chronic broken wind – advanced pulmonary emphysema – caused by the inhalation of fungal and pollen allergens. This time they agreed to have the pony destroyed and that I should do the deed after I came back from my weekend trip to Lake Rudolf.

Once again I was late to arrive as I had been shunted from hospital to hospital and from doctor to doctor as the collective medicine-men puzzled over the mystery of my truncated spine. The pony was not in pain. He was not suffering. He had the equine equivalent of a long-time smoker's cough. But the Magalettis would not wait. A neighbour had a shotgun.

While I was under the sawbones' searching scrutiny, the neighbour had cocked his gun. As he pulled the trigger the pony tossed his head in the air. The slug had hit him in the jaw, almost blowing it off. The pony screamed and rushed around the paddock, blood pouring from the wound. The syce tore after him and after him rushed the Magaletti's dogs, licking up the blood. The pony was caught. The neighbour fired again and once again missed the brain. The pony fell to the ground, but was not dead. The neighbour had only brought two cartridges. He had had to go home to replenish his arsenal. Twenty minutes later he returned to finish off the wretched pony, now almost dead from shock and loss of blood.

I received this appalling piece of news as I lay abed in the War Memorial Hospital, abridged and twitching from my at that time undiagnosed malady. I had fervently hoped that I would have no further dealings with the Magalettis for a very long time.

But at 2am on Saturday 24 April 1980 a colt foal was born to a 21-year-old thoroughbred mare, owned, yes, by the Magalettis. The birth was normal, took fifteen minutes and the foetal membranes were passed shortly afterwards. All previous foals born to this mare, four in number, had died at, or shortly after, birth. All had been colts. This, naturally, did not please the Magalettis. Four years of endeavour, at least by the stallion and mare, brought to nought. They vented their displeasure by complaining to the world at large and to me in particular, as though I had been personally responsible.

At 8.30am I received the dread summons.

'Dr Cran! You must come to see our foal, as soon as possible. All the previous foals born to thees mare have died and we do not want another to die. You must save this one! You are coming now.'

This latter request was couched in tones which suggested that I had had a personal hand in the deaths of the other four.

All too soon for my liking I was on the premises, being lectured to by Mrs Magaletti. 'Four dead foals! Thees mare, she is 21 years, do you understand? Thees is her final chance. Eh! Ze last. Eet must leeve!' It sounded like my final chance as well.

I looked at the foal. A bay colt, suckling its mother. The foal did not look strong and during the night it had passed about 6 inches of meconium, the foetal dung. Not enough. 'Thee other foals all had colic and zen zey died. Zat Cherman vet and zat African vet came and zey are hopeless! Hopeless! All died. Do you hear? All! All!' Her voice rose to Callas-like heights.

'Right. Let's have a look at him.'

The foal was bright and active, but small. I was worried, knowing that retention of the meconium was more common in colt foals than in fillies, due to the narrower diameter of the male pelvis. I asked for a bathroom scales to be brought and Mr Magaletti scurried off like a nervous rodent. The foal weighed 60 pounds. I was glad to note that we were still in the stout realm of British weights and measures and not dealing with effete continental kilograms.

'Please keep me informed. I want to know how much meconium is passed during the next few hours.'

I departed, praying that the foal would do his duty.

He did not. I was afraid of this and in anticipation had forsaken my postprandial Saturday afternoon Whitecap. I would need all of my strained wits to deal with the foal and his demanding mistress. At 5.30pm she was on the blower, giving strident tongue.

'Now 'e 'as ze colic. Ver' bad. Come!'

I came and he was very bad, distressed, rolling onto his back, turning from side to side and straining. I lubricated a finger and inserted it carefully into his rectum. At the pelvic exit I could feel a plug of rock hard meconium. The pelvic exit was so narrow it would not admit the passage of my little finger. 'Shit!' I thought, appropriately. There was no way I could winkle this out.

'I'm going to give him an enema of liquid paraffin and also the same by stomach tube to try and shift this,' I told the beady-eyed hunchback at my elbow.

'OK,' she rasped.

The syce held the little animal carefully as I slowly fed the tiny tube up the foal's right nostril, holding the end of the tube to my ear to make sure that it was in the oesophagus and not in the trachea. Air being expelled with each breath meant that it was in the wrong pipe. A bubbling sound indicated that it was near the stomach. To pour liquid paraffin into the trachea would have the animal dropping dead at my feet, followed in swift succession by myself as the signora leapt for my jugular. 'Get this right, mate,' I thought, 'or you're dead meat. This bitch will rip your guts out and serve them up like pasta if you get this wrong.' I could feel my stressed adrenals going into overdrive as I listened again to the sound from the stomach tube. Was that sound coming from the stomach or was it air from the trachea? Which was it? No, it was from the stomach. I held up the end of the tube and gave it to another syce hovering nervously behind me. A funnel was inserted into the end of the tube and 200ml of liquid paraffin slowly poured into it, flowing into the patient by gravity. Once done I did the same at the other end, inserting an enema tube into the rectum, hoisting the foal's rear end into the air and allowing 50ml to flow into what amounted to a rectal rock fall.

I gave the foal 3ml of ampicillin by intramuscular injection to ward off possible peritonitis. A lower bowel under pressure from concrete constipation could allow potential pathogens across its tensed wall and into the abdominal cavity. Reaction and pro-action. God, it was like a military campaign. Only with the Megalettis it was more like guerrilla warfare.

Between bouts of colic the foal was still suckling from his mother, but less frequently than earlier.

'Right, now we just have to await the outcome of that,' I said. 'I'll come back later this evening to see how he's doing.' The signora made a noise like an eructating dromedary. I was unsure whether this signified approval of my treatment or otherwise. I feared the latter.

At 10pm things were unchanged and the Magalettis were in volatile mode.

'Mr Cran! (Demoted from Dr to Mr I noted.) Ah, your treatment it is not working! Look, now ze foal he has stopped feeding from 'is mother. Only every three or four hours is he drinking. Hah, he will die very soon. Just like all ze others!'

'Liquid paraffin takes time to work its way through the gut and to penetrate the inspissated mass.'

'Eh, what is zat about piss, you are saying?'

'It means dried up, hardened, concrete-like.'

At 1am I could feel an 18 inch sausage-like length of rock-hard meconium filling the lower bowel, massed up against the anterior pelvis.

'Right,' I said. 'If there is no improvement and if no dung has been passed by morning, then I will have to operate.' Another grunt greeted this announcement.

The Sabbath dawned both bright and fair but I did not look forward to a Day of Rest. I tried to console myself with thoughts of the proverb which stated that the Better the Day the Better the Deed. Very well. At 8.30am I was examining the foal once again. The foal had not suckled for four hours and was rolling and lying on its back and suffering from severe unremitting colic.

I was prepared for this and had arrived in appropriate mental and physical mode. And I was not going to take any more flak from the Magalettis.

As the malignant memsahib opened her mouth, exposing her yellowing fangs, and even at this early hour enveloping me in a heart-stopping gust of garlic laden breath, I checked her gallop by saying – 'Right. Your foal is going to die unless I operate – now. We've tried the conservative, medical approach. That hasn't worked. All your other foals have died from the same problem. Now is the time to save number five. Can you please provide me with plenty of hot water, soap, towels, a clean table and bring a bathroom scales.'

Her wrinkled chops fell. Her mouth closed, opened and closed again. She looked like a newly landed geriatric cod, gasping for air. Without a word she turned and went, a shrunken deflated balloon.

The black syce holding the foal looked at me and grinned. 'Mzuri sana, bwana daktari! Endelea tu!' (Good for you, daktari! Carry on!)

The syce looked like a Nandi, a worthy descendant of the splendid warriors who, unlike those of other hypertrophied tribes, such as the overly-vaunted Maasai, did not take the advance of the Iron Snake lying down. His almond eyes glinted in his fine, dark, oval face. I could imagine them sizing up a lion or a member of an inferior tribe, both ripe for skewering on his slender spear. Perhaps even one of the Magalettis. I felt encouraged when I thought of that.

'Where are you from?' I asked.

'Chemuswa,' he said, naming a small town south-west of Eldoret.

'And your name?'

'Langat.'

'OK, Langat, I have to operate on this foal in order to get rid of the waste stuck in its bowel. I want you to do exactly what I ask and we will have a good result.'

'Ndiyo, bwana daktari,' he replied. I did not tell him, far less the Magalettis, that I had never done this operation before.

Mrs Magaletti returned, gasping and muttering under her breath. Behind her followed a retinue of servants carrying the requested items. I weighed the foal. It was still 60lb.

The table was placed outside the stable in the sun. I laid out my instruments, studying them closely to ensure that I had everything. There is nothing worse than getting halfway through an operation and then discovering that a vital piece of equipment is missing and then to have some incompetent rooting around looking for something he can't even recognise. So I examined the rows of scissors, artery forceps, needle holders, tissue forceps, scalpel, suture materials and everything else with more than usual concentration.

I looked around. A bare-footed fellow with a barrel chest, who looked like a gardener, was hovering in the background. Operations were, in my biased opinion, not a spectator sport, so I roped him in as Second Assistant. His name was Kiprono and, like Langat, he was also a Nandi.

Anaesthetic was Pentobarbitone Sodium, today regarded as antiquated as chloroform. 'Right, Langat, hold the foal's head up so I can raise the jugular vein, and you, Kiprono, put your arm round the foal's rump to hold him still while I give the injection. I don't want him leaping like an impala when he feels the prick of the sindano.' I computed the dose – 60mg per 5lb bodyweight – one ml – so theoretically 12ml in total. Using a fine needle I slipped the solution into the jugular, drew back a little blood and gave 3ml by rapid injection. By so doing I overcame the excitement which can occur should the drug be given slowly. The foal's head drooped and slumped and we carefully laid the small body onto the straw. Then I slowly injected more of the solution until he was fast asleep. Ten ml in total was enough to put him into a state of operational anaesthesia.

The mare looked alarmed at what we were doing to her baby. She stamped and whinnied.

'Right, let's lift him onto the table and get cracking. We've got about an hour to do the job so let's get moving.'

'Ndiyo, bwana daktari,' my two assistants said in unison. The lurking owner said nothing. I could feel her gimlet eyes boring into my back.

We laid the foal on the table on his right side and to protect his upper eye from the sun I covered it with a small towel kindly provided by the signora from her personal closet. It bore upon it a realistic motif of a gladiator skewering a luckless opponent with a trident. Cheering Romans, all with thumbs down, filled the background. With a razor blade I carefully shaved the left flank between pelvis and ribs and swabbed the area with surgical spirit. I draped the area and after momentary cogitation made a vertical incision midway between the last rib and the pelvis, long enough to admit insertion of my hand and wrist.

Being right-handed I went around to the back of the patient and insinuated my hand into the foal's abdomen, where I easily located the impacted rectum and lower colon, filled with its solid sausage of inspissated meconium. I glanced up. Langat and Kiprono were staring open-mouthed. Mrs Magaletti gave us a sceptical sneer. The mare snorted softly and turned to crop the grass beside the stable door. Not for the first time I thought – 'Cran, it's not the animals you got to worry about, it's the bloody owners!'

Gently I massaged the rectum and colon and broke the mass into separate pellets and slowly milked them between my thumb and forefinger through the narrow pelvic culvert and towards the open air and freedom. After twenty minutes I was done and it was time to close up. I returned to the other side of the foal and carefully stitched the peritoneum and abdominal muscles with a continuous layer of catgut. Before final closure I squeezed a tube of intamammary antibiotic into the abdominal cavity and closed the skin with monofilament nylon.

'Well, though I say it myself,' I said, 'that looks pretty neat.'

'Safi sana, bwana daktari,' said Kiprono.

'Asante,' I replied. No word from the hovering presence. I gave the patient ampicillin and prednisolone by intramuscular injection to ward off infection and to allay localised swelling. After all, the surroundings could hardly be classified as being sterile. The foal's eyelids had been abraded while rolling on the ground during the night when suffering the agonies of colic. I now applied a little skin ointment to the affected area.

Back aching, I straightened up and turned to the signora. 'Right, Mrs Magaletti, that's it. Let's lay the little fellow on the straw and let the mother come in.' Langat led the mare into the stable. She bent her head and sniffed and nuzzled at her baby. I looked at my watch – 11am. Time to go. 'Please let me know how he is at 2 o'clock.' Mrs Magaletti nodded, but said nothing.

At 2pm the phone rang. Was the foal dead or alive, I thought? I had never known the Magalettis to phone with good news. They seemed to delight in being the bearers of bad news, grim harbingers of death and disaster. I prepared myself for the worst. It was Mrs Mageletti. 'Ah dottore! Dottore! Eet ees a miracle! The foal, he ees on his feet and he is suckling from hees mother. He ees fine and there is now no colic. I am so so happy.'

'Well, so am I, signora. That *is* good news,' I replied. 'Please let me know if anything goes wrong.'

No news is good news, so they say, and so it was. The Magalettis were not the sort of people to waste money on reporting glad tidings. The phone did not ring. For the next three days I returned to give the foal ampicillin and prednisolone, visits which the Magalettis seemed to regard as financially unnecessary in view of the foal's present wellbeing. A week after birth the foal weighed 76lb, having gained 16lb, and a fortnight later weighed 95lb having gained 35lb in his first two weeks of life. There had been no recurrence of colic and dung and urine were being passed normally. The foal continued to grow and remained healthy and blooming.

The Magalettis were secretly pleased to see their foal grow and flourish and for a time I enjoyed an uncertain popularity. This did not extend to being offered entry to their mansion to partake of cappucino or cake or a glass of Campari – they did not possess the uninhibited generosity which characterised most Kenya settlers – but for a short and giddy time I was the Man of the Month.

Chapter Nine

STEERING WHEEL BLUES

In the Men's Bar at the Rift Valley Sports Club there was no such thing as Closing Time. Drinks were served until the last man standing had staggered out of the door, or been helped upstairs to lie down, cooling cloths at hand, ready to be laid across the throbbing settler brow by attentive stewards. Even in the late 70s such solicitous colonial habits died hard.

Mike Hughes lurched through the arched doorway, homeward bound. Mike's capacity for beer was such that he had his own personal mug, a huge Teutonic stein capable of holding two litres of the golden fluid, kept below the bar and brought out like a sacred priestly chalice by Maina, the head barman, whenever he appeared.

Mike had a laugh resembling the noise made by a donkey stallion when it spots a receptive female. It had a no-holds-barred sound about it and he made it now as he bade his still standing or sitting companions a raucous farewell.

Five minutes later he reappeared, wild-eyed and incoherent.

'What's the matter, Mike?' asked Roy McDougal, from his lofty stool at the bar. With his silvery hair and patrician manner he resembled an elderly eagle perched precariously on its eyrie. 'Lost your keys?'

'Shum bugger's pinched the steering wheel of my Merc!'

'What? Now that *is* serious. That's a police matter, if you ask me.'

'Too right. Maina, get me the phone.'

Maina did as he was bade, bringing the instrument on its cradle, tethered by a long rubberised line. 'Get me the police, Maina, chop, chop!' 'Ndyio, bwana!' (Yes sir!)

Despite the fact that it was past midnight the voice on the other end sounded alert and crisp and ready for action.

'Shes he'll be here in ten minutes,' slurred Mike. 'Shaid his name was Inshpector Mungai. Now why would anyone want to steal my steering wheel?'

'Is it made of walnut, or covered with bespoke yak hide?' asked Roy.

'No, it's just plain boring old plastic,' said Mike.

Ten minutes later a steward padded into the bar to announce the arrival of the inspector. Inspector Mungai marched in, cap under his left arm. 'Which of you gentlemen is Mr Hughes?' he asked. Mike introduced himself and was rewarded with a smart salute.

'Is that your Mercedes outside in the car park?' the inspector inquired.

'It is,' responded Mike.

'I've just closed the right rear door. It was wide open, the interior reeked of alcohol and although there is no steering wheel in the back there is one in the front! Perhaps it might be a good idea not to drive home tonight!'

Chapter Ten

LUMP IN THE THROAT

My previous secretary, the ever-ebullient, lovely Sophie Sinclair-Smith had, sadly, departed, lured away by the bright lights and other attractions of Nairobi. Her successor, Renata Grioni, was of Pakistani and Italian ancestry. Pale and plump, I had to admit that although she was alarmingly efficient she was not by any stretch of the imagination the powerful sexual magnet that Sophie had been, who drew the men – and even the women, clients and non-clients alike, to the surgery, like vultures attracted out of an empty sky to a succulent carcass. So I had to work that little bit harder to make up the shortfall. Whereas in the past I could sit back and let Sophie chat up the clients, now I had to get out there, paste on a winning smile and do the welcoming bit. Most people were accommodating, but some were hard work. I found that it all depended on their sense of humour. Some nationalities have more than others. The Danes, Dutch and Germans could be hard work, but once you broke through the surface crust you usually made contact with a warm inner centre, rather like biting into one of those expensive chocolates with an unexpected core of uplifting liqueur. The Australians, Canadians and Americans were on the whole always friendly and easy-going, perhaps superficially so, but they made my job easier. They were relaxed and appreciative and I liked that. Most Africans were grateful and undemanding. They knew when someone was doing their best to help them and I was happy with that. I never felt as on edge with African clients as I did with some Europeans, whose eyes you felt boring into your back as you bent over their animal. I could read their thoughts – 'Does this guy *really* know what he's doing?' 'He's trying to pull the wool over my eyes.' 'I don't believe a word he's saying, not a word!' With these people you had to get things right – first time. It was the only way to convince them that you knew more than they did. One good result and you could do no wrong, mostly, even when later things did go wrong – as they sometimes did.

On his farm at Kilombe there lived an elderly remnant of the Empire, beached when the captains and the kings departed. Brigadier Percival Marmaduke Fitz-Henry ruled his personal empire with an iron hand. An iron fist inside an iron glove. He had played a prominent part in the Burma campaign against the Japanese, had served in the Chindits under the brilliant, if eccentric, Orde Wingate, behind the Japanese lines, been captured when his headquarters had been overrun by the Knights of Bushido and had spent two years as a reluctant guest of Emperor Hirohito, toiling as a starving, malarial coolie while his prison camp companions dropped down dead on every side. Fitz survived, mostly as a result of iron discipline and by not letting his personal standards slip. If he had been in the German Army as opposed to the British he would have been awarded the Iron Cross, First Class, with Oak Leaves. His sense of humour, however, was well hidden.

The consequence of this experience had made him a man who expected others to emulate, if not match, his standards. He had no time for shirkers or clock-watchers. His workers were kitted out in smart blue uniforms with 'Kilombe' writ large on their uniformed backs. His Guernsey cows were sleek and fat, their coats gleaming, and they produced calves and milk to regular order. His dairy was a very model of cleanliness. The milk churns shone with such lustre that when, on one occasion, as I strolled into the dairy, a shaft of sunlight struck one gleaming churn I reeled backwards as I caught a distorted reflection of myself in the mirror-like metal, squat and dwarf-like one moment and elongated and grotesque the next, like a hideous image in a showground hall of mirrors. Fitz was married to Betty, who was Anglo-Irish and feisty and stood no nonsense from him, or anyone else. They had a son and a daughter. The former did not match up his father's exacting standards, being rather less than bright and as a result suffered by comparison to the daughter who was smart and good looking. Fitz could be a martinet and a bully at times. The Fitz-Henry's dining room was large and filled with dark, highly polished furniture, polished to soldierly perfection by droves of salaaming servants. The walls were festooned with hunting prints, polo mallets, ceremonial swords, Japanese as well as Imperial British, Malayan daggers, ancestral daguerreotypes, photographs of unsmiling moustachioed officers, Ghurka kukris, and the stuffed head of an unsmiling tiger.

'Cran! Fitz-Henry here! One of my best animals has a growth in her throat. It's about the size of a potato, not your local pygmy rubbish, but an English King Edward. She's not happy about it, neither am I, and I need you here soon.' In other words, now, if not before.

'Right, give me a few minutes to clear up here and I'll be on my way.'

I heard a harrumph at the other end of the line and then the rest was silence.

The Brigadier's farm at Kilombe was not close and it took me a good 45 minutes of fast driving and matatu dodging to get there. As I drove I puzzled over what this might be. Kenyan farmers did not feed their cattle on root crops such as turnips or swedes as farmers did in the UK during the winter with the resultant risk of choking on an extra large piece of inspissated forage.

When I worked in Aberdeenshire I always carried with me a probang – a long leather-covered tube with a metal ferrule at the business end, for pushing reluctant foreign objects down cows' gullets into their rumens. During the winter I used the thing so often that I took to walking around with it draped across my shoulders, rather like some doctors – and some vets – like to casually suspend stethoscopes around their necks in a mute but elegant demonstration to Joe Bloggs that here is a man (or woman) who knows what they are about.

I did not possess a probang in Kenya and since I arrived in the country in 1966, thirteen years previously, had not had the need to use one. Now I wondered whether my bovine armoury was deficient in a vital element. But I did have a horse stomach tube should push come to shove. Would that serve?

With my mind a whirl of differential diagnoses I rocketed up the bougainvillea-bordered drive to the Brigadier's redoubt and ground to a halt in a cloud of dust. When it cleared I saw the bulky figure of the old soldier glaring at me, sifting particulate matter from his moustache with a pair of nicotine-stained fingers.

'Took you a while to get here, what? Anyway you're here now, so come along. The cow's in the crush.'

The crush, I was glad to see, was, like the Brigadier, stoutly built, and not the usual ramshackle affair to be found on most Kenyan farms. A pair of dungaree-clad workers lolling in the shade jumped to their feet when they saw us approaching and gave the Brigadier a smart military salute. I was impressed. I, as a mere private, did not warrant a salute.

In the crush stood a large Guernsey cow. She was drooling and swallowing convulsively. Halfway down her neck I could see a round swelling, about the size of a large orange – or a King Edward potato. I leaned over the side of the crush and felt it – it was hard, smooth and unyielding. What was it? I tried to milk the object up and then down the animal's neck but it stubbornly refused to comply. From the way the cow was gulping and gagging it was apparent that the mass, whatever it was, was lodged in the oesophagus. I conveyed my findings to the watching warrior.

'Right. I guessed as much myself. The point is – what are you going to do about it?'

'Well, I want to try to shift it with a stomach tube, which I have in my car.'

I returned from the car with the eight foot long tube, coiled in my hand like a lariat. It had a diameter of about an inch. I also brought with me a metal bovine Drinkwater gag, named, I presumed, after a chap called Drinkwater. At least the anatomical connotations were correct. The gag was so designed that it lodged between top and bottom sets of molar teeth on one side of the animal's mouth, wedging it open and allowing sufficient space for the insertion of a hand, or, in this case, the stomach tube. I made sure that the gag was securely in place. If it slipped, the animal's sharp teeth were quite capable of severing the tube and more than one vet has felt the sudden hot flush of desperation on finding that his stomach tube is now half its original length, gone without hope of retrieval to distant gastric parts. I had tied a length of strong twine to the gag. Cows are capable of swallowing indigestible objects without turning a hair and the last thing I wanted was to see the gag on its way down the cow's gullet to join the unknown object down there.

I could feel martial eyes watching closely as I got things ready.

I turned to my two helpers, 'Aizeru, watu wote, shika kichwa ya ngombe,' (Right, everyone, hold the cow's head.) lubricated the tube with a little liquid paraffin and fed it gently into the cow's mouth and down her gullet until it came up short against the solid object. I gave the tube a measured push in the hope of dislodging the mass. Nothing happened. I withdrew the tube a few inches and tried again. Still nothing.

I turned to Fitz. 'I can pour a little liquid paraffin down the tube to see if the mass will soften sufficient to get it moving or lubricate the outside of whatever this is. If that doesn't work the only other solution is surgery. If that thing is left there for too long it will cause pressure necrosis of the gullet. And then, good night sweet prince – or princess in this case.'

'Right then, give it a try.'

Carefully I poured a cupful of liquid paraffin down the tube, raised the end to my lips and gave it a good blow. I withdrew the tube by a few inches and advanced it again until it contacted the mass and gave it a firm push. Nothing doing.

I tried again. This was hopeless.

'Brigadier,' I said. 'I think we – or rather I – should operate – now. If we wait, then if whatever is blocking the gullet doesn't move it will obstruct the blood supply to the area it is pressing on and cause death of the gullet wall. Operating may cause some constriction but this animal is going to die if we don't act fast. She is going to get bloat as well through inability to eructate. I can trocar her to relieve that but that will only be a short-term measure.'

The Brigadier was not a dilly-dallier and did not delay in voicing his thoughts. What I did not know, and should have, was that he had had a classical education. 'In rebus asperis et tenui spe fortissima quaeque consilia tutissima sunt. Livy,' he barked. I had done Latin for six years to Scottish higher level at school, but I just gaped at him. 'In grave difficulties and with little hope, the boldest measures are the safest. Get on with it, man!'

I did.

I retrieved my surgical bag from the car, and, on a clean towel spread on a bale of hay, assembled the instruments I thought I would need. The house was close at hand and one of the workers was dispatched to bring a bucket of warm water and a bar of soap. I did not sedate the cow. I did not want her head to be lowered during the proceedings or to have her producing copious volumes of saliva. While a worker elevated her head I carefully shaved a wide area around the swelling, swabbing it with spirit and infiltrating local anaesthetic into and below the skin.

I knew that the oesophagus of the cow is much wider and more distensible than that of the horse, shorter and less sinuous. This, I hoped would make my job a little easier. But apart from that my anatomical recall from my distant student days remained a stubborn blank.

'So be it,' I thought. 'It will have to be back to first principles.'

I could feel the Brigadier scrutinising me with what I considered to be unnecessary intensity.

With my two helpers cradling the patient's head in their arms I made a careful incision into the skin over the lump. 'Careful, now. Careful.' I thought. 'There are vital nerves and blood vessels in here. And God knows what essential muscles.'

Slowly, ever so slowly, I cut deeper, swabbing away as I did to enable me to see what I was doing. Using a pair of scissors I parted the muscles. I pushed aside a fat, white, worm-like nerve and burrowed underneath a pulsating artery. So far so good. But, it seemed to be taking forever to get to what I had thought lay just below the skin. 'Take it easy, lad,' I thought. 'Take it easy.' A drop of sweat rolled off my nose. A fly landed on my forehead. I wrinkled my snout in an effort to dislodge it. It stayed there, roaming freely. I could feel it stopping every now and then to rub its legs together. Soon it was joined by another. And another. They were having some sort of conference on my forehead. Probably discussing the taste of my perspiration.

At last! The oesophagus – a pale anaconda – sprang into view, bulging with its prey. I breathed more freely. I gave the lump a tentative prod. It was solid, and round, like a cricket ball. For a wild, unthinking moment I almost asked the Brigadier if he had lost one of his balls.

Slowly I cut down onto the lump, through the muscles of the wall of the oesaphagus, which parted like the opening jaws of a carnivorous plant, to reveal a round, hard, olive-coloured, smooth-textured sphere, which popped out into my grateful hand. I handed it to the hovering mandarin and turned my attention to repairing the gaping wound.

Twenty minutes later I straightened up, muscles creaking with the strain and turned to Fitz. 'That's a hairball. Your cow must have been doing a lot of grooming and licking to have formed that. They're quite rare.'

He massaged it in his palm.

'Thank you, Cran. Stout chap,' the Brigadier was almost effusive in his gratitude.

When I was next in the Fitz-Henry's dining room, some weeks later, another polished trophy was on display. There, on the mantelpiece, gleaming in a shaft of sunlight, perched on a hand-crafted plinth, stood the hairball.

Chapter Eleven

Things That Go Bump
in the Night

Opposite the surgery a beggar sat importuning the passing public for alms. He was a leper, with stumps where his hands had once been and he had no toes. Like a mediaeval monk his head was covered in a black cowl, hinting at hidden horrors beneath. Not for the first time did I think that here was the Middle Ages in modern dress. He would sit there for hours at a time. Then, when he had a few coppers in his bowl, he would, with what was an obvious effort, drag himself to his feet and lurch and shuffle away down the street.

Further up the street a blind man squatted, beating a drum, accompanying the same, never-ending tune emanating from a ghetto blaster demurely hidden beneath a crocheted cloth, nestling by his side. I did not mind the rhythmic jungle beat – I found it rather soothing – but I did mind the tinny, staccato, off-key radio-phonic screech. On and on and on it went. The surgery was some distance from where the man sat but his minstrelsy was all-invasive. It was all very well if you just happened to be passing by. If you were trying to explain and justify the finer points of a knotty diagnosis to a doubting client over and above the brain-numbing discord, it was not. But I was obviously in the minority. Hawkers peddling their wares adjacent to the source of the din seemed blessed with some efficient noise-filtering facility, denied to lesser mortals. They carried on chatting to each other, flogging their second-hand clothes and counterfeit Chinese sneakers, and slumbering in the shade, totally unconcerned by the adjacent cacophony.

These aural disturbances were all part and parcel of urban life in Africa, where, as the population multiplied and competition increased, people resorted to ever more desperate measures to earn some money.

The battle for survival had become increasingly nasty. Minibuses cruised the streets, loudspeakers booming, music blaring, advertising dubious products for sale. The pavements were clogged with shoeshine boys, vegetable sellers, pickpockets, loiterers, opportunists, whores, con men, purveyors of third-rate magazines and second-hand books – useful things like *Teach Yourself Croat in Three Months* and *Balti Cooking for the Single Suburban Mother* – pushy Somalis parading with trays of trashy watches, young men selling teddy bears and heaps of brassieres, while opposite the now defunct Stag's Head Hotel, rows of curio sellers waited for the tourists who never came. There was no room for pedestrians on the pavements. They were forced into the street, where they were at the mercy of the chaotic, uncontrolled traffic. A man stood in the road waving biro pens at indifferent passers-by. A woman stood at a corner holding up an embroidered tablecloth. She stood there every day and it always looked like the same tablecloth. The competition between matatus was fierce and they employed desperate measures to pull in more passengers. Their speeds increased, they forced more and more passengers into their foetid interiors, they overtook other vehicles with reckless abandon, on blind corners, on the left; if they indicated they were turning left it usually meant they were turning right and vice versa. Their slogans became more and more bizarre – First Violin, Coffin Carrier, Smasho. It was every man for himself and the devil take the hindmost.

Buildings were jerry built and ramshackle, walls and windows filthy with dirt and dust, curtains, if there were any, knotted and dense with grime. African architecture was utilitarian. Aesthetics formed no part of the picture.

Drains were either non-existent or open and clogged with debris. With every downpour of rain they overflowed, water coursing across roads, filling depressions and pouring into buildings.

Litter and plastic bags were everywhere, tossed aside with careless abandon by the thoughtless citizenry. Did they not see what I saw and smelt? The rubbish and the stench, and the progressive conversion of a pleasant town into an urban slum were overpowering.

Nakuru was a melting pot, bubbling and boiling with an effervescent mixture of people from all over the country – tall Luos from the Lake, squat Abaluyas from the border land near Uganda, fine-featured Kipsigis from the Kericho highlands, tough Turkanas from the far north-west, slender Maasai from the south and the ubiquitous Kikuyus, selling and bargaining and making money as hard as they could.

But the people themselves were as easy-going and as friendly and as cheerful as ever. They seemed not to notice their progressively deteriorating surroundings. But I was always glad to escape into the country, where things were just as bad but, being more spread out and diluted by space, not so obvious and in your face.

However, some forays into the 'field' – Africans for some reason loved to refer to the 'field' – made me wonder which was to be preferred: town or country.

'Miss Nguru here,' the well-modulated voice said. 'My dad says can you please go to his farm at Bahati, as there is a cow there which has been trying to have a calf for three weeks.' I glanced at my watch – half past two.

'Three weeks!' I expostulated. 'Three weeks? Are you sure?'

'Yes, but another vet came to see it two weeks ago and said it was all right, but now we don't think so, as the cow is not eating and can't stand, so can you come please?'

This I could not believe. Surely there must be a mistake? The cow must have aborted and had retained her placenta. No rush then. Still…

I asked my ever-trusty Kikuyu assistant, Moses, to make sure that there was plenty of obstetrical lubricant in the car, together with my well-worn embryotome, calving ropes, knives, etc. Hoping against hope that we wouldn't have to use them we bade farewell to Renata and set off.

We turned onto the road leading to the Solai Valley. On our left rose the brooding bulk of the extinct volcano, Menengai. On its rim was a fringe of forest, but at its base an ugly rash of tin huts was beginning to creep upwards. After a few miles the crater itself came into view, a thick anthropoidal tongue of black solidified lava licking hungrily at the base of the surrounding cliffs. Curling plumes of steam rose from vents hidden in the vegetation.

We reached the junction where the road to Bahati branched off from that which led on to the Solai valley. Here, at Lavender's Corner, I had spent my first 18 months in Kenya. The small wooden house in which I had lived was now a butchery – I could see a haunch of bloodied beef hanging in the window of what used to be my bedroom – the lawns were gone, replaced by bare earth, and the great pepper tree had been cut down. Women selling potatoes, tomatoes, beans, peas and cobs of maize squatted beside the road.

I drove on. The road was now surfaced. Previously it had been dirt and a deterrent to all but those with necessary business in the area. Now speculators and nouveau investors had converted what had been a sleepy rural lane wandering innocuously through the countryside from one hamlet to another into a busy, blacktop highway as they sped from one important appointment to another.

The farm was just off the road, up a rocky track. I drove up it and stopped the car.

A man appeared, a rough-looking fellow, with shaggy hair and unkempt clothes.

'Habari gani? Wapi ngombe nashinda kusaa?' I asked. (How are you? Where is the cow which is unable to give birth?)

He grinned, showing a mass of large yellow teeth.

'Chini ya milima,' he replied, (At the bottom of the hill) gesturing to the field behind him. 'Right,' I said to Moses. 'Let's go and look at the damage.'

At the foot of the hill we found the patient, a nondescript, cross-bred cow, looking decidedly below par. Her rib cage resembled the spars of a wrecked ship, wind-scoured and long beached on a hostile shore, her eyes were sunken in their sockets, dull and leaden, her coat was dry and rough, and she looked as though she had barely enough strength to draw breath.

'Ah, you've arrived!' I turned to see a young man, light skinned, snappily dressed, and wearing a pair of incongruous winkle picker shoes. 'I'm Miss Nguru's brother. Glad you could make it. This is apparently one of our best cows and it seems she might be pregnant. I know nothing about cows myself. I'm in banking and only flew in from London this morning. I work at Canary Wharf. Dad's around somewhere.'

'Mmm,' I thought. 'Your Dad also knows nothing about cows, if this is anything to go by.'

A spindly youth trotted down the hill carrying a battered tin bucket. It was half full of dank, dark brown water. Wordlessly he handed me a hard grey object which I assumed was made of soap. Muttering a short, fervent, prayer I sank to my knees, with difficulty lubricated my left arm and insinuated it through the patient's vulva. The tract was dry and tacky and initially I could feel nothing. I advanced my hand and reached the cervix, which on first contact seemed to be closed. Closure usually means either that what is in front is empty or is occupied by a live calf. My spirits rose. Then I insinuated an exploratory finger through the neck of the cervix and realised that there was a dead calf behind it – a very dead calf, judging by what I could feel. My heart sank.

Swivelling my head with difficulty towards the young, sharp-suited magnifico standing at my metaphorical elbow, I revealed my bleak findings – and my bleaker prognosis – 'Look, there's a three week dead calf in here, the cow can't stand, she's toxic, she hasn't eaten for days, she's lost half her body weight, her chances of survival are almost nil. Even if we get the calf out she'll probably die of shock.' There was a short silence. 'But she's *certainly* going to die if the calf stays in there, won't she?' 'Certainly, but her chances of survival are minuscule.' I didn't say that any putative struggle to get the calf out would probably make my own chances of survival pretty small as well, hoping that he would see sense. But I knew that if I refused to make the attempt the people here would think that she *might* have lived, if only I had tried.

I sighed. 'OK. But I hold out little hope. Can I now have some *hot* water, please?' 'Right away, sir.' The accent was pure East London.

Hot water came, and I got down to work – literally, as, with the cow being unable to stand, I was on my knees, grovelling in the dirt. Like a good Muslim I always used my left hand and arm for this sort of work. This was not really a very good idea. I had used my left for so long that my right had almost atrophied from disuse. It was fine for shaking people by the hand, for writing, shaving and brushing my teeth, but when it came to any sort of sustained muscular activity it was almost worthless. If I lost the use of my left arm I would be sunk without trace.

I poured a goodly quantity of lubricant over my arm and advanced it up the tract until I reached the cervix, which I had to open if the deceased occupant on the other side was to vacate the premises. The cervix felt like an iron ring, solid and unyielding. Kneading and pummelling is something best done with the whole hand. Ask any pastry cook. If you try to do it with just the tips of your fingers you very quickly run out of steam, as I found out as I tried to massage the rigid tissues into something more malleable. With fingers which felt as powerful as the contents of a packet of uncooked sausages I struggled on. After about half an hour of this I was able, finally, to insinuate my whole hand through the cervix and into the uterus. Now by opening my hand and pulling it backwards I slowly, very slowly, persuaded the cervix to open. But, could I widen it enough to get the calf out? I felt as though I was shoving my arm up a rubber pipe which had been left out in the sun for a couple of weeks. Try it some time. I poured more lubricant into the vagina and tried again. I got my hand over the calf's head. The hair was coming off. Not a good sign. I pushed my arm farther in and felt a leg. With an effort which almost disjointed my elbow I slithered my hand down the leg to below its knee and brought it up and through the cervix. With the leg through the cervix the passage was almost closed again. I had to widen it much more in order to extract the calf. So it was back to forcing my arm through the opening in order to widen it. Another half an hour passed. My arm felt like putty. I found the other leg and with eyes popping with the effort got that also through the cervix. Now only the head remained. Only! I grinned mirthlessly.

'Moses! How's the patient doing at your end?' I asked.

'She's not too happy, but holding on.'

Not too happy, eh? Well, that makes two of us.

I decided to try and loop a rope snare over the calf's head but try as I might I could not get it behind its ears. I knew that if it was not thus placed, as soon as the rope was pulled it would slip off, accompanied by tears and cries of frustration, and worse. But I could get a finger into the left eye socket. That was something.

'Moses,' I croaked. 'Can you bring me an eye hook.'

This was a sharp curved hook, rather like a huge fish hook, the sort of thing which might be useful for catching great white sharks and small whales. It had an eye at the blunt end through which I had looped a soft rope. If I could get the hook inserted into the bone of the calf's eye socket I would, in theory at least, be able to pull the head through the cervix. I cupped the hook in the palm of my hand and slid my arm in the direction of the waiting head. In obstetrical textbooks I had seen drawings of gowned clinicians doing this, casually slipping the hook into a waiting eye socket with what appeared to be ridiculous ease. They were usually wearing a small smug self satisfied smile as they did this, as if to say 'any idiot can do this, and you're certainly one if you can't.' I almost didn't as I wriggled and squirmed with the needle sharp hook perilously on the point of skewering my palm instead of the calf's eye socket. With an exhausted whimper, such a marathon runner at the very limits of his endurance might give on touching the line, I nudged the hook into the socket and told Moses to give the rope a tug. The hook bit into the bone. But one was not enough. I had to get the other hook into the other socket.

'Moses, how's she doing up there?' No point in flogging a dead horse – or a dead cow.

'Not as good as before, but still hanging on.'

'Right, can you give me another eye hook.'

As he did so he gave me a look which clearly said – 'This is a waste of time.' My sentiments entirely, but I was in too far to wade back. I felt like Macbeth, steeped in blood, drenched in gore. The next socket was further away and therefore considerably harder to reach. There was so little room that I was unable to open my hand holding the hook. All I could do was attempt to cup my fingers over the socket and then what? Struggling mightily I nudged the point of the hook over the rim and, feeling fatigued, rested before my next effort. I gave a weary grunt, a bit like that which a hippo gives when coming up for a much-needed breath of air. For some reason, best known to himself, Moses seemed to think that this was a signal for him to heave at the capstan bars as the next thing I knew my vital left palm was impaled by the needle sharp hook. 'Stop! Stop!' I yelled. He did stop, but not before I was well and truly bayoneted, with the sharp end embedded deep into my palm. 'Great,' I thought, 'if this doesn't get infected then nothing will.'

With a justifiable oath I pulled my hand back, freed myself, and with my hand throbbing like an outboard motor in overdrive, shoved the hook with the effort of desperation into the elusive socket. 'Now pull!' I instructed my alerted assistant. He did so and the hook was in.

Both ropes were looped to a baton of wood which I had brought from my car. But the calf's skull was not as it had been three weeks before. Maceration had taken place and the bone had softened, so much care would be needed to avoid tearing out of the hooks, one of which was daubed with my personal blood. I looped a soft calving rope around each available foreleg, sorted out the spaghetti-like tangle and advised in a polite but firm tone which rope to pull – 'and no bloody jerking or I'll jerk something and you won't like it!' Someone gave a nervous giggle.

Slowly, very very slowly, millimetre by interminable millimetre, the wreck that had once been a calf crept out into the fading light of day. A nose appeared, a bloated tongue, a hoofless foot and a leg with the hair coming off it. The smell was awful. With the approach of darkness the flies had retired. Now they returned.

Impasse. The vulva was too small to allow easy egress and what was worse, the hooks were beginning to tear through the soft bone.

'Moses,' I said. 'Bring me a scalpel. I'm going to have to do an episiotomy, enlarge the vulval opening. How's she doing up there?'

'She's pretty weak. She's got her head down.'

My own condition exactly.

Where the bulge of the calf's head pushed out the vulva I made a long lateral incision and told my dark helpers to gently pull. The cow was beyond sensation and local anaesthesia was forgone in the interests of speed. The head moved and then popped out. But we were not done. As the calf emerged so it lengthened to an alarming degree as its tissues stretched to breaking point under the strain. There was every possibility that at any moment it was going to sunder in two, with the direst of consequences to both the cow and to me. Once again I yelled 'Stop! Stop!'

I slipped another rope over the head and around the chest – not without difficulty – and once again monitored the pulling. The abdomen was grossly distended with the gases of decomposition and was impeding forward progress. It required urgent deflation. As soon as a portion inched into sight I incised it with the scalpel, inserted my hand – the left as usual – and removed the malodorous contents, guts and all. Now surely it would come out! Come along, come along! The men pulled.

For one horrible moment I thought its pelvis was going to jam and I would have to do an embryotomy. That, I thought, would be the end. Finis. Finito. But come it did, albeit with reluctance. When it did it came with a rush, followed by a tidal wave of malodorous dammed up uterine fluids.

The men cheered as it emerged. I did not feel like cheering. The cow did not look like cheering. In fact she looked like dying.

I creaked to my feet and turned to the young man. He was not there.

'Where the..?' I began. 'As soon as he saw and smelt the dead calf he left, quickly, in a rush,' someone said, grinning. I couldn't blame him. Canary Wharf did not prepare him for this sort of thing.

'Right, Moses, it's stitching time,' I said. 'Can you bring some catgut and needle holders.'

Half way through the stitching the cow gave a long, sad, shuddering sigh and died.

Great, I thought. Just great. Poor cow! The only consolation, if there is any, is to know I was right, but all that effort. God, all that wasted effort – and for nothing! Perhaps not even payment. A heap of dead meat. Not fresh either! Far from it! Perhaps clipping dogs' toenails or squeezing anal glands in the warm safety of the surgery isn't so bad after all. You're inside, in the dry, in the light, running water nearby, standing up, actually standing up, wearing a nice, spotlessly clean, starched, white coat, perhaps with your hands neatly enclosed in sterile gloves to keep them pure, certainly not besmirched by unmentionable fluids and crouched down in the mud and the blood and worse, like a re-branded Caliban, waiting discovery and unwelcome publicity in the gutter press for gratuitous cruelty to your patient.'

'Pole, bwana daktari, wewe lijaribu sana.' (Sorry, daktari, you really tried.)

I turned my head, besmirched as it was like the rest of my person. It was the shocked-headed Peter whom we had first met on arrival.

'Anante sana, rafiki.' (Thanks very much, friend.)

I felt better. I had tried. That was something, I supposed. Someone had noticed.

Back in Nakuru I dropped Moses off at the surgery and drove to the post office to check my mail box. By now it was 8pm and dark. With a bit of luck someone might have sent me a cheque. The street was deserted, with only one car to be seen, angle parked outside the post office. I drew in beside it and jumped out and ran into the mail box section, which was set back off the main street. The driver of the other car, an angular Irish priest with gingery hair and wearing the obligatory, ecclesiastical grey flannel trousers, was bent over, extricating a mass of letters and packages from his box. Probably pastoral bumpf from his bishop or the Pope, I thought. As these unclerical thoughts were going through my head there was the most almighty crash. I turned to see my car being propelled onto the pavement and up into the mail box section. The good father let out an unsanctioned oath and skipped nimbly aside as my 504 came to rest, front bumper inches from the row of locked mail boxes. 'What the hell.....?' I rushed to my car. The priest's car was now embedded in the left side of my Peugeot, and behind the priest's car was another car, which had rammed him in the rear.

From out of this car, a beat up Nissan with cracked windscreen and bald tyres, emerged a bemused-looking African, who gazed around him as though wondering where he was. A rank gust of beery breath, borne on the soft night air, assailed my expanded nostrils, expanded and dilated like an epidermal trumpet by a rising tide of fury.

'Harro, my flend,' he slurred, his features wreathed in a quiet, soporific, smile. 'How are you?'

'How am I? How am I?' I ground out the words between gritted teeth, hyperventilating in an effort to stay calm.

The priest stood at my quivering shoulder, gazing at the scene, stunned. Bits of his car tinkled onto the pavement with a musical clang.

'My son,' he said finally, with mild disapproval. 'Have you been drinking?'

I answered on behalf of the object of his censure.

'Don't strike a match, Father. We're likely to go up in flames if you do. Our friend here smells like a brewery. He's as drunk as a skunk.'

'My dear flends, I am not dlunk. No, no, no. Never have I dlunken a dlop. Lound the corner I came and this car was in my rawful path.'

'And so you dlo – I mean, drove into it?' I said.

'Yes, it was there, in my path.'

The logic of unreason, I thought.

This interesting conversation was brought to an unsatisfactory end by the unwelcome appearance of a policeman, summoned I later heard, by a well-meaning, if unthinking, passer-by.

I well knew that once the police were involved the situation could only go from bad to worse. And so it proved.

'You must all cam to thee porice station to make statements and then to have your vehicles inspected for roadwathiness. Fuata mimi. Forrow me.'

'Excuse me,' I said. 'Our two cars were parked and stationary at the time. The only one which was moving was driven by this –' I paused '– gentleman.'

The 'gentleman' gave a gentle smile. Was he on drugs?

'It is the raw. Afta an accident all vehicles mast be inspected. Ret us go.'

By now the usual collection of rubber-neckers and thrill-seekers had gathered and they enjoyed themselves prising the vehicles apart and trying to do as much damage in the process as they could. More metal from the priest's jalopy clattered onto the pavement. I saw his lips moving in what I was certain was not a prayerof intercession for the poor and needy. I got into my car, wound the window down and sat waiting for the priest to reverse his ravaged his car away from mine.

As I sat there, seething, I became aware of a long, thin, black arm slowly insinuating itself through the open window. It resembled the tentacle of an octopus searching for prey on the sea bed. The hand came gently to rest as it contemplated its next move. My briefcase was lying on the seat beside me. I eased a biro pen out of my shirt pocket. The hand moved again. 'Right, you bastard!' I thought and seizing the biro like a dagger drove it into the back of the moving hand. To my gratified surprise the pen remained sticking out of the hand at right angles. Its owner gave a great shriek and pounded away into outer darkness, taking my biro with him.

Biro-less, but feeling much better, I followed the two other cars to the Central Police Station.

As I followed the others up the broken steps into the gloomy interior, a police Land Rover with no working headlights roared up behind me and squealed to a halt. Two cops piled out, dragging three, ragged, hand-cuffed, men from the vehicle's interior. The men were shackled together. As they stumbled up the broken steps into the filthy-walled building, the policemen struck them with the butts of their rifles. One man fell to the ground. All three were dragged through a barred door into what resembled a large cage in a zoo, and into a room. The door was slammed shut. Thumps and screams and yells rang through the barely lit corridors of the police station.

Suddenly things had taken on a rather sinister slant.

The policeman motioned us to a door. 'Get in!' he commanded.

We got in.

A table, three broken chairs, a cracked window, curtains tied in a knot, walls smeared with a grey fungal deposit, mountains of rotting, string-tied files bursting from ramshackle shelves, a sagging ceiling and a dishevelled cap-less officer slumped in the corner, wiping the sleep from red-rimmed eyes – my heart sank as we filed in.

He motioned to the chairs. We sat down. Behind us the ash-coloured wall showed in grimy outline where previous heads and shoulders had rubbed against it.

The policman yawned and gave us each a slow, baleful stare.

Without speaking, he tossed us each a form to fill in. This was the dreaded 'abstract form', about which I had heard so much. 'Feel in all that has happened,' he ordered us.

Suddenly he looked up.

'Eh! Wat ees that smell? Eh – you, mzungu,' looking at me – 'you, you are smelling too much!' (Wewe nanuka sana, sana!)

'Sorry, officer,' I said. 'I've just been doing a rotten calving, and water was in very short supply on the farm. It's not a personal smell, but an acquired one, you understand. There is a big difference.'

'Cavving? Cavving? Wat is that?'

'Ngombe lishindwa kusaa, na njau likufa ndani ya tumbo la usasi.' (A cow was unable to give birth and the calf was dead in the uterus.)

'Ah sasa na sikia.' (Ah now I understand.)

Like the sun breaking out from behind a bank of dark clouds his teeth shone in the gloom.

'So, you are a daktari, eh?' He grinned. 'Me myself, I am from West.' – he meant western Kenya – 'We have no good daktaris there.'

'Oh dear,' I said.

'So, you mast help mee.'

'Oh yes. And how can I do that?'

'My fam it is very faa, but you can give mee good advice. I have cows, I have sheeps, I even have pigs! But they are suffering. We are suffering. My cows they cough and then they die. My sheeps they get diarrhoea and then they die. And the pigs, one day they look OK. The next, dead pok.'

He leaned across the table.

'The govment salary for us is very low.' He circled the index finger and thumb of his right hand. 'Without my shamba and my animals we would stav.'

The abstract forms were forgotten. For the next 45 minutes we were neck deep in the niceties of animal disease treatment and prevention in Western Kenya. The reasons for our being in this horrible office were lost in the intricacies of a veritable labyrinth of ovine, bovine and porcine problems of baffling complexity. Out of the corner of my eye I could see the priest shaking his watch and holding it, first to his right ear, and then to his left. The cause of our troubles sat polishing his glasses and holding them up for inspection to the fly-specked light bulb. By the time we were done I had plumbed the depths of mental exhaustion and was beginning to think that the filling in of the abstract forms would, by contrast, be pleasurable light relief. Priestly coughing, interspersed by a symphony of sighing and grunting from our bespectacled friend, indicated a degree of what I considered to be unwarranted impatience. After all, I thought, I'm the one who's doing all the hard work here, all they have to do is to sit back and take it easy.

Finally, having drained the sum of my knowledge, my interlocutor sat back.

'Now we mast attend to thees other matters. That of the cas. You have scratched my back. Now I will scratch your back! A Blitish saying! Ah, you Blitish!'

I wondered what was going to happen next. I had had enough and I could barely keep my eyes open.

'You, daktari, may go. And so may you, Father. You, broder,' he looked at our bemused, bespectacled companion, 'you mast stay to assist us with our inquiries.'

A cloud of alarm, relief, concern, and resignation passed across his cherubic features in quick succession.

Outside the police station I drew in a lungful of slightly less polluted night air.

I turned to the priest. 'I wonder what will happen to him?'

He gave a quiet smile and held up the index finger and thumb of his right hand, not encircled this time. He rubbed them together.

I understood.

Chapter Twelve

T9

In an unrecorded town, somewhere in the bleached bush of northern Tanzania, close to the Kenya border, a place so unremarkable that its name has been lost to posterity, a travelling circus had set up camp. The circus wasn't an African version of Bertram Mills – far from it. A threadbare Big Top, a duo of razor-thin gymnasts, a bony lion, a couple of jugglers, a tame zebra, a pair of clowns, a quartet of drummers and three performing dogs, it looked more than a cavalcade of tattered refugees, fleeing the latest local conflict.

One of the dogs, called 'Simba', meaning 'Lion', a yellow, sharp-nosed Basenji, had been tattooed inside the flap of his right ear. Why he had been tattooed is not recorded. Perhaps he had once been the property of an Asian or European, who had wished to stamp his authority upon his dog. But there, clearly visible in blue ink was the mark of what was to become a future byword for fear and terror – T9.

One night Simba escaped from bondage and daily beatings and fled northwards towards the border. He avoided villages as he knew that there lay danger. He ran the risk of capture, of being stoned by children, of being attacked by other dogs. But he needed food. Desperate with hunger he slunk through the tangled remnants of harvested maize fields, gnawing on rotting maize cobs, drinking from pools of stagnant water in the beds of dried up rivers, lying panting in the perforated shade of spindly thorn trees, growing thinner by the day.

Late one afternoon Simba saw a strange dog lying by itself in a patch of withered grass, munching at something hidden from view. Simba approached carefully. The dog did not move and remained where it was.

Simba crept closer, wary, but curious and drawn to one of his own kind. Now he could see that the stranger was not eating something succulent and tasty but, horrifyingly, gnawing at its own foot. There was blood on the stems of the grass. The dog looked up and stared at Simba. Its eyes had a fixed, manic, glare, red and glazed, seeing but not seeing. Simba was transfixed, terrified. Too late, he turned to flee. The dog rushed at him with a whining snarl. Simba withdrew in stumbling panic, but the stranger was quicker and as Simba slipped and scrabbled on the rough ground he was bitten on his neck. He yelped with a high-pitched squeal and ran panting with fear into the bush.

For the next few days he travelled northwards, crossing the border into Kenya near the village of Ntiramu. He felt strange and light-headed. His throat was tight and constricted. He blinked. The sun was hot, but not that hot. Anthills and bushes danced crazily in the heat shimmer. Simba began to run, stumbling through the bush, staggering and lurching over the uneven ground. He tried to focus on his surroundings but he was seeing double. He had no appetite now for food. He had no sense of direction. All he felt was an impulse to get away from whatever it was that was driving him on. There was a demon inside his head, stirring his brains with a long wooden spoon.

Sitting on his carved stool outside his hut on the outskirts of Migori, large splayed toes planted firmly on his native soil, mind pleasantly in neutral, Jackson Okambo puffed contentedly on his clay pipe. His large brood of children gambolled carefree in the dust. Chickens scratched around their feet. In the distance Mrs Okambo could be seen labouring homewards, bent double beneath a large load of firewood on her back. Smoke drifted heavenwards from neigbouring homesteads. As a loyal Jaluo, Mr Okambo was fond of fish and looked forward with keen anticipation to washing down the evening's stomach-distending repast of broiled Nile perch, prepared by his long-suffering wife, with mind-blowing draughts of the local firewater.

To protect his compound against unwanted intruders, both animal and human, Mr Okambo had three nondescript mutts, all of a singularly unprepossessing appearance. Flea-bitten, razor-thin, wall-eyed and brindle in colour, they looked like starving coyotes as they skulked and slunk around Mr Okambo's rural idyll. As Mr Okambo's thoughts passed lightly from thoughts of the forthcoming piscine blow-out to the young woman whose ripe charms he had lately been enjoying in a nearby village, his lurid full-technicoloured reverie was rudely interrupted by a cacophony of outraged yelping from his canine cohort. Frowning in irritation at his imaginary coitus interruptus, he rose to his feet.

The dogs were barking at something in the long grass at the edge of the compound. Thinking that they had seen one of the many snakes which infested the area, he seized a panga and went to investigate the cause of the disturbance.

As he strode across the beaten earth, Simba lurched out into the open, surrounded by his fellow canine tormentors. Simba's eyes were glazed, the whites no longer white but a dull red, his tongue lolled from his mouth, dry and earth-covered, his coat dull and matted. He stopped, panting and gasping, his chest heaving, and as he did so the dogs rushed at him. Simba was almost done, but as the first dog closed on him, he turned and bit the dog on the cheek. The dog leapt away, howling. Another dog rushed in, followed by the third. Simba bit for the last time. As he did so, the last thing he saw was Mr Okambo's panga descending with frightful finality onto his head.

Mr Okambo turned Simba's corpse over with the tip of his blood-stained panga. 'Eh! Wat is this?' he exclaimed. 'Hey, wife!' he called to Mrs Okambo. 'Come here! Look at this!' He pointed to the inside of Simba's right ear, where clearly stamped in blue letters could be read the mystic T9.

A month later both of Mr Okambo's bitten dogs developed the same symptoms which had overtaken the luckless Simba. They in their turn had run amok and eventually died. Before they did so they had bitten two of Okambo's children, five dogs, three chickens, two goats and one donkey. Thus a new and devastating outbreak of rabies arrived in Kenya, spread, according to the bush telegraph, by a previously unknown and terrifying species of canine – the T9. Rumour spread like a bush fire. Soon every stray dog was referred to as a T9.

From Mr Okambo's Nyanza Province, the dread contagion spread far and wide.

About three months later I was just about to remove a dangling tumour from an aged, but much-loved, labrador bitch, owned by one of the local gentry, when I was informed by Yolanda, my Italian/Pakistani receptionist, that there was a lady at the door asking to see me.

'Is it urgent?' I inquired, looking at the current patient waiting resignedly on the table.

'Well, I don't really know, but she's come a long way.'

She had indeed. The lady was from a mission based near the town of Maseno, about 70 miles due north of Migori, not far from the lake which bore Queen Victoria's royal name, and 190 miles from Nakuru. Her accent was Glaswegian, and she was small and sharp and wiry, as the inhabitants of that great city often are.

'Helloo, are yew the vet?' I confirmed that I was. 'Aye, weel, we hae a wee dug here, a dachshund in fact and he's got a wee bit o' a problem wi' his moo, I mean his mouth. At first we thocht he had a bone stuck across his teeth but after I had a wee bit o' a poke with ma finger doon his throat it appeared that he hadnae anything there, and noo he canna shut his moo – Ah mean his mouth.' She continued – 'In addition the wee fella is lame and no eatin,' so we brocht him tae ye.'

'Right,' I said. 'Bring him in.'

Moses carefully removed the labrador, who looked relieved to be no longer the centre of attention.

The lady, Miss Elsie MacTough, was not alone. Behind her was another smaller, self-effacing version of herself. This friend's accent was an impenetrable thicket of glottal stops and guttural consonants. How the locals understood her was beyond me. I came from Scotland and I could barely comprehend one word in ten. Perhaps she spoke fluent Swahili in a Glaswegian accent.

Miss MacTough placed Haggis, as her wee dug was called, on the table.

Haggis stood there, staring vacantly into space. His lower jaw hung open, slackly. With a pair of large artery forceps I pushed it closed, but he was unable to keep it closed and it sagged open again. Suddenly he tried to snap at something we, and possibly he, could not see.

'Can you place him on the floor, please?' I asked.

'That I can,' Miss MacTough said.

Haggis was able to walk, but dragged his right hind leg.

'Miss MacTough,' I said, 'I pretty sure your wee dug, I mean dog, has got rabies. There is no rabies in this area but I am certain that's what he's got.'

Miss MacTough blanched. 'So he will die, won't he?'

I nodded. 'I'm afraid so, and he must stay here. We can't let him go. He might bite someone or another dog. And you especially, and anyone else who has handled him, must get a course of vaccinations immediately. This very day. Plus any other dogs you might have.'

'He's the only one,' she said sadly. 'About a month ago he was involved in a scrap with a shenzi (stray) dog which came out of the bush and then disappeared. Just a wee nip on Haggis's foreleg. It healed up in no time. I suppose that was it.'

'Almost certainly,' I said. I phoned a doctor friend, Ehsan

Malakooti, who was an Iranian Bahai who had fled his homeland due to the Ayatollahs and their fanatical followers, and asked him to be on standby, preferably with a bilingual interpreter at his elbow. Ehsan gave a hollow laugh.

In 1981 there was no rabies in the Nakuru district. It was a rabies-free area, and had been so ever since colonial times, when a strict policy of vaccination, dog licensing and movement control had stamped it out. That happy situation was now to change.

Over the next three days Haggis declined, unable to eat, slipped into a coma, and died. Examination of his brain at the government veterinary laboratory at Kabete, on the outskirts of Nairobi, confirmed my diagnosis of rabies.

Chapter Thirteen

A DASH OF SMIRNOFF

Ten miles from Nakuru, strategically sited on the edge of a picturesque bluff, overlooking the papyrus-choked swamp of Mbaruk, Blackthorn School was no Eton or Harrow, by any stretch of the imagination, but it filled a need and provided a basic education to those able to pay its fees. Most of the pupils were the sons and daughters of European expatriates and latter-day settlers, Asian businessmen and African nouveau riche. There were two other competing schools in the area – the co-educational Christian, supportive, St. Mungo's at Turi, 30 miles from Nakuru, perched at over 8,000 feet on the wooded western rim of the Rift Valley, and Haverford House, at Gilgil, 30 miles in the opposite direction, an all-male, all-white bastion of reactionary exclusivity.

All three were prep. schools. St Mungo's clientele was drawn, in the main, from the ranks of the widespread missionary fraternity and from the established Ugandan and Rwandan aristocracy. Haverford House's pupils came from a background of wealthy white settler farms and ranches, scattered across the former White Highlands of Kenya, leavened by the occasional stray bird from northern Tanzania. Haverford gave the distinct impression of regarding itself as being more than a cut above the rest, the equivalent in its own eyes to a top grade English public school, with St. Mungo's a namby-pamby, overly religious, mediocre Comprehensive, and Blackthorn a floundering, working class, racially ambivalent Secondary Modern.

The headmaster of Blackthorn was Rudyard Rowntree. Rudy was a benign, non-confrontational individual, who steered the scholastic ship with a surprisingly elastic hand. On occasion it appeared he took his hand off the tiller entirely. Clad in a dove-grey suit, silver hair neatly combed and parted, Rudy was a picture of suave elegance, something which, alas, could not be said of his socially inept wife, Nina. Her dress sense was such that it looked as though her clothes had been flung onto her bulky frame with a dung fork. Her insistence on wearing short, tight skirts and exposing what shouldn't be exposed was a constant source of embarrassment to her husband and to the school. On Speech Day she would sit on the stage, legs wide apart, with pupils and parents seated below squirming in distaste and discomfort, like horrified rabbits mesmerised by a menacing serpent.

Despite his many years of living in Kenya, Rudy's linguistic knowledge of Swahili was scant indeed, being limited to precisely one word – 'mzuri', meaning 'good', pronounced in his fruity accent as 'mezoori'. Whole sentences would be constructed around this single word. 'That's not very mezoori,' he would say to his gardener who'd just made a hash of pruning the rose bushes, or to a slacking African pupil – 'could you perhaps make that a bit more mezoori by tomorrow?'

Rudy's teaching team was more than a little bit suspect. On what seemed like a regular basis teachers would mysteriously disappear, never to return. Others, although possessed of formidable brains and considerable teaching talent, seemed to teeter along a narrow tightrope between normality and dangerous eccentricity.

Frank Pinchbeck, the peripatetic woodwork teacher, was known to all and sundry as Effing Frank, because of his excessive fondness for the adjective. Mike Dewing, of the science department, kept poisonous snakes in his bedroom and had a volcanic temperament, which would erupt without warning and would finally lead him into some very hot water indeed. Kaftan-clad, larger than life Susan Small of the catering department, had a peculiar body shape and even more peculiar digestive preferences, if rumour was to be believed, owning up, apparently, to a personal predilection for ripe ticks, which she swallowed as though they were succulent grapes.

History teacher Mervyn Rusk combined his love for his chosen subject with a desperation to sow his seed by ferrying a succession of compliant whores on the back of his motorbike the ten miles from Nakuru to the school and thence to his study-bedroom. After a night of pleasure and not much study the chosen lady of the night would be smuggled out before dawn and trundled back to the town. Little wonder then that the classroom recipients of Mervyn's wisdom fared less than well in their exams, prompting another exhortation from Rudy to ask them do more mezoori next time.

And then there was Magdalena Slominski, daughter of Polish refugees settled in Kenya.

I first met Magda when called to attend to her spaniel, Smirnoff, a cantankerous individual who only understood Polish, of which I knew not one word. Magda was a statuesque, striking blonde in her mid-twenties, resembling an off-stage slimmed-down Brunhilde in the early stages of her operatic career, with a voice to match. Magda was employed as a matron at the school. Why, I never discovered, as there was nothing in the least bit matronly about her. Perhaps Rudy took her on as a platonic foil to offset the ever-looming presence of the unlovely Nina.

Magda's ground floor flat connected with the junior boys' dormitory, the better for her to keep a closer eye on her pre-pubescent charges. As I disembarked, late one afternoon, from my Peugeot I could hear through the half-open door of the flat a torrent of expletives more suited to the barrack square or to the poop deck of one of Nelson's ships going into action against the French, than to the supposedly restrained environs of a prep. school.

'You fucking little insects! Stand up straight when I talk to you and get that insolent smirk off your horrid pasty face, Jones! Do that once again and I'll tan your revolting backside!'

'Yes, miss,' I heard a piping voice exclaim.

'What do mean, yes miss?'

'I mean, no miss.'

'That's better.'

A door banged shut and there was the sound of inanimate objects being kicked around.

I approached the door and gave it a tentative rap.

'Yes? Who is it?' the perpetrator of the recent tirade bellowed.

'It's the vet, come to see your dog, as requested!' I replied.

There was a short pause and the door was flung wide and Miss Slominski stood there, clutching in her hand a tumbler, brimful of a clear liquid. I did not think that it was water. She was breathing heavily.

'I've just about had enough of those little squirts! Enough! Give me dogs and horses any day! They may bite you and kick you and shit on you but at least they don't give you cheek and play the fucking fool all the time.'

She grinned. 'Come on in and have a drink.'

'Right,' I said. 'But I'd better have a squint at the patient first. I gather he's dripping blood from his prepuce.'

'Yes, randy little bugger. He's probably been fucking the local bitches and caught a dose. Serve him right but I can't have him messing up the carpets, can I?'

'No indeed,' I agreed. 'Right, can you hold him while I have a glance at his offending organ?'

This apparently innocuous request seemed to cause Magda inordinate amusement as she gave a high-pitched laugh of alarming volume, sounding like an inebriated hyena. Judging by the speed with which she was downing her drink I reasoned it wouldn't be too long before she was inebriated as well. There was no time to lose before her powers of assistance were rendered null and void by further infusions of whatever was in her glass.

Smirnoff was not in a cooperative mood. He retreated beneath a table, growling softly. I glimpsed sharp, white fangs and a retracted, corrugated lip. This, I could see, was not going to be easy.

Magda spoke to Smirnoff in Polish, English and Swahili. She spoke softly and gently. She shouted and she swore. Smirnoff was having none of it. His low growl took on a higher, more menacing note. Magda had another slug of firewater.

I could see that this was going to take all night. Were it not for the fact that it was late afternoon and that I had no further calls to make, I would have told Magda just what she could do with Smirnoff, including that which she was busily gulping. I had noticed a half empty bottle, emblazoned with the special 'guaranteed-to-blow-your-head-off' blue label round its capacious circumference, lurking behind a convenient flower pot.

'Magda,' I said. 'I've got a sedative in the car. Acetylpromazine. If we can get it into him we've a chance to look at him. If not, then this is a hopeless mission. But it's got to be given by intramuscular injection so we'll have to get a lead round his neck and you'll have to hold him while I inject him – OK?'

'Righty-ho,' she slurred.

I repaired to the car, filled a syringe and returned, to find Magda topping up her glass.

She rooted around in a drawer and after a good deal of cussing came up with a mildewed leather collar and lead, with which, after what seemed like an age, she managed to encircle Smirnoff's neck. He did not take too kindly to this and submitted with a pretty poor grace, with much growling and teeth showing.

'Now,' I said. 'Your front door looks like the usual, hopeless, ill-fitting school variety with a big gap at the bottom to let the wind and the rain and the rats in. Thread the lead under that and go outside, shut the door and pull the lead as tight as possible. Smirnoff may choke a bit, but that's his fault for being so uncooperative. I hope that collar's not loose. If he gets away he'll be on *my* jugular, not yours!'

Magda gave another of her hyena impersonations.

She did as requested and hauled away with might and main. Smirnoff did not appreciate this, snarling and leaping and twisting and voiding copious amounts of faeces and urine. But by grabbing his tail in mid-twist I got the needle in and emptied the syringe into his hid leg.

'Right,' I shouted, 'you can let go now!'

Magda let go and Smirnoff subsided in a heap, panting.

Magda came in and surveyed the mess on her floor.

'Shit!' she expostulated. 'I'm not sure I don't prefer the blood on my Persian carpets!'

'This,' I replied, 'is a one-off. The blood is not. It's not going to stop unless we do something about it.'

By the time we had cleaned the floor and got rid of the smell, Smirnoff had slumped into a semi-conscious heap. I rolled him onto his side and extruded his offending organ to reveal a revolting cauliflower-like mass of growths along the shaft of his penis.

'Ugh! What on earth is thaaat?' Magda grimaced in disgust. 'God. That is repulsive! I need a drink!' Putting action to words she downed the rest of her glass in one impressive swallow.

'That, Magda, is the notorious transmissible venereal tumour, which is caused by a virus and spread when eager males such as your Smirnoff copulate with infected bitches. The virus is transmitted by friction.'

'OK, OK, I've heard enough. How do you get rid of it?'

'Cut it off – the tumour I mean. Anti-tumour drugs are also successful but hard to get here so it's the knife. But not here in your sitting room or there'll be even more blood. Bring him in soon and I'll do it in the surgery. There'll be some seepage for a day or so as it's not possible to stitch the wounds but after a few days that'll stop and he'll be as good as gold.'

'I doubt that, but yes, I'll bring him in.'

I washed my hands in Magda's minuscule bathroom, which was difficult as the place was a veritable thicket of suspended articles of female underwear, hanging like dangerous throat-throttling lianas, through which I had to fight my way to the minute hand basin set in a small clearing in a jungle of intimate foundation garments. By the time I emerged I was perspiring freely and in dire need of a drink.

'Right,' I said as I was proffered a brimming beaker of Russia's best, 'before we get totally smashed, let's move the patient to where he can recover in peace.'

'Good idea,' said Magda. 'Let's move him into the kitchen. I'll take his head and forelegs while you hold his hind legs.'

We bent to our task. That I had the less dangerous end was soon made obvious when the somnolent Smirnoff, reacting violently to being handled, turned like a striking cobra and seized Magda's left hand in his jaws and gave it a good worrying.

'Shit, you ungrateful bastard!' Magda yelled, dropping her end. 'That's all the thanks I get for trying to help you! Now there's my blood as well as yours on the carpet!'

As Smirnoff tumbled to the floor, he staggered to his feet and was propelled through the half-open kitchen door by a forceful boot from Magda's toe. She slammed the door shut.

Magda was nothing if not verbose and for the next two hours, pausing only to fill her glass and mine, she gave me chapter and verse on the manifold deficiencies of school and staff. Like the wedding guest held in thrall by the Rime of the Ancient Mariner I too sat spellbound as she related an epic tale of gossip, innuendo and scandal with no-holds gusto, peppered with words seldom heard in polite society.

Finally, reeling from a surfeit of vodka and Magda's verbal bombardment, I arose, a wiser man, and carefully made my way towards the door, which now seemed to be at the end of a long dark tunnel. This short journey was up what appeared to be a perilously steep treadmill, up which I clawed my way like John Bunyan's hero Christian surmounting Hill Difficulty. I could not understand why I had not noticed it when I entered. In the kitchen I could hear Smirnoff blundering around, knocking down empty bottles and generally making a nuisance of himself.

Being incapable of coherent speech, I mouthed a silent farewell to Magda, and, with due diligence, snailed home.

A week later Smirnoff was presented and I duly removed his tumours. As I returned him to Magda later in the day, she turned and said 'Oh, by the way, I'll be away all of next week. It's half term and I've got to get away from the place or I'll go bloody well mad. For my sins I look after the school horses. I've asked one of the teachers to keep an eye on them until I get back. So if there's a problem she will call you.'

'No problem,' I said. 'What nationality is she?'

'Irish.' She gave a hyena laugh and was gone.

Chapter Fourteen

A Touch of the Irish and a Night on the Bare Mountain

I had just finished spaying a ridgeback bitch owned by Jolyon Molesworthy. I had always thought that Molesworthy, even Jolyon, was a name only to be found within the pages of comic fiction, but this one was a real person, if a trifle odd and twitchy. One of those chaps who are always smiling quietly at nothing in particular. Not for the first time I wondered if a name had a bearing on a person's character. Would a Hector, for example, be more manly than a Clarence? Would a Jeremy be more cerebral than a Clint?

The phone rang. My appellative reverie was disrupted.

'Hello, my name is Bernadette Quinn. I'm phoning from Blackthorn School. I'm a friend of Magda Slominski, who asked me to phone you if we had a problem with a horse.'

Ah, the Irish teacher.

No Irish accent here though. Instead a rather attractive, upper-class, faintly aristocratic, home counties intonation. But Bernadette? Wasn't that what nuns were called? Serious, plain, virginal, self-effacing, humourless nuns clad in wimples and button boots. Hmm.

'One of the horses is acting strangely.'

'Acting strangely?'

'Yes, you know, salivating, straining, biting the stable door, attacking the other horses, that sort of thing. He even had a go at the syce.'

'What's happening now?'

'Well he broke out of his stable, but the syce managed to get him back in again. That's when he was almost bitten. But now the horse is standing quietly. But every now and again he gets the urge.'

'That sort of thing, as you so quaintly describe it, sounds like rabies. Just as well it's half term and the kids are on holiday. Do nothing, leave him in the stable, keep people away and I'll be along shortly.'

'Right, I'll wait for you at the swimming pool. It's half term, the sun's shining and it's on the way to the stables.'

Some people, I thought, have all the luck and she didn't sound like a nun either.

Getting out of the surgery was never easy. In theory it should have been simply a matter of pushing open the batwing doors, taking a couple of short firm strides to the car, getting in and driving away. That never seemed to happen. Either the phone would ring just as I got to the street, or someone would drive up just as I was driving away, or a passer-by would decide that he had urgent business which could not possibly wait. On this occasion it was Ian Cuthill, dragging a black labrador dog behind him. Ian was fond of his beer, very fond, and it showed in his massive gut, which preceded him wherever he went. Like the bows of a battleship moving majestically and effortlessly through an ocean swell, crowds, through which lesser mortals such as myself had to battle their way, parted like the Red Sea before the inexorable pressure of the Cuthill paunch. Ian was short and, like many short men, forthright, belligerent and argumentative. 'Mr Cran!' he bellowed from several yards distance. 'Don't run away! Sambo here needs you! Urgently! He's gone and got his wedding tackle entangled in his chain and if you don't free him he's a done dog!' Finesse was not part of the Cuthill makeup.

I looked more closely. Sambo's dog chain was wrapped closely around his lower abdomen. The rest I could not see.

'Right, bring him in and let's have a look at him.'

Ian's anatomical impedimentum prevented him from helping, so Moses and I hoisted Sambo onto the table.

'Right, turn him onto his side.'

'Good Lord!' I exclaimed. 'How on earth did *that* happen?'

The snap link at the end of the chain, instead of being clipped into a loop on the chain, was now snapped tightly around the base of Sambo's penis, which was extruded from its sheath to its uttermost limits, swollen to the size and consistency of an overgrown, prize carrot, beetroot in colour, and looking distinctly well past its sell-by date.

'What on earth happened?' I asked Ian, as I examined the damage more closely.

'I was about to give him – more correctly the house boy was about to give him – his weekly wash in tick dawa – and had him on a chain for easier handling, when Sambo smelt a passing bitch, got all randy and worked up, tried to get at her, got entangled in the chain et voilà!'

Voilà indeed!

I tried to prise open the snap link. It was like trying to open a can of beans with bare fingers. Not to be done by mere mortals. Quite apart from the apparent impossibility of accomplishing this, was Sambo's non-compliance. I would have thought that with a metal tourniquet clamped tightly round the base of his most vital member all sensation further down the line would have been rendered null and void but seemingly not so. He did not like it and all my best intentions were rudely rejected, with bared teeth and antisocial lunging.

'Right,' I said to Ian. 'We'll have to knock him out and use a hacksaw. If we try to do this with him fully conscious there'll be blood, probably mine, and maybe bits of Sambo's penis all over the walls.'

Ian winced.

'Yes, I can see your point,' he replied. 'Not good for the décor.'

It was always pleasing to have an understanding client.

After weighing him and deducting the weight of the chain, I gave Sambo his computed dose of pentobarbitone slowly and methodically into the vein on his right foreleg until his eyes flickered and closed and he lay quietly on his side, oblivious to strangulated penises and beckoning bitches.

'Right, Moses,' I said, 'bring me the hacksaw.'

Out of the corner of my eye I could see Ian wincing again.

We laid Sambo on his back so that I could get access to the snap link, and get the blade onto the offending clip. The metal seemed to be offensively hard and before I finally sawed through the last millimetre and removed the chain, my honest brow was beaded with drops of honest sweat.

'Now, Ian,' I said, 'we have to see if what is out will now go in.'

Ian gave me a wary look, obviously wondering if such levity was not misplaced. Several important inches of his dog were where they should not be.

He need not have worried. After a few minutes of purposeful penile massage, aided by some timely lubrication, Sambo's now flaccid member was decently hidden from view within the confines of his prepuce.

'Right, Ian,' I said. 'Leave Sambo here until this afternoon to allow him to recover from the anaesthetic and then take him home. Apart from a bit of understandable bruising he should be fine. Sorry, I've got to rush – there's an Irish colleen out at Blackthorn with a sick horse and she's been waiting for hours and by now she must be absolutely raging!'

I broke no speed records on my way to Blackthorn but I did not dally either. As I arrived at the wicket fence surrounding the seemingly-deserted swimming pool I was almost disappointed to see no impatient figure striding up and down, shaking its wrist and peering at its watch in obvious irritation and impatience. Instead, as I pushed open the gate into the pool area, I saw, on the far side of the blue water, a prone female form lying at obvious ease on a sun-lounger. She was clad, if that is the correct word, in dark glasses and in a barely-essentials-covering, psychedelic bikini and was evenly tanned to the colour of well-seasoned mahogany. That, I thought with admiration, must have taken many hours of dedicated effort. No sign of a wimple.

Eyes goggling, I stood, momentarily transfixed, hormonally unhinged, rooted to the spot by this mesmerising vision of female pulchritude, all thoughts of why I was there banished from my re-routed consciousness.

I shook my whirling head and coughed discreetly.

The vision removed her sunglasses and opened one amused eye. 'Ah, Mr Cran?' I nodded mutely. 'You've arrived! I'm Berna, that's short for Bernadette by the way. I was beginning to wonder what had happened to you. There's a limit to the amount of sun a person can take at a sitting, you know.'

'Sitting?' I thought. 'Surely you mean lying!'

I decided that, at first acquaintance, it would be politic to forgo a detailed resume of exactly why I was late. You never know how the fair sex will react to lurid descriptions of cutting and incising, and until you do, it's best to remain mum.

'Ah, yes indeed,' I said. 'Quite so. Right then. We'd better have a look at the horse. Sounds pretty serious to me. How's the syce?'

'A bit shaken, but otherwise OK. And I have to tell you that I know absolutely nothing about horses. I rode one as a child, got tossed off, broke my arm and haven't been near one since, until today. And I don't want to get too close to this one.'

She rose gracefully in one fluid movement. I always wished I could do that. Whenever I got up from one of those loungers it was more like the mechanical unhinging of a wooden toy, accompanied by attendant on-stage creaking sounds and utterly devoid of any grace. She pulled a long tee-shirt over her perfectly formed head and over her perfectly-formed body. My heart rate steadied.

At the stables I leaned over the door and looked at the horse, a small, dark brown mare, called Molly. She was standing quietly, gazing abstractedly into the middle distance. I noticed that she had a curious nibbling twitching of her lower lip, from which hung a dribble of saliva. Every now and then the mare propped herself against the stable wall, as though to rest herself. She raised her tail as though to pass dung, and strained, but nothing appeared.

'What do you think?' my companion asked. I noticed that the syce, who had now appeared, kept well back, a furtive figure, lurking nervously in the shadows. Once bitten...

'Hard to say,' I said. 'Could be rabies, might be tetanus. I'd like to see her take a few steps.'

Without thinking I opened the stable door and stepped inside. In view of what had recently happened to the syce, this was not a clever move, but it just goes to show what happens to an otherwise perfectly normal chap when under the all-powerful influence of a gust of adjacent female pheromones. He just ceases to think in a rational manner. As I entered the stable Molly gave me a distinctly unfriendly stare, uttered a hoarse, un-equine grunt, and, with teeth bared and clattering furiously like a flamenco dancer's castanets, came at me like a fighting bull targeting the matador's fluttering cape. I made a frantic convulsive leap to one side as her great yellow incisors met with a horrid snap by my left ear. A tsunami of hot horse breath smote me in the face and a torrent of cold sweat rushed down my spine.

Wildly I looked for a way out of the stable which now seemed to be filled to bursting point with demented horse flesh. In a flash I envisaged my lifeless form lying on the straw, flayed, pulped and flattened beneath pounding hooves. Desperately I searched for the exit door, but that was now firmly blocked by Molly's rampaging bulk. In the corner of the stable stood Molly's food trough and in one despairing, hip-dislocating jerk I levered myself up and onto it as she whirled furiously towards me. As she tried to cut me off at the knees I spotted a roof beam which, under normal circumstances would have been far beyond my mortal reach, but at which now, propelled by a red-hot pint of molten adrenalin, I leapt like a demented jack-in-the-box. As my outstretched fingers closed over the beam, Molly collapsed onto the stable floor, leaving me suspended like an exhausted gibbon, swinging limply over her recumbent, tooth-snapping form.

As I hung there, panting, pondering my next move, a disembodied, well modulated voice spoke from the safety of the other side of the stable door – 'Well, Mr Cran, have you reached a diagnosis now?'

'Yes,' I replied with some difficulty. 'Yes, I'm pretty sure we could classify this as a case of furious rabies.'

'She certainly looked pretty annoyed to me,' came the reply.

Another understatement. Miss Quinn seemed to like the low-key *bon mot*.

'Yes,' I answered, 'more like homicidal from my current coign of vantage.'

She gave a silvery laugh.

It was time to descend. Molly seemed unable to stand and lay on the stable floor, lips twitching and teeth chattering. Down, but certainly not out.

I took a chance and dropped lightly onto her manger, hoping it would bear my uncontrolled descending weight. It did not. Whoever had built it had not designed it with this contingency in mind. As my feet struck the woodwork there was a splintering crack and it collapsed, catapulting me backwards in an unedifying parabola to land with a sickening crash on Molly's recumbent rump. She did not appreciate my sudden arrival one bit. With a snoring snort she staggered to an upright position. At this moment Miss Quinn, no doubt intrigued and curious to know what on earth was going on within, opened the stable door. Through this I was unceremoniously ejected to land at her very feet.

'Welcome back!' she said. 'I say, you do seem to lead an adventurous life. Does this sort of thing happen often?'

Being seriously winded and mildly terrified I was temporarily bereft of speech. Gasping for air, making a mental note to answer Miss Quinn's inappropriately-timed question at a later, more convenient, date, I clawed myself to my knees, dragged myself to the vertical and lurched across to the stable. Molly had collapsed again.

For the next three days she lay there, dying during the evening of the fourth day.

Getting someone to transport and deliver an entire horse's head, weighing half a hundredweight, to the Veterinary Research Laboratory at Kabete on the outskirts of Nairobi was not an easy task. But in order to confirm the diagnosis it was essential. While I, alone, in leper-like solitude, gloved and booted, single-handedly decapitated the late Molly, Miss Quinn spoke nicely to one of the school drivers, a jolly fellow with the unlikely name of Septimus Joyful Wachira. For a small consideration Septimus agreed to deliver the goods...

A week later, after the usual telephonic skirmish, involving what appeared to be a squadron of dead or dying telephone operators, the diagnosis was confirmed – rabies. Everyone who had been in close contact with Molly, including the nearly-bitten syce and myself, endured a costly vaccination course of five injections at varying intervals. Fortunately the days of painful injections into the abdominal muscles were over and the ones we were given were mere pin pricks by comparison.

But this proved to be only another opening round in a long series of encounters with this terrifying disease.

— ✳ —

At the southern end of Kenya's share of the Rift Valley lay Lake Magadi, a petrified soda lake, whose dazzling white contents were a valuable source of revenue to the company which mined it. Being only 2,000 feet above sea level the climate was stinking hot and the atmosphere from the lake itself was powerful enough to bring tears to your eyes.

To the south-east of the lake rose a mountain called Shompole. From a distance it looked much like any of the other innumerable humps and lumps which littered the landscape. Indeed its summit was more than a thousand feet lower than the bed in Nakuru to which I retired each night. But from the vantage of Lake Magadi it assumed almost majestic proportions, rising like a breaching whale from the surrounding flatlands to a mysterious, dimly discernible summit. Like the carcass of a petrified monster it lay there inviting closer inspection. Sharp rib-like ridges leading steeply up to a forested summit plateau reinforced its resemblance to a sleeping beast. No one of my acquaintance had been near it, far less climbed it.

Had I more sense I should have wondered why not.

The thought of climbing a virtually untrodden peak stirred my fevered imagination. Included in that technicoloured vision of striking the colours in the unknown was the enticing Hibernian stunner at whose shapely feet I had so ignominiously fallen. Here was a chance to retrieve my lost laurels and perhaps gain another. Quite apart from being well-endowed in all departments she looked like a game sort, ready to take the rough with the smooth, equally at home in the bush as in the salon, or the classroom, for that matter. Together we would ascend to that far summit and return to the sound of music, quietly triumphant in our shared achievement. But first I had to ask her. Perhaps climbing a mountain was the very last thing she wanted to do. Especially with a virtual stranger.

'An unclimbed peak you say?'

'Well, almost unclimbed – no one's been up it for years.'

'Why not?'

'Well, it's a bit off the beaten track.'

'And you say there's a clear route to the top?'

'Look's like a lovely ridge walk right to the plateau.'

'Good views, eh?'

'See for miles, right over Magadi and Lake Natron.'

'And not too hot?'

'Mediterranean, balmy, we won't even need a tent.'

'Mosquitoes?'

'None, they don't venture above the swamp at the base.'

'Wild animals?'

'The odd gazelle.'

'You mean like Bambi?'

'Yes, something like that.'

'Sounds idyllic.'

'So, you're on then?'

'Let me sleep on it and I'll let you know.'

Well, wasn't that just like a woman, to keep a chap hanging on, tantalizing him with thoughts of romance in the wild with me as the noble leader and she as the tamed proud beauty, awed by my bushcraft and manly leadership.

Days went by. Mobile phones lay in a distant and unimaginable future and contact required more effort then than it does in today's world of constant chattering communication. I estimated that we would need three days to knock this mountain on the head – one day to drive to the base, another to get to the top and day three to drive back. We would go in my Peugeot 504, which could tackle almost anything bar a six foot deep river. No one today goes into the bush in a saloon car, but 30 years ago one just slung in an extra jerry can of fuel and tossed a couple of spare tyres onto the roof rack and thought nothing of it.

In the meantime I was not idle. I drove to Lake Baringo to stitch up a camel which had fallen into a cesspit. One night I had to call out Nakuru's decrepit fire engine to winch a donkey out of an abandoned pit latrine. A cow on a farm near Nakuru fell 40 feet down a cliff into the Njoro River, breaking its back on a pile of jagged rocks. Why these variegated species should have chosen to indulge virtually simultaneously in activities normally more associated with lemmings and Gadarene swine cudgelled my brain for a while.

But not for long.

Periods of quiet were to my mind to be regarded with more than a mite of concern. They usually presaged an imminent emergency, an eruption from the wings of something guaranteed to get the adrenalin flowing. A lull before the much clichéd storm. Like a dog sensing an approaching tsunami I would be on edge, but unable to flee. Some clients invariably phoned just as I was packing up to go home, after a peaceful afternoon, spent, if not in quiet contemplation, in nothing more exciting than routine vaccinations and spayings. A cheerful voice would boom from the receiver – 'That you Hugh? Look, we've got a horse here with colic. We've given it colic drench, beer, walked it around, stabbed it with what's its name and it appears to be getting worse. Started last night. Can you swerve by?' Swerving in my dictionary was a sideways curving movement, sometimes sinuous, even sensual, but involving minimum effort on the part of the swerver. Not so. Right-angled bends and backward motion were usually required in order to arrive at the source of the distress signal.

As it was shortly after the mass leapings into the abyss.

At ten minutes to six on a Wednesday evening the phone rang.

'Allo! Daktari? Allo? Allo? Can you hear me? Allo? This is Pelican Stud at Elementaita. We have a horse heya who has banged his head on a tree in tha field and he is having much effusion of blood from his head and now his nose and we need you to come right away, sir. It happened at three sir, but now we are wanting you to attend.'

I recognised the voice as that of Eric Kiptanui, head syce of the thoroughbred stud owned by fellow tribesman, Samson Korir. Both were Kipsigis, originating from the highlands overlooking the mighty lake which, even in this post-colonial era, still bore the name of the Great White Queen. At one time Samson had been a thin, undernourished jockey working for a white horse owner. Rumour had it that his imperial master deliberately kept him on half rations to keep his weight down and so increase his chances of winning races. Undernourished no more,

Samson now exuded an air of varnished opulence. He shone in the sunlight like an ebony beacon. He always wore a three piece charcoal suit and an extravagant tie. His shoes were brightly burnished and his gold watch was as big as a ship's chronometer. Oversized rings bedecked oversized fingers on hands which he waved around like signalling semaphore flags, while starveling jockeys and obsequious grooms circled in his wake like scrap-searching seagulls following an ocean liner.

By the time I reached the stud gates it was almost dark. On the way I had almost run into a tractor. As I came round a corner it was there right in front of me, on my side of the road. I swung the wheel with some violence and as I did so I noticed that a) the tractor had only one valid front wheel, the other being entirely absent, and that b) the driver had only one arm. For one brief alarming moment I thought he was going to give me a cheery wave but he thought better of it. He did give me a huge grin as did the man sharing his seat and the two others perched on the mudguards. I shook my head in disbelief and carried on.

The askari at the gate was having difficulty opening the lock, fumbling and fiddling in the semi-darkness. Finally in apparent frustration he gave up. He seized the post to which the gate was attached and lifted the whole thing out of the ground and, cradling both gate and post in his arms, swung wide the portal. He was a big man but I was impressed.

I drove into the stable yard. The horse, an enormous dun-coloured gelding with a hogged mane, held by a syce, was standing there quietly, blood trickling steadily and remorselessly from his left nostril, dropping with worrying regularity onto the sandy ground. I manoeuvred the car until the headlights shone on the horse's head, walked across and examined him more closely. With apprehension I read the name on the brass plate on his head collar: 'Crazy Horse'. There was a slight trace of blood on the forehead, above the eyes. Not much else to be seen. I laid my hand there and for reasons I was later unable to explain, gave the short hair a slight tug. Horrors! It was like opening a trapdoor into the workings of the horse's inner cranium! The frontal bone swung open to reveal the whole of both frontal sinuses, white and red and daubed with blood. Quick as a flash I closed the door, but the horse was not appreciative of my unauthorised entry into his cerebral sanctum and reared skywards with a deafening whinny, lashing out with both forelegs. One steel-shod hoof caught my shirtsleeve and almost tore it from my shoulder.

I wasn't having that. Shirts don't grow on trees, neither do arms or shoulders. I returned to my car and filled a syringe with a potent sedative.

Xylazine, marketed under the trade name Rompun, was designed for use in cattle, in which small doses are extremely effective. Much larger doses – up to ten times – have a similar effect in horses. Thus armed, I returned to the waiting patient and infused a 20ml dose into his jugular vein. Five minutes later he was to all intents and purposes – mine at least – putty in my hands. His lower lip drooped, his head hung conveniently low, and he stood spaced out and stupefied, rooted to the spot.

I requested water and it duly arrived, appropriately enough, in a horse bucket. I inspected it for cleanliness. Sterility was out of the question but I was averse to dead flies floating on the surface and suspended foreign bodies lurking lower down. It passed muster. Not without difficulty, using a razor blade, I soaped and shaved Crazy Horse's skull, revealing an impressive longitudinal wound some nine inches long, adjacent and medial to his left eye and running up almost as far as his ear. From here it made a sudden 90 degree turn and passed horizontally towards the right ear with a similar wound just below the eyes. The underlying bone had suffered a huge rectangular fracture, but the skin on the right side of the horse's head was not broken, allowing me to lift the skin and bone and peer once again with anatomical interest into the exposed frontal sinuses.

'Kumbe!' exclaimed the syce holding Crazy Horse's head collar, 'na weza ona bombo ya farasi!' (Wow! I can see the horse's brains!)

I sincerely hoped not.

I flicked away a black beetle marching purposefully towards the cranial cavity. Carefully I cleaned and disinfected the edges of the wounds, tapped the frontal bones back into place and infiltrated local anaesthetic along my projected stitch line. Not having needles strong enough to stitch bone, I concentrated on the thin overlying layer of muscle, followed by the skin. There is no spare skin on a horse's skull so every little counts. In order to avoid incurring too much tension on the final closed wound I placed single interrupted stitches about a centimetre apart. Too many and too close together and the blood supply is compromised. Everything looks wonderful for a day or so and then things start to come apart and the end result is tears and a disgruntled owner.

So I took my time and made sure that there was no undue stretching or pulling.

Finally it was all done. I stepped back to admire my handiwork. As I did so the patient stirred and raised his noble head. With his shaven skull and Mohawk mane he did look rather like an equine Red Indian. I gave him an injection of antibiotic and tetanus antitoxin. There is not much point in spending hours and hours in fabulous cosmetic reconstruction only to have your patient succumb to tetanus ten days later because you neglected to take basic preventive measures.

As I was engaged in returning my gear to my car and washing the blood off my hands, there was a throaty metallic roar and powerful lights swung into the yard. It was Samson at the wheel of his Merc. Clad in a high-collared leather jacket with brass buttons and wearing black knee-length riding boots, he was a dramatic, if almost invisible, figure.

'Ah, Dr Cran! Finished the work I see. How was it? Looks quite a small wound. That will mean a small bill, eh? Ha ha!' His rings flashed in the headlights.

I knew from bitter experience that whether the bill was large or small an uphill battle lay ahead before I saw the fruits of my nocturnal labours. Samson was one of those charming rogues who made his money, in part at least, by delaying payment for as long as possible, using other people's money to fund his numerous projects, giving his fawning minions the task of fobbing off requests for payment while he swanned around the world, flying in pampered comfort from one race meeting or thoroughbred sale to another.

'Indeed it will be – by your standards, anyway! I'll be back in ten days to remove the stitches. If there are any problems in the meantime let me know.'

'We will, don't you worry!'

We both laughed.

By the time I reached home my major domo and cook, Njoroge, who had grown grey and cirrhotic in my service, had almost given up hope of my return. Almost, but not quite. As I drove up to the back door, I saw that the lights in the kitchen were still on and that the windows were grey and opaque with steam.

Gently I opened the door. Njoroge lay on the floor, mouth agape, spread-eagled upon his back, bare feet pointing at the ceiling, thorax rhythmically rising and falling. The sour smell of rancid beer hung heavy in the thick oxygen-deprived atmosphere. Upon the stove a pot bubbled furiously, emitting acrid gouts of pungent smoke. I glanced at its contents. The charred mess being reduced to unrecognisable ashes was, I assumed, the morbid remains of my evening meal.

I tapped the horny soles of Njoroge's feet with a conveniently sited broom handle.

He stirred momentarily, pursed his lips, his eyelids flickered and he relapsed into the overused arms of Morpheus.

I tapped harder. Njoroge's eyes opened and he saw the Bwana standing there, looking stern and displeased. Njoroge sniggered, let rip with a stentorian belch and scrambled with difficulty to his feet.

He looked at the smouldering remains in the pot and casually switched off the gas. Swaying gently he levelled an accusing finger in my approximate direction.

'Wewe, *wewe*, na chelewa!' (You, *you*, are late!)

So, it was all my fault that my much-anticipated meal had been reduced to an inedible mass of indigestible carbon.

I sighed. In his present state of inebriation argument and remonstration would be merely an exercise in applied frustration. I would have to seek alimentary solace in a beer and a sandwich.

'Any messages?' I asked.

Njoroge puckered his brow, scrunched up his eyes and scratched his pate. He thought hard and long. 'Come along, come along, my man,' I thought. 'You've only been on 'duty' for about three hours.'

'Hapana. Ngoja. Ngoja. Ndiyo. Memsahib moja mzungu, nafikiri mwalimu lisema, lipiga simu. Lisema tapiga simu mara ingine. (No. Wait. Wait. Yes. A European lady, a teacher I think she said, phoned. She said she would phone back.)

'Any message?'

'Hapana, hakuna' (No, none.)

'Right then, you'd better take yourself off before you do any more damage. You can clear up in the morning.'

Njoroge seemed to regard his dismissal as an affront to his professional status. He flounced out with a stagger and a hiccough.

I opened the windows to get rid of the all pervading reek of burnt offering and stale beer.

As I did so the phone rang. 'Not another blimmin emergency!' I thought, resignedly lifting the receiver. 'Hello, is that Hugh Cran?' the voice said. 'This is Berna. You know, the Irish teacher from Greensteds. You threw yourself at my feet, remember?'

Trying to remain cool and collected, I replied, 'Yes indeed, an involuntary prostration. One of the hazards of the trade.'

There was an unrestrained, slightly mocking, burst of laughter at the end of the line.

'My cook told me that a teacher from Greensteds had rung and I was racking my brains as to who that might be. He only speaks Swahili. Most of you teachers are expats or 'two year wonders' knowing little more than 'jambo bwana,' if that, so communicating with my man would have been a serious struggle.'

She laughed again. 'I was brought up in Tanzania, and went to school there and also in Nairobi, so I probably speak Swahili as well as he does. But I have to say that I had a bit of a job getting through to him. He sounded totally smashed, utterly rat-arsed, if I may use a vulgarity. Is he often like that?'

'I'm afraid so. It's almost time to bid him goodbye. But I'm sure you didn't phone up to discuss my cook's drinking habits.'

'No indeed. It's half term next week, so what about that mountain you were talking about?'

—✽—

Ten days later we were rounding the southern shoulder of the Ngong Hills, known as Corner Baridi or Cold Corner. Behind us the four humped summits of Karen Blixen's beloved hills marched towards the Nairobi suburb which bears her name. A chill wind buffeted the car. Herds of cattle and flocks of sheep, tended by Maasai boys, grazed the steep green slopes. We stopped the car. High above us a pair of augur buzzards circled and yelped to each other in the clear blue sky. To the south the land swooped steeply downwards, dropping, dropping, into the hazy depths of the Rift Valley. Up here the grass was sweet and green. Down there it was yellow and sere, a harsh land of rocks and thorn trees, dry river beds and unrelenting heat. There was no sweetness down there.

'So then, where is your mountain?' inquired my companion.

I pointed southwards to where a small, barely perceptible bump broke the skyline. 'That's it there. Looks small from here but we're about 3000 feet above its summit. It'll get larger as we get nearer!'

'Can't wait!'

When we had stopped the car the landscape was empty of humanity, apart from distant totemic figures, red cloaks fluttering in the breeze, tending their antique herds. Now, seemingly out of nowhere, uninivited and intrusive, knots of supplicants and mendicants, merchants and trinket-sellers rose unbidden from near and far. Within minutes the car was surrounded by a heaving mob, begging for alms and pleading with us to buy beads, bangles, bracelets, clubs, spears, necklaces, shields, gourds and crude carvings of noble lions and proudly silhouetted warriors.

'Time to go I think!' I said, as a group of ochre-bedaubed hags began to jiggle their withered paps by my right elbow. I started the car and moved gently forwards. Outstretched hands clutched at us, mounds of beaded tribal artefacts were thrust through open windows, prices dropped dramatically, voices rose in simulated despair, and as I moved into second gear the whole mob broke into a uniform trot in order to keep pace with our gathering speed. Gradually, as we coasted downhill, the less agile fell behind until we were left with a knot of hardened youths brandishing their wares at us and howling their diminishing prices. As I broke into top gear we were left with one panting finalist, frantically trying to sell us a rather nicely polished knobkerrie. Knowing that we would have to return eventually by the same route and not wishing to have to re-run a gauntlet of hostile, waiting bead-sellers I fished a fifty shilling note out of my pocket and proffered it to the gasping runner. He accepted it with alacrity, I grabbed the club and onwards we sped.

I passed the club, or rungu, as it is called in Swahili, to Berna. 'Here,' I said. 'This might come in handy, in case we meet anything unpleasant on Shompole, like snakes or scorpions, or rabid jackals.'

'Thanks,' she said, 'but I thought you said that the mountain was free of all antisocial elements.'

'Just a sensible precaution.'

The road descended in a series of steepening loops, swooping round un-signposted corners and uncambered blind bends and dropping sharply without warning down narrow unexpected clefts. Thanks to the self-interest of the Magadi Soda Company the road was tarmac and smooth. We voiced our grateful thanks. Very soon the cool highlands and closely cropped green grass of the Ngong Hills were distant memories, far in our rear. Now there was no grass, just bare khaki-coloured soil, scattered thorn trees, black volcanic rocks, bony hills and increasing heat. A pair of dik dik dashed across the road, a ground squirrel raced madly along the tarmac before jinking into the verge. Thin cattle lunched apathetically on non-existent herbage and fat goats with mad yellow eyes eagerly nourished themselves on a diet of gravel and bare leafless twigs, standing on their hind legs to dine off the spindly roadside bush. A pair of hornbills lurched overhead, red bills like the noses of heavy drinkers. Now we were on a flat desiccated plain. The air shimmered and dust devils rose in the heated air. Far ahead we could see a pair of tiny black figures marching along the road. As we approached they separated until one was on either side. Both were carrying long Maasai spears. They stopped and turned to face our approach.

Berna turned to me. 'I say,' she said. 'What *are* those chaps up to?'

'Who can fathom the mind of man in Africa?' I facetiously replied.

As we drew nearer, the two men, clad in little more than wisps of scarlet chiffon and decorative beads, slowly raised their six-foot long spears.

'Right,' I thought. 'This is it. The bloody end of a romantic weekend in the bush. Over before it's even begun.'

Berna looked faintly concerned, but, as I learned then, and later, she was a cool kid. A slight furrowing of the alabaster brow, but no more.

The spears were now at shoulder height and it was too late to stop. I depressed the throttle and we shot forwards. As we rocketed through the mini-gauntlet, two gleaming spears arced high over the car. I glimpsed two rows of gleaming teeth as their owners doubled up with laughter. In the rear-view mirror I saw the spears embedding themselves in the dry earth and the two scantily clad comedians slapping their ebony thighs in unrestrained glee.

I glanced at my companion, who merely raised her eyebrows and pursed her lips. She was, after all, an Old Africa Hand.

At a slightly slower pace now, we pressed on. To left and right, stony mountains crowded in on the narrow road. Pools of stagnant water in a dry river bed were surrounded by herds of skinny cattle and flocks of sheep and goats, monitored by their languid Maasai owners.

As we dropped further into the Rift Valley the temperature rose in shimmering, juddering waves. There was no sign of permanent habitation. Occasionally we passed old abandoned manyattas, the low, grey, chest-high huts falling to pieces, the circular thorn barricades crumbling. On our left was a mountain which I had identified on the map as Olorgesaille. It appeared to be strewn from base to apex with football-sized boulders and vegetated with leafless bush from whose naked branches protruded an array of thorns of intimidating aspect.

Would Shompole be any better?

The road ascended a steep hill and there, far distant, glittering white like an incongruous tropical snowfield, lay the solidified soda surface of Lake Magadi. An hour later we rattled over the railway line built long ago to transport the mined soda to civilisation. On either side of the road were shallow odiferous ponds in which pink and white flamingoes sieved frantically.

'Ye gods!' said Berna. 'The heat! The stench! I think I'll bag some of it on the way back and take it home to school for science teacher Mike Dewing to analyse!'

We came to a barrier across the road, adjacent to a police post. A forbidding sign in red and black informed us that the Company took no responsibility whatsoever for the well being of anyone proceeding beyond this point and that should anyone find him or herself in difficulties no rescue should be expected as none would be attempted. We looked at each other and raised our eyebrows. I signed the book in the police post. The on-duty constable looked as though he couldn't have cared less whether we returned or not. In slow mo and suede safari boots he strolled out of his booth, languidly raised the barrier and we continued on our way.

The houses of the Magadi Soda Company were built along a high ridge running due south, overlooking, and parallel to, the lake. The better to catch whatever little breeze there was, we surmised, and also perhaps to make sure no worker down at the mine was slacking. We could imagine the manager sitting on his verandah, cold gin in hand, binoculars pressed to gimlet orbs, scrutinising the mine buildings in the centre of the lake for any dereliction of duty. Out there the heat would be terrific. Where we were was little better, so when we passed the entrance to the Magadi Club and caught a fleeting glimpse of a blue swimming pool I slammed on the anchors.

'I'm parched,' I said.

'Likewise,' said Berna, 'my throat feels like the sands of central Sahara, and this may be our last chance for a cold drink until we get back.'

We levered ourselves out into the furnace, and strode purposefully towards the club entrance.

'Hey,' said Berna, 'I say, that looks a bit unfriendly,' pointing towards a shaded sign – Magadi Club. Private. Members Only – in foot high letters.

'Well,' I said, 'we can but try.'

I pushed open the gate into the club and we sauntered across to admire the pool, which was surrounded by about an acre of velvety green lawn, upon which little sprinklers were softly showering a benison of cool water. Small umbrella-shaded tables were scattered around, seemimgly awaiting just such as us. The place was empty.

'Excuse me, sir and madam? Can I help you?' A uniformed African flunkey popped up beside us, materialising out of nowhere like a genie.

'Yes, indeed,' I replied. 'We were passing and wondered if we might be able to refresh ourselves in your charming establishment before pressing on into the wilderness?'

'Are you membas?'

'Why, no!'

'Then I am afraid you must leave. This club is for membas only.'

'Can we speak to the manager, the secretary, the gaffer?'

'Hello James, having trouble? Can I help?' Another voice, aristocratic, plummy and male, entered the conversation. The owner was tall, middle-aged, with too smoothly combed iron-grey hair, wore baggy shorts commonly known as 'empire builders', knee-length socks (a bad sign), a short-sleeved shirt and a cravat (another bad sign). He also sported, if that is the correct word, a rather aggressive moustache in the style formerly called a 'soup strainer'. James seemed to shrink visibly in size before this new presence. I pasted on my most winning smile.

'Good afternoon sir,' I said. 'Delighted to meet you. We're on our way to tackle Shompole and were wondering if we might be able to have a short pit stop here, buy a cold drink, use your facilities, perhaps even have a dip in your pool?'

He stared at us, seemingly not delighted to meet us, taking in our travel-stained attire, Berna's micro-shorts, my tattered hat, our dusty boots. He glanced through the gate at my 504. His lips pursed, his nose wrinkled. 'My name's Fortescue. I'm the club manager. I'm sorry, but this is a private club, for members only, who are, in the main, employees of the Company. It's not a hotel or a lodge. We just can't allow in any passing wayfarer who decides that he, or she, would like to take advantage of what we have here. And, in addition,' staring fixedly at Berna's shorts in particular, 'there are certain sartorial standards we insist upon. You can probably buy a Coke in the village shop. A warm one, but better than nothing, ha! Good day and good luck! With that car you may need it! James will see you out.' He gave a high-pitched barking laugh and turned on his heel.

With the departure of his boss James re-inflated himself and with an air of self-satisfied enjoyment escorted us back to our car.

'Thank you, James,' I said, as I opened the car door. 'Nothing like a bit of good old-fashioned hospitality to set a chap up for the day, eh?' Of course, it was grossly unfair of me to say that. He was just doing his job and probably didn't really relish turfing out stray Europeans any more than the next man. But then why the smug smile? That vanished at my remark and he glared at us as we drove off.

'Well,' said Berna, 'we won't be calling in *there* on the way back, will we? We'll be lucky not to get a rock through the windscreen from Master James and as for that jumped-up popinjay Fortescue...' She was lost for words. We fussed and fumed as we rattled past the Magadi golf course, which was unique in that it was totally devoid of grass. The fairways were gravel and the greens smooth, hard packed sand. The rough was just that – bleak bony outcrops of bare rock and impenetrable thickets of grey thorn, into which no self-respecting golfer would dream of entering. Here a sliced ball was a lost ball. There was no sign of any golfing activity.

'Bloody cheek, casting aspersions on our car,' I said. 'He probably tools around in an air-conditioned Land Rover which has never been off the tarmac. Pompous ass.'

The track descended to bare baking flats at the southern end of the lake. Hot springs boiled busily near the prominent landmark of Bird Rock. Flamingoes with asbestos legs guddled nearby in the steaming water. Ahead we could see dense green stands of elephant grass and papyrus. We were now entering the great swamp which lies between the southern end of Lake Magadi and the northern shore of Lake Natron in Tanzania. Here the river Easo Nyiro from Kenya winds its sinuous way in glittering serpentine coils before sliding into another inhospitable soda lake, to have its fresh waters diluted and lost in a shimmering expanse of alkaline ooze.

The track was dwindling, getting more and more difficult to follow. This was no through road. On the map it went to a village, also called Shompole, at the foot of the mountain. After that it went nowhere. Even now it was only a tenuous dotted line, bisected by unnamed watercourses entering the swamp. We pressed on, hoping for better things, but expecting at any moment to come across some undriveable impasse. In the distance we could see cattle and their Maasai attendants. For miles now we had been so intent on the track or lack of it to pay any attention to our distant objective. Now I glanced up and there, filling the dusty windscreen, was the vast western flank of the mountain, riven by gullies and transected by narrow steep ridges.

'Ye gods,' exclaimed Berna. 'So this is what you've brought me to? What do you think I am? A mountain goat?'

'Calm down, dear!' I replied. 'Calm down. These things always look steeper when you look at them face on.'

'Well, we're not looking at this one face on, but from the side and it looks damn steep to me!'

I let that one pass and concentrated on the remnants of the track in front of me. Fortescue's assumed Land Rover, with or without air conditioning, would have been useful here, I had to admit. On more than one occasion I had to ask Berna to nip out to modify the track, shift boulders, lift fallen branches and test the depth of the occasional rivulet. By the time we emerged from the swamp and saw the distant shacks of Shompole village, cowering below its eponymous mountain, we were getting a mite desperate.

'I wonder if there's anywhere here where we can get a drink?' wondered Berna.

I gave a mirthless laugh. 'Fat chance,' I said. But, as we trundled up to the ramshackle collection of windowless cabins to which the usual collection of colourful, blanket-clad locals had been magnetised, we saw, emblazoning one ochreous shack, the familiar faded Coca-Cola logo, and, above it another sign – Hotel Hargeisa. A small flock of goats was gathered at the door, as though seeking entrance. I headed towards it and ground to a halt. As we stopped a tall elderly Somali gent with a hennaed beard appeared in the doorway. We got out and pushed our way through the goats. The Somali smiled. 'Welcome to Shompole! Come in! My name is Mohamed Yusuf and you are very welcome. Enter! Enter!'

Well, this was a change from the Magadi Club. Inside there were a couple of plastic tables set on the dirt floor and little else as far as we could see. From behind a beaded curtain came a beautiful Somali girl with a plate of samosas which she placed before us. She brought cups which she proceeded to fill from a large thermos flask – hot, spicy tea. Coca-Cola was forgotten as we sipped the enriching brew. The girl gave us a dazzling smile and disappeared behind the curtain.

Mohamed Yusuf dragged another plastic chair across and sat down. 'Where you from?'

'Scotland' I said, 'and Ireland,' said Berna.

'Ah yes. Originally, so, but here for long I think? I can tell those here for short and those for long time. You, the way you walk, the way you look at things, how you dress, yes you are from Africa.'

We sipped our tea. 'Me, myself, I come from Blitish Somaliland. So Hargeisa Hotel, ha! Long time ago. Before me here was Indian duka wallah. Uhuru come, Kenyatta say to Indian 'get out.' So I come. I was askari with Blitish forces. Good times. Left, right, left, right! Yes sir, no sir! But now things are bad there. Now we have govment from Mogadishu. Pah! No discipline. They are mafia. What can you expect, when the country before was run by a gang of wops! No discipline!' He laughed. 'Hey, Fatma! Bring me that bottle of Johnny Walker! To drink a toast to my Blitish fliends!'

We raised our collective eyebrows. Weren't Muslims supposed to eschew alcohol?

Not this one, it seemed. Fatma returned bearing a tray upon which stood three glasses and the bottle of Johnny Walker, Black Label appropriately enough, and whose level, I noted, was well below the Plimsoll line.

Mohamed Yusuf sloshed a generous measure into each glass.

'Chin! Chin! as the old Colonel used to say! Ha! Ha!' He tossed his drink back. We sipped ours.

'So why are you here in this dump?' asked Yusuf.

'We want to climb Shompole,' I said.

'Shompole!' he laughed. 'Hey, Fatma!' he shouted, 'they want to climb Shompole!' Fatma reappeared. She also laughed. Berna and I looked at each other.

'No one. No one,' said Mohamed Yusuf, 'climbs Shompole.'

'Why not?' I asked. 'Is is it some sort of sacred mountain?'

He laughed again. All this laughing was beginning to get on my nerves. 'No, it's because it is impossible. It's covered with wild sisal, cactus, elephant grass, it's too steep, it's infested with mosquitoes...' Berna looked at me. 'You told me...' she began.

'What about the Maasai? Don't they know the way up?'

'They won't go near it. Not good for their cattle and goats. They don't like the hills anyway. They prefer the flat ground. Easier on the legs.'

He gave another laugh and knocked back another slug of whisky. There was a commotion at our backs and a musky smell. Two Maasai had entered, tall, handsome young men, wearing red shukas over brown shoulders, copper ornaments swinging in their ears, beaded bracelets on their slender wrists, leather sandals on their feet, knobkerries in their hands. 'Soba!' they greeted us. 'Eba!' we replied. They smiled, an open honest smile, showing white, glistening teeth, moist with spittle.

Mohamed Yusuf talked to them in Maa. We heard the word Shompole mentioned. Much tut tutting, shaking of heads and tinkling of ear ornaments.

He turned to us. 'They say they will point out the way but they won't go up with you. By the way, what do you both do?'

We told him. We heard the word mwalimu (teacher) and daktari (doctor) mentioned. The Maasai looked at us. More talking in Maa.

Mohamed Yusuf turned to us. 'They say that if you have a look at their animals they will go a bit further with you up the mountain and look after your car while you are up there.'

'Right,' we said simultaneously. 'Where are the animals?' I asked.

'On the way,' Mohamed Yusuf replied. 'They have a manyatta at the foot of the mountain.'

We knocked back our drinks and emerged blinking and stumbling into the afternoon sunlight. 'Bloody hell!' I said, *sotto voce*, 'whisky at 2 o'clock in the afternoon! That was not such a good idea!' Berna appeared to be bereft of speech.

We wrung Mohamed Yusuf's horny hand, pledging eternal amity and promising to call in on him on our way back to civilisation. Fatma grinned from the doorway. Was she his daughter or his wife, we wondered?

The two Maasai made as though to get into the Peugeot, but stopped when they saw that the rear seats were encumbered with spare tyres and camping gear. 'Wapi manyatta?' I asked. (Where is the manyatta?) 'Huko,' one indicated with his chin. (There) About a mile away, in an open glade in a fold of the mountain. By the time we had got ourselves into the car and started the engine they were half way there, loping in easy strides across the veldt.

As we neared the thorn-enclosed boma Berna regained the use of her tongue. '*You* told me that this mountain was going to be a doddle. Now I gather it's shunned by all of mankind. What have you got to say for yourself?'

'Regard it as a character-forming exercise. At least you don't have to teach their kids differential calculus!'

'Are you suggesting that my character *needs* forming?'

I had no time to answer this one as by now we were surrounded by a mixed mass of goats, sheep, cattle, men, women and children, and several billion flies. We tumbled out of the car, anxious to do our duty and be on our way. Already the hour was late and if we were not careful we would be kipping in the manyatta. We noticed that there seemed to be some sort of ceremony in progress. By an earthern wall sat a group of old men. In front of them was a large metal sufuria, or cooking pot, filled with an amber fluid. Young men were approaching in a reverential manner, bowing respectfully to have an ancient hand placed on their heads and then given a cupful of the drink to imbibe.

We moved among the livestock, prodding and poking, examining and suggesting. I scrutinised infected eyes, peered at runny noses, gave advice on deworming, counselled on the control of ticks and tsetse flies, mosquitoes and midges, lifted hooves, and rectally examined a few cattle, testing for pregnancy. Flies were everywhere. The people seemed not to be bothered by them, as they crawled into their eyes and covered their faces. They drove us mad. We flapped our hands in vain. They paid no attention.

Finally we were led into a small hut. There lying on a cowskin bed lay a boy of about ten. His right arm was bent at an abnormal angle, the elbow locked and the wrist drawn in towards his forearm. He had been bitten by a puff adder six weeks previously. The arm had swollen hugely. He had almost died and when the swelling had subsided the tissue damage caused by the haemotoxic venom had destroyed the muscle tissue leaving his arm a useless withered wreck. There was nothing we could do and we doubted whether anything could be done. We advised his parents to take him to the hospital at Magadi to have him examined by a doctor. But if they had not done that in the six weeks following the bite, what chance was there now? The boy stared at us with huge pleading eyes. What use am I now with only one arm, he seemed to say? Feeling helpless and hopeless we shuffled out into the afternoon sun.

As we did so we were ushered towards the knot of ancients dishing out whatever was in the pot. One of the young men told us that this was a ceremony to initiate a junior elder, his father having recently died. The recipient of this honour was seated on a stool, wearing a rather fetching skin cloak and having a pair of bead anklets stitched onto his ankles by a couple of giggling, nubile young women. The new elder looked about 35 and was slightly drunk, swaying gently from side to side. His shaven head shone with red ochre. He looked benignly at us. 'Come, come and sit,' he said. We were given stools and sat. 'Drink!' he commanded. We stared at the massive metal dixie, almost as big as a baby's bath, filled with what we assumed was some sort of beer. Struggling across its khaki-coloured surface was a host of semi-submerged flies, feebly breast-stroking their way to alcoholic oblivion. As we tried to keep our thoughts to ourselves we were handed huge plastic mugs, both of which looked as though they could have done with a good wash. One of the attendant elders plunged a large dipper below the active surface and came up with about a pint of fluid and a pound of moribund flies. This, we thought, was too much. Help was at hand though. In his other hand the lop-eared geriatric produced an appropriately sized sieve which he placed with a theatrical flourish over our mugs before decanting our portion of booze. Hundreds of flies were left struggling on the mesh, rather like a shoal of netted herrings untimely lifted from the North Sea. Relieved, we lifted our mugs to our lips.

The stuff was surprisingly good, which probably explained why there was such a convivial gathering milling around the manyatta. People had trekked for scores of miles to be there. Some had even crossed the border from Tanzania. It all went to show that the world over people will travel miles to go to a good party.

The drink was some kind of honey beer, innocuous to taste but lethal in its effect. When I was a student I spent a summer vacation near Aix-en-Provence in the south of France, ostensibly building houses, but, as it was under the umbrella of M. Ricard, the latter-day absinthe king, spending rather a lot of time sampling the produce of his vats. The first time I did this was almost my last. I had never tasted the seductive, aniseed drink before. Sitting comfortably in a pavement café, in cool shade under a striped awning, chatting with drinking friends and watching the Provencal world go by, I tossed back beakers of the stuff until it was time to go. I stood up and walked out onto the sunblasted pavement. Next thing, to the sound of blaring klaxons and shouted Gallic oaths, like a beached jellyfish, I was floundering in the gutter. This, I felt, was very soon going to happen again, if I did not exert my iron will and get up and go. I turned to Berna to signal that enough was enough. To my consternation she was deeply into the niceties of Maasai ritual and the role of women in Maasai society with her nearest neighbour, a handsome young buck, who spoke startling English with a clipped BBC accent. Several frantic signals and two plastic mugfuls of Maasai mead later and we were back at the car, shouldering our gear and wondering how to set one foot in front of another, let alone breast the slope ahead of us.

Anxious to get away before we were persuaded to participate in some esoteric tribal rite I shoved whatever came to hand into my rucksack. In went a plastic tub of limp, leathery sandwiches, several oranges, a couple of Mars bars, two hard-boiled eggs, a large bottle of water, a camera, a battered P G Woodhouse paperback, a packet of crisps, a pair of plastic mugs, a small gas cooker, and some tea and sugar encased in small plastic tubs. For good measure I forced in a can of baked beans. I strapped a karrimat to the outside of my sack and we were ready to go. The karrimat was only big enough for one person to lie on, but we could sort that problem out later. The main thing was to get going. It was already past 4pm. As we were leaving, I saw the Tilley lamp which for some reason we had packed along with all the other stuff. I grabbed it and we set off. Bent almost double beneath my load I staggered after Berna, who, more lightly encumbered, exhorted me to get a move on, we hadn't got all day to potter around and whose idea was it anyway to pub crawl around the foot of the mountain? The Maasai, deep in their cups, seemed to have forgotten us. I, for one, heartily wished I hadn't drunk any cups at all.

The going was open and, in the now-declining temperature, could almost, but not quite, be classed as pleasant. The mountain was not exactly Alpine though, more like a stony, tilted slag heap. We kept on barking our toes on the ubiquitous boulders with which the ground was littered. We headed for the base of a wide, seemingly-bare ridge, which snaked its way up to the summit plateau. Trying to avoid the boulders we stumbled and weaved our way between the scattered thorn trees until we arrived, panting and perspiring, at the foot of our chosen ridge.

Berna gazed upwards at our intended route. 'So – this is the start of the lovely ridge walk, eh? I wonder what the dormitory facilities will be like?'

'Pretty spartan I'm afraid,' I replied. 'We'll just have to hope for some soft rocks!'

The temperature had certainly dropped but it was far from cool. It just wasn't hot. By the time we had toiled upwards for a thousand feet or so we, or certainly I, had sweated away most of the alcohol so intemperately imbibed down there on the foothills.

By now the sun was sinking in the west. The ridge, though still wide, was getting narrower. We paused to take stock. Far below us now, the swamp, which stretched towards the distant blue and purple Nguruman Escarpment and the far side of the Rift Valley, was lit up by the declining sun. The river winding through it was a silver snake, coiling and twisting, a headless serpent with no end and no beginning. The swamp looked smooth and soft and inviting, as though a person could walk across its level green surface, but we knew that the papyrus was ten feet tall and that the ooze was bottomless.

Below our desert boots the boulders were now reduced in size to unstable gravel. The gradient had seriously steepened and we pussyfooted our way upwards, slipping and sliding on the unattached surface. Darkness was fast approaching and we had to find somewhere to lay ourselves down while there was still a modicum of light.

We stopped below a medium-sized tree and examined the ground beneath. After clearing away a couple of inconveniently sited rocks, we decided that we were unlikely to find anywhere better. 'Right, Cranman,' said Berna. 'So this is it, is it? The Alpine chalet you promised me? The snug bedroom, the rose on the pillow, the flower-bedecked dining room, the friendly waiters, the sumptuous menu, the… what the hell was that?' Out of the gathering gloom came a harsh, hostile bark, which echoed backwards and forwards from the neighbouring ridge. It was followed by another and another until the air quivered with the sound. 'Baboons,' I said. 'There must be a troop of them over there on that other ridge and they've seen us. They'll settle down once it gets dark. Nothing to worry about.'

'Nothing to worry about? I've seen baboons and they've got great big teeth and they go for defenseless young women like me. Carry them off to their dens. I saw a film once…hell! A mosquito! I've just been bitten. You told me that there were none here, that they never ventured from their swamp.' Sure enough I could hear the maddening whine and feel the sting as one landed on my neck.

We spread out the karrimat, lit the Tilley lamp and sat down to enjoy our alfresco dinner before we turned in for the night. 'What'll we have first? A warm sandwich or some soggy crisps, a liquefied Mars bar or some bashed baked beans – you didn't forget the tin opener did you… did you…?!' At least we hadn't forgotten the matches and were able to brew up some tea. As the light faded and the spindly thorn trees stood silhouetted against a pearl-grey sky, there came the yip of a jackal and then far below, the mournful oooooup call of a hyena, almost immediately answered by another. But nearer at hand, as the darkness closed in, there was another sound – the low hum of a rising squadron of voracious mosquitoes. I rolled down my shirt sleeves. Berna wrapped herself in her kikoi. I pulled my socks up and pulled my hat down. I re-sited the Tilley lamp, hoping that the insects would be diverted to the attractive yellow light but they seemed to prefer living flesh to the flickering flame. We swatted and we swore. Berna mostly swore at me. It was all to no avail. There were only two of us. There were millions of them. We were bitten half to death.

'As the temperature drops,' I said, 'they'll shove off.' The temperature never did drop and the insectivorous torture continued until the distant dawn, when, like another blood-sucking fiend, they vanished.But now it was barely past evensong and we had the whole livelong night before us. Tea drunk, we nibbled on the leathery crisps and sucked at the sour oranges and stared into the darkness.

'Well,' I said. 'Look on the bright side. At least we'll both have an early night for a change!' Berna laughed. 'Let's read that PG Woodhouse book. I saw it in your haversack.' I dragged it out, now bent and battered and only fit for the bin, but for the next couple of hours we were with Bertie Wooster and Jeeves and the Drones Club in the carefree days of pink champagne and toffs and forelock-tugging subservients.

I peered at my watch. 'Good heavens! It's almost ten o'clock! Doesn't time fly when you're having a good time!' 'I'll say!' said Berna, 'right, now *I'm* going to snuggle down on this comfy karrimat, which, sadly, has just enough room for little me, and no one else. Good night! Sleep well!' So saying she wrapped herself in her kikoi and stretched herself out on our one and only karrimat.

I lowered the wick of the Tilley lamp until the flame was barely visible and then retired to my own quarters. Cleared of rocks and rubble, the ground was now ready to receive me. A hole for my hip I had already excavated, and, by curling up in the time-honoured foetal position and by exerting a good deal of imagination it was just possible to convince oneself that one was moderately comfortable.

Sleep however was slow in coming.

Those who live in towns often think that 'out there', in the sticks beyond the last urban speed limit, all is quiet and peaceful and that at night a holy hush falls on the slumbering land.

Far from it.

The creatures of Shompole which had spent the daylight hours lurking silently in holes and crevices now emerged en masse in search of prey. Twigs cracked, bushes rustled and pebbles were dislodged as unseen animals rooted and snorted and delved in the undergrowth. With one's ear millimetres from the ground all noises were magnified to proportions which made the scuttle of a scorpion and the tramp of a foraging ant sound like an approaching herd of wildebeest.

Night birds called loudly to each other, hooting and screeching. Others seemed to spend an excessive and seemingly unnecessary amount of time fluttering their feathers and clapping their wings as they folded them in preparation for sleep. Dry vegetation crackled as invisible bodies, magnified by overwrought imagination to the size of buffalo, pushed their way through the thickets. Seed pods in the thorn trees decided that this was the night to fall noisily to the ground. Other sounds were more furtive, a low snuffling, a stealthy footfall, a sinister scratching. What *was* that? A snake? A leopard? A monitor lizard? Reason told one that it was probably nothing more alarming than a small self-respecting mouse, going about its nocturnal business. But listen! What was *that* noise? That low keening, scraping sound, rising and falling, rising and falling, then fading away into a sort of bubbling, strangulated sob? *That*, I finally realised, with a mixture of relief and indignation, was the sound of the fully fledged female Irish snore. God, how could she sleep through all that racket? I hadn't had a wink for hours.

I must have fallen asleep at last though, because I suddenly came to, finding myself being rudely shaken awake from a most delightful dream of delicious realism in which, in the company of Bertie Wooster and Jeeves, I was being given a intimate body massage by a unclad young lady of singular physical attributes.

'Wha..! Wha..!'

'Cranman! Wake up! Wake up!'

'What? What's up?' I testily inquired.

'Listen!' I did and heard it. The unmistakable, coughing grunt of a lion. It came from the swamp, the distinctive, heart-stirring, soul-wrenching sound of wild Africa. We sat in the warm darkness, oblivious to the clouds of mosquitoes, as the lion asserted his dominance. 'This is *my* land! This is *my* land!' he roared. We agreed.

'I say,' said Berna, 'he's not going to come up here is he?'

'Oh no, definitely not,' I said, 'not a chance, but maybe we should stay very close together, just in case he does.' Which we did, and have done so ever since. The lady of my technicoloured dream was replaced by the even more singular lady of my real life.

The sound of doves, cooing in the thorn trees, awoke us. Stiffly we rose to greet the dawn. My back felt tingly. No wonder. I had more than 80 mosquito bites, from shoulders to lower back, through my shirt. Berna counted them. 'If I don't get terminal malaria after this,' I said, 'I never will.'

'And you said that this was a mosquito-free zone!' she laughed. A baboon barked across the ridge.

We brewed some tea. 'Time to go,' I said, 'while we're still in the shade on this side of the mountain. Once the sun hits us it'll get really hot.' I shouldered my pack and we set off, plodding up the ridge. 'If things are anything like yesterday,' I said, 'we should be up in no time.'

Things were nothing like yesterday.

As the ridge steepened still further we came to a band of wait-a-bit thorn. As with the tin opener of the night before, I had neglected to bring a panga with which to cut through such irritating obstacles. The result was mortifying from every point of view. The shirt which was no deterrent to the proboscis of the frail mosquito now fell victim to the wicked hooks of the innocent-looking bush. Once caught in the excruciating tangle there was no question of going forwards. The only way out was by reversing, leaving shirt material and skin behind. More blood was shed and the mountain rang with cries of anguish and words no young lady should ever be forced to hear. 'Mr Cran! Is that really necessary?' inquired my companion. Yes, it bloody well was.

Shirt in tatters, streaming with blood I could ill afford to lose, I finally emerged, backwards, in ignominious retreat. Only by slithering down the precipitous side of the ridge above an alarming drop did we manage to circumvent the thorny barrier.

As we regained the ridge the sun emerged above the eastern rim of the mountain. A bateleur eagle, with its short chestnut tail, black belly and white ventral wings, glided smoothly over Shompole's inaccessible ridges. Wheeling, it turned, probably checking to see if we were worth a second look. Deciding not, it quickly vanished in the direction of the as-yet invisible Lake Natron.

More wait-a-bit lay ahead and yet more blood was shed. This, however was but the beginning, the *hors d'oeuvre* before the main course. Soon we met the first of a veritable forest of wild sisal plants. Anything from 2-6ft high, these fleshy horrors are tipped with black, needle sharp spines, capable of transfixing a leg or arm, or puncturing an eye. Single plants are bad enough, but when they occur in clumps or, worst of all, are hidden among dense stands of 10ft high elephant grass, the situation becomes serious. With a panga it is just possible to hew a path through. With bare hands, forward progress becomes a high-stepping pantomime, without the laughs.

We scouted to the right. We scouted to the left. Finally we reached a tiny clearing and collapsed. We had advanced about ten feet.

'Clear route all the way to the summit, eh?' said Berna.

'We just need to get past this lot and we'll break out onto broad, sunlit uplands,' I replied, ever the optimist.

'They're sunlit, but that's about all they've got going for them,' was the answer to that.

Two hours later and we had climbed little more that a couple of hundred feet and we were now confronted with a veritable battlement of cactus, twelve feet high, solid and impenetrable, extending over both sides of the ridge. Getting through this without an army of machete-wielding press ganged navvies was patently impossible. The only way now for us was down.

As we turned to go I caught a fleeting glimpse of the elusive Lake Natron, peeping round the southern corner of the mountain.

Hours later, after fighting our way back through the thickets of thorn, wild sisal and elephant grass, we were down where we started. I looked, and felt, as though I had been attacked by a lion and had barely survived. I was covered in scratches and bedaubed with blood, shorts and shirt rent in a dozen places and unfit to be donated to the meanest beggar. Berna, by contrast, was without a mark on her and her attire, such as it was, unblemished. Her coiffeur was unruffled and not a bead of perspiration marred the alabaster brow. How did she do it? She did not, however, refuse the proffered jumbo-sized bottle of Whitecap, warm though it was, which I retrieved from the car.

The Maasai ceremony was over, and the manyatta was empty except for a few children and a couple of goats basking in the late afternoon sun.

As we approached the Hotel Hargeisa we could see the voluptuous form of Fatma, leaning against the door post, a mocking smile on her lips. We decided not to stop. We gave her what we hoped looked like a wave of quiet triumphalism and trundled on past.

Well, I mused, that's that. Hardly an episode worthy of inclusion in the Annals of the Alpine Club. More like an ignominious rout than anything else. On the other hand, I thought, looking at the superlative stunner in the seat next to me, there was some consolation in defeat.

Four more assaults and several years later, I finally reached the summit of what has been well-dubbed 'the nastiest mountain in Kenya', if not in the world.

Chapter Fifteen

WEDDING BELLS

Berna and I were married in St. Christopher's Anglican Church in Nakuru on 3 April 1982. As Berna was an Irish Catholic and I was a Scottish Presbyterian certain ecclesiastical difficulties arose and so we devised our own wedding service, welding both faiths into one with the help of the two officiating clergy, the Rev. Geoffrey Ochana and Fr. Martin O'Connor. With both a black and a white clergyman at our wedding we felt that we were taking political correctness to a higher level and quietly burnished our metaphorical haloes. The fact that these two opposing clerical factotums had agreed to come and work together was in no small part due to the hypnotic effect Berna was able to exercise over all the men she came in contact with. With an unrestrained laugh and personalised eye contact she soon had them trotting at her heels and doing her bidding with anxious eagerness. Her youth and beauty may also have had something to do with it. She was only 25. I, being ever so slightly past the first flush and not nearly so good looking, lagged behind when it came to charming deacons and padres out of the trees.

The service was a home-made affair. We selected the hymns and the readings, typed up the sheets and sent out the invitations. We hired tents and chairs. The reception was held at the home of Judy and Lofty Drews, on the slopes of Menengai crater. Food and, most importantly, drink, was provided by cordial Alex Jennings, the manager of the Midland Hotel in Nakuru. Ladies supplied flowers for the church. Claire Doig, a blue-blooded Lady of the Realm no less, produced a wedding cake, fashioned by her own aristocratic hands, whose iced marvels included entwined thistles and shamrocks. None of our relations in the UK were able to attend but we did have 350 guests who came from all over the country. A Polish friend and, appropriately, celebrated rally driver, Nick Nowicki, drove the bridal carriage. Matron Victoria Fanshawe, whether mellowed by age or transfixed by Berna, seemed to have forgiven my past transgressions, and appeared at one of the pre-nuptial church rehearsals to give unsolicited advice on carpets for our feet and cushions for our knees.

'And my dears,' she gushed. 'I just know how dreadfully nervous you must feel. We all did! You wouldn't be human if you didn't! I do suggest that a couple of hours before the ceremony you each take a Valium tablet to settle your nerves. Then you can relax and really enjoy yourselves!'

We thought about this, and decided that a drug trial, a dummy run, might be advisable. After all, we didn't want to fall asleep in the church as we were making our responses. So one Saturday afternoon we each popped a pill. Two hours later we were both snoring on the sofa, dead to the world. Next morning we still felt as though we were surfacing from an anaesthetic. We moved slowly, legs leaden and numb, enunciated our words with difficulty and our tongues felt like lumps of unrisen dough. We decided to do without the Valium.

Berna's bridesmaid, Linda Pella, was the daughter of Pat and Damo. Damo was Italian and a trumpet player of note and both were known for their addictive loquacity. At the appointed hour, smartly suited in fetching grey worsted, I stood at the church door, best man Edmund Hemsted and ushers Trevor Dixon, aka Clever Trevor, and Chris Hughes, aka Groper, in close attendance. I glanced nervously at my watch. 2.30pm. The congregation was seated and chatting away and organist Paul Frith was hard at work exercising his talents on the keyboard.

'Time to get to the front,' said Edmund. The Front, I thought. Ominous word! 'Yes indeed,' I replied. 'Berna's coming from the Pellas. I hope the car hasn't broken down or had a puncture!' Edmund raised his generous eyebrows. 'It wouldn't be the first time!' he laughed.

Paul Frith's repertoire was wide and varied, but by the time he thundered out the bridal march I was almost an expert on the minor cantatas of Johann Sebastian Bach and the more popular works of George Frederick Handel. The congregation ceased their chatter about the lack of rain, the abysmal price of steers, the pathetic performance of the new Fordson Major tractor, the inordinate cost of house-servants, the price of petrol and who had run off with who. With a great shuffling of shoes and safari boots everyone rose and turned as Berna, on the arm of her surrogate father, the redoubtable Maurice Frost of Thika, paraded serenely down the aisle. A vision in white, she looked stunning. She took up her position next to me and whispered, 'So sorry I'm late. Got chatting to the Pellas and Nick. You know what they're like. Gas, gas, gas! I looked at my watch and we were already ten minutes late! A runaway Irish/Italian/Polish chin wag!' I laughed.

'I thought for a moment that you might have changed your mind!'
'Not likely!' she smiled.

A piper welcomed us to the reception at the home of Judy and Lofty and the guests poured into the garden, which Judy had been watering for weeks, desperately trying to turn dusty brown earth into smooth green lawns. The marquees quickly filled with chattering, laughing, drinking guests. Weddings and funerals in Kenya are the great opportunity for far-flung friends and acquaintances to meet and catch up. All too soon it was time for the speeches and toasts. Anticipation for the untried speaker is usually much worse than the actual event, especially when the bulk of the audience is well oiled with drink, and once upstanding, my speech gathered pace, each remark greeted by ribald comments and impertinent advice and roars of laughter. Beakers of champagne were drunk. The party was due to carry on for many more hours but Berna and I had to leave. We were spending the first night of our honeymoon at a lodge in Lake Nakuru Park and the gates closed at dusk. Changed from our finery into more mundane wear and bedaubed with shaving foam sprayed onto our persons by well-wishers, tin cans rattling from our bumper, we left the merry throng to their drinking devices and made our way to the park.

By the time we had passed through the gate it was quite dark. We drove slowly through the forest which fringed the northern shore of the lake. Eyes reflected in our headlights glowed hot and menacingly in the darkness. Shapes moved in the thickets. An antelope dashed across the track, a porcupine scuttled into an antbear hole, a jackal loped along in front of us, turning its head to make sure we weren't getting too close. I slammed on the brakes. There was some sort of ditch right across the track. 'What the.. !' I said. 'I'll nip out and check,' said Berna. She was back in a trice, panting. 'It's a ruddy great python. It's so big that its head is in the grass on that side and its other end is still on the other side!' In the darkness what had looked like a depression was in fact the giant snake's body, slowly moving to cross the road.

I switched off the engine and we waited on the python's pleasure. When its tail had vanished into the vegetation we drove on to the lodge.

We spent our honeymoon on the Island of Lamu, off the north coast of Kenya. A microcosm of Swahili and coastal Arab culture, it was the perfect place to get away from it all. There were no vehicles on the island apart from a Land Rover owned by the DC and why he needed one when there were no roads was hard to understand. Perhaps he just sat in it, solar topee perched on his head, and imagined going somewhere important. The alleyways in the town were so narrow that two donkeys could not pass each other. The tall narrow houses with their ornately-carved doors overhung the shadowy lanes and almost touched in the middle. At the waterfront small dhows were tied up, some laden with mangrove poles, others with sand and cement. At the head of the creek a much larger ocean-going dhow was under construction. But no one seemed to be in any hurry. Whatever work was being done seemed to be done in slow motion. Skull-capped men, clad in ankle-length kikois and embroidered waistcoats, sauntered past, hand in hand. Knots of women, wrapped from head to toe in the all-enveloping black bui-bui, bold and evocative eyes rimmed with kohl, chattered their way to market. The only ones who moved with any speed were the children, laughing and running along the edge of the sea and diving into the water.

We stayed in a house at Shela on the outskirts of the town, a three-storey Arab mansion owned by Dr Anne Spoerry, who had given us the run of it, together with a resident cook and houseboy, as a wedding present. Anne was a legendary flying doctor, Franco-Swiss by birth, who flew her light plane all over the north of Kenya, tending to the ailments of the nomads in their isolated settlements. Her wartime experiences in the Resistance, and in concentration camps, were taboo subjects, never to be broached, unless one wished to be on the receiving end of Anne's rough French-accented tongue. I knew her from tending to her dogs and cows on her small farm in the Subukia valley and liked and respected her for her forthright ways and blunt good humour. She always dressed like a French peasant, in coarse blue canvas trousers and rough safari shirt. All she lacked were the sabots, beret and string of onions. The only time I saw her in a skirt was at our wedding.

We swam in the warm sea and walked along the empty beaches, sipped expensive gin at the Peponi Hotel and even more expensive beer at Petley's Inn, watched the sun rise, huge and red, over the Indian Ocean, lounged on the roof of our Arab house as lateen-rigged jahazis slipped silently down the passage between Lamu and the island of Manda towards the open sea, and imperceptibly slipped silently into the lotus-life which has seduced so many others. Some were ensnared to an alarming degree. Halfway between Shela and Lamu, just above the high tide mark, was a low, gnarled tree, in whose twisted branches lived a mop-haired hippie. His vacant expression and distant benign smile suggested that attractions other than tropical ennui held him in their grip. Young, and far from young, white women wandered by, arm in arm with beach boys and unemployed fishermen.

On Lamu beach one day we saw a wild figure gesticulating from the surf. Thinking that this was our chance to save a drowning man and have our name in lights, we sprinted across the sand. As we approached, instead of trying to struggle towards the beach, he retreated into deeper water. 'Please help!' he yelled. 'I've left my clothes on that dune and there's an askari coming!' We turned, and in the far distance we could see a uniformed figure striding purposefully along the strand. 'If I'm caught in the buff like this, I'll be put in the cells! Please, they're all strict Muslims here you know! Please!' Berna was wearing a kikoi over her bikini. She raised her elegant eyebrows. Slipping her feet out of her sandals, she trotted into the waves. Removing her kikoi she tossed it to the man, who had now ducked down so that only his head was visible. The askari approached and looked carefully in our direction, before walking on along the beach, in search of other prey. When he had disappeared I retrieved Berna's kikoi and left the naked bather to his own devices. He was pathetically grateful.

One day we went out fishing in a mashua, one of the small wooden sailing craft which looked so picturesque, gliding gracefully over the blue seas, the helmsman lounging nonchalantly in the stern, the rope to the lateen sail clamped between his horny toes, the rest of the crew asleep in the shade. 'Come aboard! Come aboard!' they called. 'We will take you feeshing! We will catch feesh! Red snappa! Parrot feesh! Even groupa!' The thought of hauling one of these exotic creatures out of the deep fired our imaginations and we clambered aboard. Within about five minutes we knew we had made a serious mistake. The boat was devoid of all creature comforts. The wooden seats bit into our backsides. In the bilges stale water slopped to and fro, together with bits and pieces of unidentifiable detritus. The water in the bottom of the boat seemed to be rising. And even with the sea breeze, it was as hot as hell.

As we ventured beyond the shelter of the land things began to get a trifle choppy. Waves began to approach us from several different directions at once. In this unwarranted turbulence the boat appeared to be pitching, rolling and yawing all at the same time. Our crew appeared to be totally unconcerned. One fellow did a bit of casual baling with an old tin can. The others lay with relaxed limbs and drooping eyelids. Only our gallant helmsman seemed to be looking towards his front.

Other waves were soon assaulting us. The first horrid wave of nausea struck us both simultaneously. If there had been a rail we would have moved rapidly towards it. All we could do was to twist and retch over the side. The crew was highly amused. They offered us limes, a sure-fire cure, they assured us. 'Sure-fire, my ass!' Berna said later, when we finally staggered onto the jetty.

We caught no grouper, and no other fish either.

Lamu was infested with cats. They were everywhere, thin, scrawny and famished. At night they screeched and howled from the rooftops and fought pitched battles with one another. Their caterwauling even drowned out the nocturnal wailing of Lamu's numerous muezzins, calling the faithful to prayer. By day they skulked through the alleyways and congregated on rubbish heaps and stole scraps from hotels and restaurants. Dead cats, washed to and fro with the tide, floated in the harbour, entangled with seaweed, plastic bottles and discarded rope.

One balmy evening Berna and I decided to have a meal at a small, outside restaurant, near the waterfront. It was a secluded place, a charming courtyard surrounded by a high stone wall. There were only four tables. The menu was short and select, mostly seafood. The Swahili staff were attentive and polite and we chose lobster and wine. Perfect. The crickets were singing, soft Arab music drifted on the humid air from the town, and the moon was in its ascendancy. We had just finished our meal and were pleasantly relaxed, sipping our wine and enjoying the evening, when another couple came in. They spoke French and nothing seemed to please them. Everything was 'mal' or 'mauvais.' Their table was 'très sale', the waiter was 'trop tard', the chairs were 'extremement dur' and they berated the girl who brought them their carafe of wine. 'What iz zis? Zis iz not wine! Zis rubbish from California! Wine! More like horse piss! Allez op! Bring ze soupe! Vite! Vite!' They laughed loudly at the poor girl's discomfiture.

Their table backed into a corner of the courtyard. Above them and directly above their table were the entangled branches of a tree, growing over the wall. Strangely, the two irritable epicures found the soup to their liking and they bent their heads over the broth and sipped away with insatiable Gallic gusto. In a pause between slurping they looked at each other and nodded, as if to say, with mutual surprise – 'Pas mal!' At the same time our eyes were caught by a movement in the branches above.

Almost hidden in the half-darkness were two cats. One was formidably male, judging by the size of his gonads, now revealed as he turned his rear towards us. As we watched, and before we had time to close our sagging jaws, he raised his tail and ejected a fine spray of urine into the air over the soup-sippers' table. It drifted down, unseen and unnoticed by the two diners as they bent their heads to their bouillon.

It was time for us to leave.

Chapter Sixteen

THE EYES HAVE IT

Back in Nakuru, the first casualty of the New Order was major domo Njoroge.

He had always worked, if that is the correct word, for bachelors.

His tasks were light. His hours, although often erratic, were not of an arduous nature and supervision of his labours by his employer virtually non-existent. Bizarre notions such as regular dusting and the scouring of pots and pans for no obvious reason were totally foreign to his nature. Bed-making was slapdash and slovenly. His cooking was basic in the extreme and the presentation of his offerings at mealtimes resembled that commonly-seen in truck stops and school canteens. He was a covert and, at times, overt alcoholic, and on occasion I would return in the evening after dealing with yet another emergency to find the kitchen windows steamed up, a pot at its last gasp on the hob, noxious fumes seeping below the doors and Njoroge prone on the floor, snoring the sleep of the well-established inebriate.

This had to stop, or Njoroge had to go. But you can't teach an old dog new tricks and old Njoroge was a stubborn set-in-his-ways Kikuyu. His rhubarb crumbles and meat pies however were almost as good as those made by my mother, and so I persuaded Berna to give him one last chance.

One night Berna and I were invited out for a meal. We returned about midnight to find a note by the telephone inscribed in pencil in Njoroge's dishevelled script – 'Night Girl phoned – wants to speak to Daktari.' I could feel Berna's eyes boring into the back of my head as I read, and re-read, this alarming missive. 'This,' she said through gritted teeth, 'needs explaining!' My head awhirl, I stared wildly at the grubby piece of paper. I saw a phone number written in one corner. Berna also saw it. Njoro 32Y1. 'Right,' she said in a steely voice, 'let's have a chat with 'Night Girl', shall we?' After an interminable delay the sleepy voice of the operator came on the line and he put the call through. By now it was getting on for 1am. Whoever we were phoning wasn't going to be too pleased at being roused at this hour. Finally, 'Hello! Hello!' It was a man's voice, muffled and semi-coherent, as though he was speaking with a pad of cotton wool over his mouth, or had forgotten to put in his dentures. Well, thank goodness for that, I thought. 'Bruce Nightingale here. Can I help you?'

'Sorry to trouble you, Bruce, but did you phone earlier?'

'Yes, I did. One of our dogs is not too well and I would like Hugh to see him in the morning.' Relief all round and another small nail in Njoroge's coffin.

Not long after this I was summoned to Bruce's broad acres near the best-avoided bidonville of Njoro to examine one of his horses, which had an eye problem. I rattled up the rutted tree-lined drive to the stables, trying, and failing, to avoid the minefield of potholes which reduced my speed to snail's pace, until I was being overtaken by old grey-haired women tottering along with loads of firewood on their aged backs and by mewling weanlings barely able to walk. 'Deters undesirables such as income tax inspectors and officials collecting for the latest non-existent charity,' Bruce told me. I nodded knowingly, and was envious of his rural isolation. Lurching over a few hundred potholes was a small price to pay in order to escape from the deafening chorus of financial entreaty.

The patient was a large grey mare, wheeled out by an aged syce, wearing a pair of hundred-year-old, wide-winged corduroy jodhpurs, the sort favoured by British cavalry officers during the Great War. Their antique effect was slightly marred by his non-existent socks and his red plimsolls, through which his big toes protruded, like the heads of small impudent brown mice.

My heart sank when the horse turned, for, jutting from her left eye was a large, ulcerated pinkish mass.

'Ye gods, Bruce,' I said. 'How long has that been there?'

Bruce was small and brown and wiry, a bit like a beached Ancient Mariner, without the long grey beard and glittering eye. He had been born and bred in the Highlands of Kenya and was a consummate farmer, breeding Friesian cattle, rearing racehorses and growing wheat and maize.

'Well, it was quite small before we went off skiing in Switzerland – that was for three, no, I tell a lie four weeks – and then when we got back we had to dash down to the coast for another two weeks with relations and when we got back a couple of weeks ago it was like that.'

'I see,' I replied, peering at the protrusion more closely. 'Well, it's a squamous cell carcinoma, probably sun-induced as she's a grey and the only option is surgery. It's too big to excise from what I can see. So the eye will have to come out.'

'Right. Can you do it now?'

'Yes. I'll have to knock her out with Xylazine and Ketamine, so we'll need a nice soft grassy field. Plus some reliable helpers.'

'We've got plenty of those and my son Oliver is here between Gordonstoun and college and he'll be able to assist as well.'

'Great! Great!'

Gordonstoun eh? I thought. Full of active, practical lads, and now lassies as well, swinging from ropes and crossing raging torrents and rowing at high speed up and down the Moray Firth in flimsy coracles.

'Well,' said Bruce, 'I'll leave you. I was up all night with a foaling mare and must go and lie down, before I fall down.'

'Good idea,' I said, wishing I could lie down now and again.

I drove my Peugeot into a large field and prepared for surgery. I laid my instruments out on a clean towel on the bonnet. As I did so a tall, dark, good-looking young man appeared. 'Hi, I'm Ollie. I'd like to see what you're doing, and if I can be of any use, please let me know.'

'Many thanks, Ollie. I may ask you to hold some instruments when I get going, so stand by.'

'Right, ready when you are.'

With the patient now standing in the field, I asked the ancient syce to raise her head so that the jugular vein became more prominent when I placed my thumb in the jugular furrow. Slowly I injected a computed dose of the sedative Xylazine into the vein and stood back. Two minutes later the mare's head was drooping at the level of her knees. Good. Now for the anaesthetic Ketamine. This I injected fairly rapidly. Within a couple of minutes the mare started to crumple and slowly collapsed onto her side.

'Gosh!' said Ollie. 'That stuff's effective.'

'Yup.' I said, 'but we may need to top it up if we don't finish the job within 15 or 20 minutes. It's pretty short-acting but it's reliable and safe.'

I dropped to my knees. Ollie stood by me. Working swiftly, I cleaned the skin around the eye, disinfected the eyelids and then clipped them together with a pair of Allis tissue forceps. As the teeth of the forceps bit into the skin I heard Ollie gasp. 'OK up there?' I asked.

'Yes, fine,' came the reply.

'Right, now I'm going to cut along the edge of the eyelids, below the forceps, and peel them back so that we can then dissect out the whole globe of the eye.'

'OK,' came a rather guarded reply.

'Here we go then.' With a super-sharp scalpel I incised along the length of both eyelids and, using the side of the blade, peeled the skin back to expose the eyeball, snapping another pair of tissue forceps onto the top and bottom layers of skin. A few arteries spouted bright red blood. I clamped them off.

There was a sort of sigh and a groan and a wheeze behind me followed by a thump.

I glanced around. Ollie was lying on his back in the grass, out cold as far as I could ascertain. A couple of spare syces scurried to render assistance. Being otherwise engaged I pressed on, clamping and cutting. I was just at the point of severing the muscles attaching the eyeball to the bony orbit when I heard a scrabbling sound at my back and, out of the corner of my eye, I could see Ollie on his knees, scrambling to his feet. 'Hi Ollie!' I said, 'welcome back!'

'Gosh! Sorry about that! Don't know what came over me. One moment I was OK, the next out for the count!'

'Don't worry. It happens to the best of us. You'll be fine now. Take a deep breath. Anyway you haven't missed much. I'm just about to cut the muscles at the back of the eye. There may be an interesting bit of blood here.'

Inserting the blade of the scalpel between the eye and the bone I cut round the back of the globe. Blood immediately gushed up as I knew it would. Taking a pair of large curved scissors I inserted them behind the globe in order to cut the large optic nerve. There was a confirmatory crunch as I severed the nerve, followed almost immediately by a metallic clang and a slithering sound.

Once again I turned my head, to see Ollie, his back against the side of my car, sliding slowly to the ground, eyes closed. This time he lay there quietly, in the shade of the Peugeot, chest rising and falling, as I staunched the blood and stitched the eyelids together. The syces looked at each other and smiled quietly in conspiratorial satisfaction.

By the time the mare was sitting up, prior to struggling to her feet, Ollie was in a similar state of recovery, blinking for the second time and wondering again what had happened.

I was relieved to see that my sturdy Peugeot had borne its unexpected buffeting well, and was, as far as I could see, unscathed. For a while I was unsure if the same could be said about the robust reputation of Gordonstoun, in view of the multiple swoonings of one of its alumni at the mere sight of a drop of blood, but as time went by it became apparent that this was not a constant of Ollie's character. Indeed the experience almost seemed to galvanise a cathartic addiction towards the manly sports of field and stream, involving the use of gun and rod, in which the shedding of blood was not infrequent.

Chapter Seventeen

PESTLE AND MORTAR

In the event we did not have to give Njoroge his marching orders. Unable to take any more of what seemed to him to be a dictatorial regime of cleaning and polishing and cooking under the eagle eye of the new memsahib, albeit on an irregular basis, he threw in the sponge, and lurched erratically, wild-eyed and muttering, out of our orbit. His replacement, Peter Gichane, was an improvement, although this was not immediately apparent. When he cleaned our silver cutlery set, a treasured wedding gift, with wire wool, his future, not to mention his life, hung precariously in the balance.

Berna continued to work at Greensteds School, commuting the 15 kilometres, initially on her motorbike, and then in an open plan, canvas-topped Mini Moke until she graduated to a Mini Minor.

Ken Penn, the tall and craggy headmaster of Nakuru Secondary School, was leaving, moving back to his roots on the rocky shores of Cornwall. Prior to his departure he asked me if I would take over the role of Honorary Correspondent for the Nakuru area, reporting to the British High Commission in Nairobi, a role which he had filled for the past several years. 'Nothing to it, old boy! Nothing ever happens. Haven't filed a report of consequence for years. And you get a yearly invitation to the Queen's birthday bash at the Residence, plus an embossed Christmas card every December signed by His Excellency the High Commissioner himself!' His Excellency! Well, that clinched it. It was a no-brainer.

One month after I had been inducted into the lowly ranks of the unpaid untermenschen attached to the High Commission, there was, on 1st August 1982, an attempted coup. Sections of the Kenya Air Force had attempted to overthrow the government by force. Within hours I was overwhelmed by scores of Britons of every hue, mostly unknown to me, bellowing on the blower, begging for timely and immediate assistance. The helpful advice from the High Commission was to stay inside, keep your heads down and to stock up on essential foodstuffs, a difficult task when most shops were barricaded shut or being looted by vandals.

On the radio, Strauss waltzes were being played *ad nauseam*. The *Blue Danube* is captivating when heard for the first or even for the second or third time but after that it definitely begins to pall. In the event the uprising was quickly and brutally crushed by the Army and the General Service Unit, the crack paramilitary police, and things returned to chaotic normality.

Another month later I received a call from the High Commission saying that a British citizen had been admitted in a critical condition to Nakuru's Provincial General Hospital and would I please attend.

The Provincial General Hospital was the sort of place most people avoided if they possibly could. Only the very poor went there and of those who did, many did not return. Drugs were few, facilities were basic, limited bed space often resulted in two patients per bed, the wards and corridors were dark and sepulchral and if there were curtains on the windows they were filthy and tied in permanent knots. The doctors on duty were often there, not of their own volition, but because of a compulsory posting following their graduation. As a result many did their work with reluctance and resentment. They couldn't wait to leave and make their fortunes in private practice.

So it was with a degree of foreboding that I parked my Peugeot in the decrepit car park and walked into the foyer. Behind a grubby desk sat a clerk, hidden behind, and obviously engrossed in, the *Tropical Inquirer* ('We Tell It How It Is'). I scanned the day's headlines – 'Man dies in dog rescue drama,' 'Farmer cuts off organ,' 'Lethal brew kills 100.' From the intensity with which the clerk was studying the inner pages I could tell that the centrefold held even more titillating excitement. I coughed. With exquisite deliberation the clerk slowly lowered his paper.

The clerk was small and ferrety, wearing an oversized shirt and a hideous yellow tie. 'Ndiyo?' (Yes?) he asked. 'Natafuta mzungu,' (I'm looking for a European) I said.

'Iko ndani,' (He's inside) he said, jerking his head backwards, indicating the corridor behind him.

'Thanks.' He returned to his paper.

Despite the fact that it was mid-morning, the corridor was so dark and gloomy I could not see its end. The walls, formerly white, were now khaki, overlain with a greasy sheen. In various small rooms off the corridor furtive individuals lounged on chairs, drinking cups of tea, chatting to each other or studying their newspapers. None took any notice of my passage. A porter appeared out of the shadows, trundling a metal trolley with an ominous sheeted shape hunched upon it. The wheels rattled and squealed as he shoved his load towards me and the exit. The wheels of his cart were not in alignment, so he had to push sideways in order to get the thing to go forwards.

As he approached, the trolley made a sudden swerve in my direction. With a frisson of alarm I skipped nimbly to one side. The grisly gurney rumbled past, enveloping me in a cloud of formaldehyde fumes. The porter gave me a horrid leer. 'Rafiki yako iko ndani,' (Your friend's in there) indicating whence he had come. A grey hand hung limply below the sheet. It swung to and fro.

At the end of the corridor I came upon a small desk with a white-coated doctor seated behind it. I waited until he had dealt with a couple of supplicants and put my case to him.

'Ah yes: Mr Adam Harker. He was brought in a couple of days ago. He was on his way to Kaimosi when his car was hit by a lorry near Eldama Ravine. RTA – road traffic accident. The police took him to the local mission hospital there and when they were unable to cope there he was sent here. Came in the back of an open pickup!'

Ye Gods, I thought – Eldama Ravine was over 40 miles from Nakuru.

'He arrived unconscious and in a bad way. At first we didn't know who he was. Then we got a call from his school in Kaimosi. He was on his way there and didn't turn up so they had been calling around. I'll get a nurse to take you to him.'

I followed the small, black nurse into the ward. At the entrance I stopped. I was looking at a scene which might have been transposed from the Crimea. Here were no orderly rows of beds, with patients lying quietly within snowy bed sheets, crisply uniformed nurses moving with obvious efficiency from one to another, bearing trays of pills and potions, stethoscopes slung round well scrubbed necks. Instead there was chaos. Beds seemed to be strewn everywhere, in all directions. Families seemed to be camped between the beds, brewing tea, cooking pots of maize, feeding patients. The noise and smell were overwhelming.

'How on earth,' I thought, 'is anyone going to get better in here?'

Above the hubbub I could hear a ghastly, rasping, choking sound as though someone was on the verge of asphyxia.

The nurse led me to a bed with side rails, rather like an oversized baby's cot and as soon as I saw those rails I knew that things were bad. The sound was coming from here. I approached with trepidation. I could cope with any number of sick animals, but this was different. I looked over the side of the cot and immediately I knew that Adam Harker was dying. It was horribly obvious. He was unconscious, gasping, wheezing, his arms and legs moving feebly, his eyes rolled up into his head, almost out of sight. Whether anything could have been done to have saved him was now immaterial. It was too late. A man in an adjacent bed saw me looking at Adam Harker and shook his head in sympathy.

But I couldn't just leave him like that.

I walked back through the mayhem to the white-coated doctor.

'He's dying,' I said.

'No, no, I don't think so. He's got concussion and shock, no more, possibly some internal haemorrhage.'

'Well, I'm going to phone the Flying Doctors to try to get him to Nairobi.'

He shrugged his white-coated shoulders.

I tore back to the surgery and got onto the phone and spoke to an extremely efficient African nurse in Nairobi who said she would arrange for a plane to be dispatched within the hour to the airstrip at Lanet.

As I put the phone down it almost immediately rang. Adam Harker had died. A later post-mortem revealed that he had died of a ruptured liver.

Now I had to deal with the consequences. I phoned the British High Commission. During the course of the day they managed to contact the deceased's widowed mother. He had been unmarried which meant that there was no one to help with the inevitable formalities.

His mother wanted him to be cremated and she wanted the ashes, encased in a tasteful urn, to be sent to her at Mullion-on-the-Moor, Derbyshire, she wanted a Church of England service to be arranged, in Kenya, to commemorate his passing, she most positively wanted his signet ring, a precious family heirloom, encircling the third finger of his right hand to be retrieved and kept in safe custody and dispatched to her at the earliest opportunity and finally, she wanted Her Majesty's Representative dealing with these matters to write to her frequently, keeping her fully abreast of all matters relevant to the terminal affairs of her late son.

First I had to get that ring. I drove back to the hospital. I strode into the ward. The cot was empty. Adam Harker was gone. As was the doctor. 'Ye blimmin gods!' I thought.

I collared a passing orderly. 'What's happened to the European man who was here?' I asked.

'They took him to the mortuary,' he replied, giving me directions. He did not offer to accompany me.

The mortuary was sited apart from the main hospital buildings. A squat, stone structure with a heavy door, it exuded an air of lurking menace. Not previously having had any good reason to visit a mortuary I did not look forward to this new experience with much enthusiasm.

As I approached the door, it opened and a low-browed, thickset, unshaven individual shambled out. He squinted at me and gave me a cunning grin. He pointed a thick finger at me. 'Ah, Mr White Man, I know why you are here. Your friend is in here. But I will make him look nice and respectable. At de moment he is not respectable. No, no. You just give me two tousand shilling and I will do good job. Make him look like new!' He tittered. His eyes were yellow and he staggered slightly. A rancid beery gust reached me. 'Come,' he beckoned, turning, and opening the door. There was that choking formalin smell again. A sheeted body lay on a zinc covered table. Another, that of an African, lay unsheeted on the stone floor. A skeletal leg protruded round a corner. I breathed deeply.

The man lifted the sheet. Adam Harker lay there. He did not look at peace. My eyes went to his hands. His fingers were ring-less. The man saw me looking and smirked, through broken, blackened teeth. 'Looking for samthing, Mr White Man?'

Before I could answer, I heard the sound of rapid steps behind me. I turned. It was the doctor. He glared at the man. 'Go!' he hissed. 'Go!' He went. 'You shouldn't be here,' he said to me.

'I came for Mr Harker's ring. His mother especially wants it sent to her.'

'I have all of his effects in my office. Things tend to disappear in a place like this.'

During the next few days I came to learn a bit more about Adam Harker, through students and teachers who now began to call from Kaimosi. He was greatly respected by all who knew him. He had sponsored more than one young African student through college. Being single, living in an area of the country where fleshpots and other Europeans were sparse, he had directed all of his celibate energies into the school.

Berna and I drove to the scene of the accident, went to the police station at Eldama Ravine and drove back again.

At the church service, which Berna and I had arranged in conjunction with our friend, the Rev. Geoffrey Ochana, the pews were full of Adam Harker's former students and teaching colleagues, who had travelled hundreds of miles to attend. Geoffrey rose to speak and did not mince his words. 'Who?' he thundered at the quivering congregation, 'Who among *you*, is going to replace Adam as financial supporter of so many young and promising Africans?' The congregation hung its collective head. Answer came there none.

Adam Harker was dead but we were not yet done with him. His mother wanted him to be cremated and his ashes sent to her in distant Derbyshire. The machinations of sending the body to an up-market crematorium in Nairobi didn't bear thinking about. He would have to be cremated in Nakuru.

Nakuru had no crematorium, but it did have a large Hindu community, who, I knew, regularly cremated their own dead on funeral pyres, down near the shores of Lake Nakuru, just as was done every day on the banks of the Ganges. When I thought about Hindus cremating their dead it brought to mind technicoloured visions of the burning ghats in places like Varanasi, with Mother Ganga sliding past on her way to the sea. Against a background of exotic temples, ash-smeared sadhus and crowds of colourful devotees, the bodies of the departed were consumed on great pyres of sandalwood. Skulls popped like exploding mortars in the heat of the flames, smoke rose in billowing clouds and, to the accompaniment of priestly chanting, the charred remains were cast into the holy waters.

Of course, a few moments thought would have made me realise that the vast majority of Hindus could not possibly all be living beside the Ganges, even though most might want to be cremated there. Most had to do with what they had got. Spare a thought for the Hindus in Huddersfield and Halifax.

Many of Nakuru's Hindus were my clients. I phoned one of the most prominent, Bipin Shah. I put the problem to him. Bipin did not hesitate, he was like that. 'Sure, no problem. Leave everything to me.

Just get the body down to our place near the lake and I'll do the rest. As soon as you've got the death certificate let me know and I'll get things ready. And don't bother with a coffin. It's not necessary. Just put the body in the back of a pickup.' Just as well Adam Harker's Mummy can't hear this conversation, I thought. 'Great,' I replied. 'I'll be in touch as soon as I've got that piece of paper.'

Getting the death certificate was far from easy. First I had to get the post-mortem report, which took an age, and then take that to a government office to get the vital certificate, followed by another giving permission to bury, or in this case permission to cremate. Lots of people seemed to have died recently, judging by the queues waiting for death certificates in the grubby office where a harassed woman was besieged by hordes of impatient, bereaved relatives, all talking at once.

Finally, three days after Adam Harker had died, I hired a pickup and drove to the mortuary to collect the deceased. Berna was at school, teaching, so she missed this part. I had thought about using my 504 saloon, but decided that having a shrouded corpse propped up in the back seat was not quite the done thing. A few of the students and teachers from Kaimosi were still in Nakuru. They came along to lend a hand loading the body into the back of the pickup.

The sinister mortician sidled up as I stopped the vehicle. Reeking of beer and formalin he giggled, 'Now, Mr White Man, you have to pay me to have da body of yo broder released. But I will give you a proper receipt, do'n you worry!' I was in no mood to argue. I was desperate to get away from the ghastly place. I gave him what I knew was probably double the going rate on the assumption that Mummy would pay me back. He looked at it, started to speak, saw the look in my eye and changed his mind. He scribbled an unofficial receipt and shoved the money into his pocket.

Adam was lying on a slab, wrapped in white sheeting. We shuffled into the room, trying not to breathe, no one wanting to make the first move. 'Right,' I said, 'let's get this over with.' Four of us lifted him off the slab and staggered out into the sunlight. He was lumpy and weighed a ton. I tripped on the sill of the door and almost dropped my 25 per cent.

Sweating and panting, we loaded Adam into the back of the pickup and set off. Half the Kaimosi contingent was in the back with him. A pedestrian walking along the road heard us coming and turned and thumbed a lift. I almost stopped but thought better of it.

After about 20 minutes we emerged from Nakuru's foetid underbelly and saw, in the distance, on a grassy plain, two walled enclosures. A dirt track snaked along the edge of the forest which bordered the lake. I drove along it, the mourners and Adam bumping up and down in the back. A marabou stork launched itself off a thorn tree as we rattled past.

The track ended between the enclosures. I stopped. Bipin appeared at the entrance to one. 'Welcome!' he said. 'Have you got the death certificate and the burial permit? Good! This is the Hindu crematorium. That one is for the Sikhs. Come!' I followed him. Inside the walls, in the centre, on a lower level, was the pyre, with other huge logs, and some sawdust, to one side. A small fire was burning in a corner. Above the pyre was an open-sided corrugated iron roof. Two African attendants were hard at work sweeping and tidying.

Under the direction of Bipin we unloaded Adam and carried him into the enclosure and laid him on top of the logs of the pyre. He felt even heavier and lumpier. I stumbled as we stepped down into the central reservation. We retired to our places around the walls, wondering what was going to happen next.

The two Africans now carried the massive logs across to the pyre and arranged them around and on top of the body. There was a sharp intake of breath from one or two of my companions. By the time Bipin's men had finished all that could be seen of Adam was one big toe. That toe was significant.

Bipin busied himself throwing sawdust into the openings between the logs and pouring ghee from large tins onto the wood. He beckoned to me. 'If anyone wants to say a few words or prayers let him step forwards.' I turned questioningly to the small knot of students and teachers. Their spokesman, a serious-looking, bespectacled, individual, gave a short eulogy and then a student said a prayer. Bipin spoke to me again. 'Now, I would like you to walk three times round the pyre and then light it where the toe is sticking out. There's plenty of ghee so it should catch right away.'

'Right,' I replied. Feeling a total fraud I marched solemnly round the logs. Bipin gave me a burning faggot from the small fire and I lit the equivalent of the blue touch paper. I noticed that Mr Harker's toenail was in serious need of trimming. Well, poor chap, I thought, you won't need to worry about that once we're finished with you. Immediately the wood caught fire, went up like a Roman candle and in no time the flames were feet high, the logs were crackling like pistol shots and the heat intense enough to sear off my eyebrows. Nor wanting that to happen, I, and everyone else, moved back against the wall. Ye gods, I thought, is this when the skull explodes? Bipin seemed unconcerned by any imminent detonation and moved leisurely around the conflagration, tossing sweet-smelling herbs and condiments onto the flames.

'Makes everything smell nice and fragrant,' he shouted above the noise of the burning wood. The fire was so fierce that there was hardly any smoke. I noticed that Adam's toe had disappeared. I was not surprised. 'Look,' said Bipin. 'The fire will burn for several hours. My guys will keep an eye on it, so unless you want to stay, that's it.' I explained about the mother wanting the ashes. 'No problem. Just come down in the morning and collect what you want. One of the chaps will be here to give you a hand.'

I thanked Bipin for his help. We turned to go. I felt almost disappointed that there had been no cranial explosion. Perhaps that would come later.

Early the following morning I was back. The weather was cold and grey. The place seemed deserted. I wandered into the scene of yesterday's bonfire. There, where the pyre had been, was a large pile of ash. It was as if Adam Harker and the great pyre had never been.

I felt the ash. It was warm, but not hot. The fire had been so intense that everything had burnt right down to the ground and the night had been a pretty cold one. I heard an approaching sandal-shuffle. It was one of the attendants. He was wrapped up to his nose in a toga-like blanket. He looked like an over-done Roman, a burnt umber senator who had spent rather a lot of time staked out at the lido.

'Habari ya asubhui?' I asked (How are you this morning? – literally, what news of the morning?)

'Mzuri tu.' he replied (Just fine.)

'Mimi nataka majivu ya mzungu sisi lichoma jana.' (I want the ashes of the European we incinerated yesterday.) God, it sounded so damned heartless and impersonal, a bit like asking for an early morning, freshly baked bun, none of your stale old rubbish, thank you very much.

He didn't turn a hair. I might have been asking for a cup of tea. 'Talete kijiko.' (I'll bring a spoon.) A spoon? A few minutes later he returned with a trowel. Just the job for early morning ash-sifting.

The sun was now up and the toga had been discarded, revealing a rather natty pair of cut-offs, more torn-offs in fact, and a military style bombardier jacket with smart name tabs on the chest – US NAVY inscribed on the one bosom and GOMEZ on the other.

I thanked 'Gomez' for the trowel and bent to my task. It was at once obvious that there were two types of ash here – wood ash – and the rest – i.e. Adam Harker. The former was light in colour and in weight. The latter was the opposite, dark grey and pretty heavy. What I really needed was a pair of bellows to blow the lighter stuff away. Winnowing the stuff, by tossing it into the air and thereby separating the wheat from the chaff so to speak, seemed a bit irreverent. So it was a matter of sorting the sheep from the goats with the trowel.

I had hoped to find the relevant ash to be as fine as talcum powder or pumice, but in this I was quickly disabused. Quite a lot of it was lumpy and irregular, hard and angular. Help, I thought, I can't send it like this to Adam's old lady. She might want to toss the stuff onto the lake where Adam had fished as a lad. It would make the most almighty splash. I then thought about sending a pot of the wood ash, but she might have prior experience of this sort of thing and get suspicious.

There was only one thing for it. I turned to my companion in crime.

'Gomez, my friend, can you bring me one of those empty ghee tins? A dry clean one, if you please.' 'Gomez' was a sharp lad and quickly realised that I was referring to him. He nipped off and came back with the requested receptacle. I trowelled it full of Adam's ash and carried it carefully to the car. Thanking 'Gomez', I handed him a well-deserved pourboire for his pains, and drove off.

I arrived at the surgery just as right-hand man Moses was opening up. He looked at me suspiciously as I surreptitiously carried the ghee tin inside. I had to get this job done before secretary Renata Grioni arrived. Her Catholic sensitivities might not appreciate the presence of human remains on the premises, even if they were dry, sterile and odourless.

'Right, Moses, can you please bring me the big pestle and mortar. I've got a bit of grinding up to do. Don't ask me what for, but it's not horse cough electuary!'

Moses heaved the heavy earthenware bowl onto the table and gave me the pestle and I got going, pounding poor old Adam to dust. It was hard work. He had strong bones. As I was bashing away the phone rang. The door opened and Renata entered. Damn! She looked hard at me and at the bowl. 'Mike Sugden's on the line. Sounds urgent. He wants to speak to you.' She stared again at the bowl.

Mike was a well-built Yorkshireman with a farm not far from Nakuru. On it he grew maize, reared Ayrshire cattle and had a string of racehorses. He also had a string of African wives, not all at once, but in succession. He seemed to favour Nandis, and as a result spoke the language with much fluency and vigour. This vigour extended to the fields of procreation and, despite his bulk and advancing years, Mike seemed to possess an acrobatic virility denied to many a younger man. Seven children owned him as their father.

Which mother was mother to which children and how many of them there were was an ongoing mystery. In addition to his procreant powers, Mike was endowed with a voice which enabled him to give orders to his syces and garden boys without even getting out of bed. He would lie there in his Lamu four-poster, a fez-like nightcap perched on his head, lolling back on the pillows like a dissolute Turkish pasha, and issue orders and instructions to quivering minions lined up at the door twenty yards away.

On one occasion his foghorn-like bellow was more than useful. It was literally life saving. Mike had incurred the ire of one of his wives, a sprightly young thing, who, on observing him enter the lavatory for the usual personal reasons, quietly locked the door, before setting the house on fire. Sitting there on the throne, pondering on the state of the universe and his bank balance, Mike suddenly smelt the smell of smoke and heard the crackle of flames. Trousers at low tide, Mike leapt to his feet and roared for help through a small open window. A distant syce heard the summoning call, came running, doused the flames and freed his perspiring employer.

Mike's lady wife in the meantime, had done a runner and was seen no more.

Now Mike was on the blower. Pedestrians passing in the street outside could hear every word. They slowed their steps and cocked their ears. 'That you, Hugh? What are you up to, eh? Doing anything important?' I hesitated before answering. 'Well, whatever it is, drop it and get here fast. A foal has just torn its jugular vein in half and time is of the essence!' All delivered in a broad Yorkshire accent.

Torn its jugular vein in half? Then why isn't it dead? 'Right,' I said, 'I'm on my way.' It was a blessed relief to stop what I was doing and get back to some semblance of normality. I covered the mortar and its morbid contents with a clean cloth, called for Moses and set forth with all possible speed.

Mike's place was only six miles from Nakuru and in no time at all I roared into the stable yard and screeched to a stop.

In the middle of the grassy area in front of the stables stood, in profile, a large chestnut foal of about 9 months. One syce, facing me, was holding the foal by its head collar. Another stood, with his back to me, his arms spread like a conductor about to bring an orchestra to its feet for the final bow. From where I had stopped the car I was unable to see the foal's neck and its all important jugular. I walked across for a closer look.

'Holy mackerel!' I expostulated. 'How on earth did that happen?' There was a huge open wound about a foot long in the middle of the foal's neck. With his fingers the syce was holding closed the open ends of the foal's right jugular vein. 'I'll tell 'e 'ow it 'appened!' a voice boomed behind me. It was Mike. 'Blooody syce tried to bring too many 'osses at same time through blooody gate, didn't he? So there's a roosh and some booger 'as left a blooody great bolt stickin' out on fence post and so foal twangs its neck on bolt with the result ye see before ye.'

'How it didn't exsanguinate itself is a miracle. There's about a foot of jugular missing. That syce showed presence of mind, eh, grabbing the ends like that,' I said.

'Blooody syce knew full well 'e'd be exsanguinated if he didn't grab 'em!' said Mike.

Quite so. 'Right,' I said to the hovering Moses, 'bring the surgical bag and plenty of catgut and nylon and let's get this mess stitched up.'

As there was no way to bring the two ends of the jugular into apposition without having the foal's neck bent at a right angle and looking back over its shoulder, I tied off both ends with strong catgut. I knew that in time an alternative blood supply would take over. Repairing the open wound was more difficult. At first it looked well-nigh impossible. I gave the foal a sedative into its remaining jugular, infiltrated local anaesthetic and got going. About an hour later the wound was closed. It was hardly top-notch plastic surgery but it would do.

'OK Mike,' I said, 'that's it. I'll pop in tomorrow to check how it is. Should be OK. But you can never tell. It might go blind in the right eye, or get oedema of the brain from damming back of the blood, or have a stroke, so digits crossed! I'd better get back to what I was doing.'

'Oh aye, an' wot were that?'

'Just a bit of pestling and mortaring.'

'Right then. Off ye go.'

Back at the surgery I retuned to my grisly task. By the time I was finished I was quietly pleased with the result. Adam was now a light, smooth, scatterable, powder, of which his mother should be proud. Berna had had a local fundi make a small, polished, wooden casket and into this receptacle I reverently tipped Adam, parcelled him up, and, together with his ring and other personal effects, dispatched the lot by safe carrier to the High Commission in Nairobi. I enclosed a covering letter of commiseration to his mother, giving only brief but essential details. Alas, all my efforts were in vain. I received neither acknowledgment nor thanks.

In days to come I attended many a cremation and collected many a pot of ash down at the burning ghats, but in only the first did I have to indulge in personal ash grinding.

Next day I returned to check on Mike's foal. It was pottering about, suckling from its mother and nibbling hay. Ten days later I removed the stitches and a month later you could hardly see a scar.

Chapter Eighteen

CHALLY

St. Mungo's Prep. School, sited on its chilly broad acres at Turi, had, in addition to its piebald mix of pupils, a mixed bag of ponies and indifferent horses. These were there to provide those children who wished to have, and sometimes those who did not wish to have, extracurricular activity, in the form of riding lessons. I was frequently asked to attend to these equine inmates. Sometimes this was to vaccinate them against African Horse Sickness and Rabies, sometimes to rasp teeth, stitch wounds, treat colics, geld colts or to give the coup de grace to those past their prime. This latter task I usually performed out of term so as not to upset the little riders. Those who rode against their will would probably not have been too upset to have seen their mounts go to the happy grazing grounds. In those days the riders were indeed little. Nowadays they might be best described as bulky.

In charge of this motley collection of quadrupeds and their young jockeys was riding-mistress Jean Chalcraft. More commonly known as Chally, she was a small grey-haired widow of indeterminate age. Accompanied by her faithful companion, a large male rottweiler called Lobo, Chally would stand bellowing instructions to her pupils. 'Use your seat, Pricilla!' 'Squeeze with your thighs, Amanda!' 'Heels down and toes up, Joshua!' 'Push with your bottom, Phoebe!'

There seemed to be a lot of emphasis on the undoubted value of posterior power.

Chally was fond of cigarettes and beer. Usage of both was strictly forbidden during lessons. Chally took an elastic view of this, to her mind, unreasonable edict. Whenever possible she would light up a Sportsman, and puff away as she put her charges through their paces. On one occasion the head appeared without warning, mid-lesson. Chally swiftly stood in the accepted, military, at-ease position, hands crossed behind her back, and smiled disarmingly as she replied to various searching questions concerning the progress of the lesson. The head also smiled but said nothing about the tell-tale grey plume rising like a Comanche smoke signal above Chally's shoulders.

Chally's wardrobe was limited. Her gabardine, bell tent skirt was only worn on very special social occasions and when on the job she invariably wore khaki shorts of the empire-building variety and on her feet well-worn flip flops. With her short hair and ever-present fag drooping from her lower lip, or hanging limply from nicotine-stained fingers, children were to be excused if they had an initial spasm of gender confusion. 'Mummy,' one worried child was heard to say at the parents' visiting weekend, 'Mummy, is Miss Chalcraft a mummy or a daddy?'

Chally's command of Swahili was fluent, if ungrammatical. Eleejah, a turbaned syce, later consigned to the cleansing of the school lavatories after having been found drunk on duty, was a frequent recipient of Chally's ire. 'Eleejah!' she would trumpet, 'Kwisha sema! Shika bloody farasi!' (Eleejah! I have told you! Hold the ... horse!) Such linguistic mangling had the syces in stitches and they would imitate Chally behind her back or when she had nipped home for a lunchtime beer. The pupils rolled on the ground, convulsed with glee at the uncanny resemblance as the syces strutted up and down, mimicking Chally's every physical foible.

The syces knew how to irritate Chally. On one occasion a syce called John pretended not to hear Chally as she bellowed at him to bring one of the horses to the stable for grooming. He stood, about a hundred yards away, gazing blankly and innocently into the middle distance, apparently communing with nature and deaf and blind to the verbal outrage being directed at him. Finally Chally could take no more of this dumb insolence. Grabbing a riding crop she leapt aboard a convenient horse and galloped up to John, who turned with an expression of mild surprise at the sudden appearance of this mounted virago, who proceeded to apply the whip with more fury than force upon his blameless shoulders. John smiled benignly and ambled gently towards the stables. The watching pupils almost burst into a cheer. One up for John!

In the tack room Chally would hold forth to her frequently bored captive audience. She would show them a variety of bits – snaffles and martingales – she would demonstrate how to polish a saddle, explain the difference between a stifle and a splint, between a crupper and a croup and wax lyrical on the beauty of the rising trot. In the tack room Chally was able to puff away to her heart's content, secure in the knowledge that she would be undisturbed by undesirables such as passing heads.

One hot dry afternoon, Chally, having sucked her last Sportsman dry, tossed the still smoking butt out of the window and lit another. The room was stifling and the jodhpur-clad juniors nearly asleep as Chally droned interminably on about girths and gaskins, withers and windgalls. Suddenly one junior, a little blonde girl with a pudding bowl fringe, piped up, 'Miss, what's that smell, miss?'

'What smell? I can't smell anything. Now shut up, Prunella, and listen to what I'm saying.'

'Yes, miss.'

A few minutes passed. 'Miss, I can smell it again, miss, and what's that smoke outside the window, miss?'

'Heaven's sake, child!' Chally grunted and turned towards the window. 'Good Lord,' she exclaimed as flames now leapt across the window. 'Outside everyone! Outside!' Like stampeding wildebeest the embryo riders burst their way through the door, followed by a wheezing Chally, a pursuing lioness long past her prime. A large bush into which Chally's smoking butt had fallen was burning busily, flames threatening to put an effective end to further tack room lectures. Several singed horse-blankets later and the fire was out, with Chally threatening the pupils with unmentionable punishments should the word get out as to the origin of the fire. 'Spontaneous combustion, that's what it was. Happens all the time at this time of year. Now, repeat after me....' Which they did. They were very fond of Chally, as she was of them.

Wednesday afternoon was Berna's half-day and as I had a call to St. Mungo's to check on a lame horse, she came along for the ride. By the time I had examined the animal and half a dozen others which had been wheeled out for inspection – 'as you're here,' – it was almost dark. 'Come in for a spot of dinner and a noggin,' said Chally.

'Thanks very much,' we chorused in unison. 'Love to!'

Chally's house was on the school compound and was not so much a house as a collection of shacks, which in any civilised country would have been condemned and torn down as unfit for human habitation. In one was a sitting-room and a bedroom, in another a bathroom and store-room and in the third a primitive kitchen. We followed Chally into shack Number One. No sooner had we entered than there was a power cut and all the lights in the school went out. There was a back-up generator, but this only supplied the main school buildings and dormitories. We remained standing in Stygian darkness, unable to see a hand in front of our faces. Had we known anything of our immediate surroundings we might have preferred to have remained in the dark. 'Not a problem,' grunted Chally. 'Soon get the old Tilley lamp working.' Chally was the school expert on generators and Tilley lamps.

Whenever there was a power failure and light was urgently needed the call would go up, 'Call for Chally!' Within a couple of minutes the yellow glow of the lit lamp cast a flickering chiaroscuro over what appeared to be the authentic set of *Steptoe and Son*. A car battery stood on a table next to a couple of fan belts, together with a bit and bridle, a pile of dog-eared riding magazines, a non-working clock, a two-way radio which looked as though it might have been hand crafted by Marconi himself and a box-like phone with a quaint handle to one side, which, when cranked, supposedly aroused to activity a distant slumbering operator. In a gloomy corner stood a car wheel, propped against a large hessian sack of dog biscuits. Other unidentified items were lost to view in the shadows.

Lobo followed us in and with a canine sigh flopped down on a moth-eaten carpet. 'Sit ye down,' commanded Chally. We flopped down on a sagging horsehair sofa, which under our combined modest weight now almost touched the floorboards. 'What'll ye have?' asked Chally. 'I've beer, gin, whisky and brandy.' I asked for a whisky. Berna had a gin and tonic.' 'I've already had a couple of beers so I think I'll have a brandy,' said Chally. She gave a throaty laugh. She brought our drinks and sloshed a generous measure of brandy into her own tumbler.

'Now, I'll just light the fire and then I'll go and get supper. It's school food. I hope you don't mind. I'm allowed extra portions for guests. No idea what it'll be but it's usually OK. By the way, do you mind if Snowy eats with us? He's my cat and likes company when he's at the trough.'

'Good Lord, no,' we chorused. 'Be delighted.'

Having lit the fire, Chally rooted around in a hidden corner and emerged holding a tin tiffin carrier, with which she vanished into the night.

Five minutes after she had departed in search of dinner, the lights came back on. We surveyed our surroundings with interest. The two-way radio emitted periodic plaintive whines and squeaks. The mantelpiece was littered with ornamental beer mugs, rosettes won at horse shows, ancient Christmas cards, old wedding invitations and piles of dusty receipts and bills. Nestling among the general debris was Chally's brandy.

In one corner of the room it looked as though an internal combustion engine was being assembled.

By the time Chally had returned we had almost finished our drinks.

'You're in luck!' she said. 'It's stew and dumplings with mashed bananas for dessert. Yummy! It could just as easily have been mealies and sago pudding! And we've got light!' I did not mention that I hated bananas in any shape or form.

'I'll just check the radio to see what's going on out there. I'm a bit of a radio ham!' She shoved ear phones over her head and twiddled a few knobs and fiddled with some dials.

'Jimmy, Jimmy do you read? Jimmy, Jimmy do you read?'

Jimmy apparently did not read. She hung up.

'Right, now let me call Snowy.'

She gave a high-pitched yelp through the open door and Snowy, a large unprepossessing moggy with a square head, came at a run. He looked around with a questioning air as if to say – 'Well, where is it then?' *It* wasn't long in coming. Chally reached behind her chair, grabbed *it* and whacked a large mole rat onto the carpet. Lobo shifted position as though he knew what was coming, but Snowy went for the mole rat as though he had not been fed for days. With a low pitched growl to warn off interlopers he worried the carcass and in a trice had the innards, guts and all, spread out juicily on the carpet.

'Yes,' we said. 'We *will* have a top-up now, if you don't mind. Thanks very much.' We picked at our dumplings and sipped our drinks as Snowy wolfed his dinner. He certainly had a healthy appetite. As he was about to swallow the mole rat's head the lights went off again.

'Damn!' said Chally. 'Back to the Tilley.'

Once again we sat in semi-darkness, listening to the crunch and slobber as Snowy finished his evening repast. Concealed by the lack of light I slid the unwanted bananas to one side. What with the fire and the feline munchings it had become quite warm in Chally's shack.

I glanced up at the mantelpiece where Chally's brandy stood waiting to be imbibed. The surface of the drink appeared to be curiously and violently agitated, as though by some hidden inner force. Then I realised that a large moth had found its way into the glass and was now frantically trying to escape.

'Er Chally…' but before I could complete my sentence Chally had reached up, seized the tumbler and tossed the lot back in one impressive swallow.

'Gosh,' she gasped. 'That brandy's got a lot of body!'

No wonder, we thought, holding back our laughter, as we stumbled out to the car, having thanked Chally profusely for an unforgettable evening.

Chapter Nineteen

THE QUEEN OF THE JUNGLE

'Appalling', 'painfully inept', 'irresistibly silly'. Such were the reviews which greeted the arrival on the silver screen of 'Sheena, Queen of the Jungle', a colourful biopic wholly shot in Kenya. It told the wildly improbable tale of a white girl, a 'golden girl-child', who becomes the head of an African tribe, following the tragic death of her parents in a natural disaster, an unexplained volcanic rock fall. 'When paradise became a battleground she led the fight for survival.' So ran the hyperbolic credits. It sounds totally cringe-worthy but in the eyes of simple culture-starved post colonials, such as ourselves, it was the stuff of legend. It was so bad that it was good. And we had a minor role in its making.

The star of this epic was Tanya Roberts, a stunner if there ever was one, and one not afraid to doff her kit when the need arose, which seemed to happen quite frequently as the story progressed. Apart from her in-your-face physical attributes, Tanya/Sheena's other unique asset was her ability to summon the creatures of the wild to her aid by the mere power of her mind, a totally unbelievable affinity with Nature used to exaggerated effect in the film. When not revealing all, Sheena's entire wardrobe seemed to consist of a tattered leather bikini, to emphasise her solidarity with the members of her adopted tribe, who were also sparsely clad in animal skins.

Playing a lesser part was Princess Elizabeth of Toro, former foreign minister of Uganda, cast in the role of a sinister soothsayer. How are the mighty fallen, we thought.

Shooting took place in Nakuru town, on the shores of Lakes Nakuru and Naivasha, Amboseli, on the Aberdares and at Thomson's Falls.

The first I heard about the film was when I received a call, out of the blue, to attend to a lame horse on Crescent Island, Naivasha, where the various animals involved in the film were quartered. On a previous occasion I had been briefly involved in a film also being shot on the aforesaid island. That was 'The Flame Trees of Thika.' I had been asked to anaesthetise a Boran bull such that it appeared for cinematic purposes to be dead. It was all far too realistic for the owner of the bull, a geriatric buffer with a colossal upper-crust English accent and possessing the most un-English surname of Ratzenburg, who tut-tutted and clicked his tongue and sighed and gasped at my elbow throughout the proceedings, until he almost convinced me that the animal *was* dead.

With the faithful Moses at my side I crossed the rustic causeway which led onto Crescent Island. We pottered along the track which led to the far end of the island, passing small herds of impala, scattered waterbuck, a family of erect-tailed warthog and a giraffe, which drifted away with its smooth, rocking-horse gait. Then under distant trees we could see collections of large trucks, wired enclosures, a tethered elephant, zebras in pens and lions in cages. A sign advised us that all of these were 'Animal Actors of Hollywood'.

I stopped the car and stepped out.

A shaggy fellow with a pony tail and a baseball cap on back-to-front was passing and I hailed him. 'Hello, I'm looking for a lame horse. I'm the vet from Nakuru.'

'Hi there buddy, the name's Gus. Follow me. I look after some of these critters. I'm an animal trainer. We've got chimps, leopards, lions, hawks, even elephants. Trouble is, for this film we gotta have African elephants, with the big ears y'know, and unlike the Indian jumbos they're noivous. Tend to crap on stage! And when they crap, they crap! Wheelbarrow loads! Real pain in the ass! Right, here's the patient.' We had stopped at a pen containing a couple of zebra. 'But,' I said. 'I thought I had come to see a ....Wait a moment!' My companion grinned. I looked more closely. They looked like zebras. The stripes were exactly those of any wild zebra, right down to the fine markings on the head. But the mane and tail were not quite right. A zebra's tail is like that of a donkey, with a brush at the end, and the mane stands up, and doesn't lie flat. The tails of these animals were smooth and silky, as were the manes. 'Yup, they're Arabs, painted with hair lacquer to resemble wild zebras. They fool most people who've never seen a zebra before. They're the ones Sheena rides in the film – lucky brutes!' He gave a lascivious grin.

I examined my patient. The make-up artists had done an amazing job. Even close up the detail was incredible. I was impressed. I ran my hand down the lame leg and had the horse, a mare, trotted along the track, after having flexed the leg for a couple of minutes. I applied hoof testers to the hoof. The Arab flinched when I applied moderate pressure. With a hoof knife I removed a thin layer of horn from the sole. Streaks of blood appeared below the horn, indicative of bruising. 'Right, Gus, she's bruised her sole. Probably all the standing and travelling she's been through to get here. But with rest it'll be OK in a week or so.'

'That's all right then. We don't start the riding for another three weeks – on the shores of Lake Nakuru in fact. Let me show you what we've got here.' Gus went into the lions' cage and scratched their ears, he tickled the leopards' tummies, he wrestled with a big male chimp and at his command the elephants raised their trunks and trumpeted. 'We can take the wild animals back to the States,' he said, 'but the horses will have to stay here. Regulations about African Horse Sickness won't allow them back in. So good news for someone here who likes Arabs. Won't be painted like this though. Just be your regular Arabs, but very smart horses, trained by Animal Actors of Hollywood, and ridden bareback by Sheena, Queen of the Jungle! So they're special!' He gave that grin again.

Moses was dumbstruck by all of this. When he regained his tongue on the return journey it was to express amazement at yet another Western wonder, tempered with the respectful inference that most wazungu (westerners), myself included, were more than a little mad. He shook his head for most of the drive back to Nakuru.

A month later I was again summoned to the Sheena set. Another Animal Actor required my attention. On this occasion the patient was a rhino and the location was a clearing in the forest, 10,000 feet up on the Aberdare Mountains.

For some inexplicable reason the rhino had been housed in a pen next to another Animal Actor, a fully-grown lion. Not appreciating this particular arrangement, the rhino broke out of its enclosure and took off. Entering into the spirit of things the lion followed suit and leapt out of its pen and catapulted itself onto the rhino's back. Not unnaturally the rhino vigorously objected to this unwanted free rider and ran even faster. By rushing through dense thickets and through matted groves of thickly interwoven mountain timber, the rhino finally divested itself of its burden when it tore under a low branch, which, although low enough for the rhino was not quite high enough for the lion.

Both animals had been born and bred in captivity. Now they were in totally unknown and frightening territory: forest and moorland full of wild, unpredictable animals. They wanted out. The lion, bruised and battered from its encounter with the inconvenient branch, limped back to the pens, where, at the command of its keeper, it slunk inside, glad to be back home.

The rhino kept on running, until it emerged from the forest and onto the open moorlands. With its poor eyesight it had no idea where it was. It blundered and staggered among the tussocks, falling into mudholes and stumbling into icy streams, panting and gasping in the thin air.

The rhino ran for two breathless miles before coming to a trembling halt, heaving from its exertions. In hot pursuit came its anxious keepers, armed with dart guns, lorries, binoculars, two-way radios, trackers, ropes, nets, and all the other paraphernalia of the chase. Whether the lightly clad Sheena was included in the party was not recorded. This rhino was worth a fortune and was critical to a vital and heart-stopping sequence in the film. Its loss would have been irreparable.

Luckily the rhino conveniently stopped near a track. If it had gone down a valley or into the forest it might have been lost forever. As it was, it was able to be darted with a tranquilliser and slowly herded into a large crate on the back of a lorry and driven back to the scene of the escape.

But it was in obvious shock, which was where I came in.

A phone call brought me to the Nakuru Aero Club, where a Beaver aircraft was waiting to fly me to the patient. The Beaver was an impressive machine. With its massive radial engine, tail wheel and lurid yellow paint job, it looked like a giant hornet. This beast meant business. This was a real plane. Like a Land Rover with wings. Made in Canada and used for landing on dirt strips in the Far North, it could also be fitted with floats for landing on rivers and lakes, and with skis for landing on snow and on glaciers. I regarded it with due reverence.

I ran the pilot to earth in the club, propped against the bar, sipping a Coke – I sincerely hoped it *was* a Coke – chatting to the ever-present Abdul, a non-teetotal Muslim who seemed to be a permanent fixture of the place. It was 10am and Abdul was *not* sipping a Coke.

I introduced myself.

The American pilot had a hard bony face, stubbly gum-chewing jaws, flinty blue eyes and a crew cut. He was lean and wore a button down shirt and blue jeans and cowboy boots. Abdul was overweight, wore a suit and tie and looked soft and playful. He smiled and crooked his little finger at the barman who scurried to refresh his drink.

I shook hands. The pilot's dry grip was bone-crushingly painful. He stared into my eyes and grinned, wondering if I could take the pain. I grimaced back. Abdul's hand was limp and moist and flabby, like fondling a slab of lukewarm cod.

'Good t'meet ya,' said the pilot. 'The name's Wriggle, Jim Wriggle. San Antone, Texas.'

Wriggle? *Wriggle?* My image of the Lone Star State, the Alamo, rugged cowpokes, longhorns, endless horizons and endless big-finned Cadillacs slumped.

'Good t'meet ya,' I replied. 'Cran, Hugh, Scotland.' It didn't have the potency of San Antone, Texas, but at least it wasn't Wriggle.

'Right, shall we go?'

Abdul stroked his moustache and gave us a thumb's up.

I put my surgical bag and a selection of drugs behind my seat. We clambered into the cockpit. The firewall/instrument panel in front of us was so high I could barely see over it. This was the sort of plane you flew by looking out of the side window. We strapped in.

'Right, let's go!' said Jim, and cranked the engine. There was none of the endless fiddling around checking and re-checking innumerable dials, muttering into the mike, waggling the ailerons and flaps, stamping on the brakes and shoving the throttle in and out, which I and others religiously went through prior to take-off. This guy knew what he was about. He was a professional.

There was a deafening roar, the engine rocked in the slipstream and without hesitation Jim turned onto the runway. In what seemed like seconds the tail was up and we were airborne. As soon as the plane was off the ground Jim pulled the plane round in a sharp gut-wrenching turn and pointed it directly towards the eastern wall of the Rift Valley over which we had to ascend in order to reach the Aberdares. We roared over shacks and gum trees at suicidal height. Flocks of sheep and goats fled in wild panic, open-mouthed peasants stared upwards, poultry scattered, shedding contrails of plumage, cyclists wobbled and toppled into the dust. Jim grinned and tossed me a stick of gum.

The wall of the Rift Valley was close, only a few miles away. The crest was over 9,000 feet high, 3,000 feet higher than our present altitude. We seemed bent on a kamikaze mission, heading straight towards the side of the valley. I glanced at the altimeter. We were rising, but were we rising fast enough? Jim's jaws suggested that we were. They munched steadily and rhythmically, like those of a contented ruminant. Covertly I watched those jaws, knowing that any interruption to their tempo, any stoppage or acceleration, might indicate imminent crisis. There was none. Most pilots would have circled to gain height. Not this one. Ahead of us I could see a small gap in the fast-approaching tree-covered ridge. We hurtled towards it. Now we were lower than the trees on either side. I glanced down at the treetops flashing by just below us. In one I could actually see a ragged nest with open beaked fledglings gaping pinkly upwards. From another burst a pair of black and white hornbills. Then we were through and it was back to roaring at tree top height over farms and fields, rocketing over thatched huts and dirt tracks, skimming over woods and streams until we were above the watery expanse of Lake Olbolossat. The shallow lake was a magnet for wildfowl and landed gentry who came in droves to slaughter the former. Shotguns would boom out across the lake, retrievers would dash into the water to retrieve the downed birds, iced gin would be sipped, liver pâté sandwiches would be nibbled and a jolly good time would be had by all. Now, apart from a few apprehensive shore birds, the lake seemed deserted. Further out, though, outraged hippos plunged and snorted as we invaded their airspace. Cormorants dived for safety and ducks frantically took to the air.

The river that flowed northwards out of the lake fell, after a few miles, over Thomson's Falls, a dramatic plunge of hundreds of giddy feet into a narrow gorge. No less dramatic was the scene in the film, shot over those very falls. Sheena, manacled hand and foot by cruel chains, her non-garments rent and torn, lay struggling in the back of a small helicopter while an evil pilot flew her to a known fate. Sheena, however, by exerting her extraordinary powers, summoned up a flock of homicidal flamingoes, who darted with daring courage at the pilot and pecked out his eyes. Cockpit full of feathers and flapping birds, the helicopter went into a graveyard spin. Sheena seemed doomed to go down in flames, but, at the very last, edge-of-the-seat minute, in a series of erotic wrigglings, she slipped her bonds and free-fell several hundred feet to land unhurt on the cushioning tops of a grove of convenient trees, perched on the very edge of the falls.

The Aberdares were now looming up before us, dark and forbidding. Jim removed his gum and stuck it behind his right ear. This looked serious. I need not have worried. We rose as in an elevator up the mountainside and over the tangled tops of the forest. Higher now, we sped towards our goal, the base of a distant conical hill, which rose above the rest of the range. I peered down, wondering, not for the first time, where we might put down in the event of an emergency. The bleak answer, was – nowhere. One's only possibility would be to hope that the treetops had enough padding to absorb the plane's impact without killing the occupants. Fat chance. As we flew over a clearing in the forest two elephants raised questioning trunks as if in mocking salute. In another a group of buffalo stampeded for cover.

Craning over the instrument panel I could see the landing strip ahead. It looked ridiculously narrow, a mere thread snipped out of the jungle. Jim did not land in the same cavalier fashion as he had taken off. He flew carefully over the strip, looking and making sure that there were no unwanted intruders obstructing his touchdown. Impact with a buffalo or bongo would bring our errand of mercy to abrupt finality. All seemed well and we steamed in on full flaps and full power, nose up, as slowly as possible. After touchdown the comforting rumble of wheels on terra firma is always a pleasant sound, allowing one to satisfy oneself that one has, once again, survived the perils of the heights.

We trundled to the end of the strip where I could see a vehicle waiting. Jim came to a stop and closed the engine down. 'Thanks, Jim,' I said. 'That's the way to travel! Going by road would have taken all day!'

'Sure thing, doc. Pick you up when you've zapped that rhino!' He popped another stick of gum. His jaws began to move again.

A cheery African carried my bag to a mud bespattered Toyota pickup and I hopped into the left seat. 'Jambo!' he said, as we shook hands, 'I am Ezekial. I will take you to the rhino. We managed to get him into a crate on the back of a lorry, but he is pretty shocked, trembling and a bit cold. He ran and ran and that is never a good thing.'

'Yes, indeed,' I replied. 'Capture myopathy or post-exertional myopathy can be fatal. Excessive forced muscular activity can result in acute death from a sudden fall in the pH. Lactic acidosis from glycogen breakdown seems to affect just about every organ in the body. But as this rhino is used to people, the stress factor may be less than if it were wild. Let's hope so.'

'Yes, he was born in the States, so he's more used to people than animals.'

Chasing wild animals at high speeds over short distances of up to two kilometres, resulting in intensive and concerted use of nearly all muscles simultaneously, may cause a catastrophic drop in body pH. Stiffness, lameness, twisting of the neck, prostration, the passage of brown urine, coma and death may be seen. Many organs are damaged –heart, liver and muscles. The lungs are often congested and the windpipe may be full of froth. Longer less intensive pursuits are less dangerous and cause less damage. It appears that the condition is not due to exhaustion but to the excessive and sudden attendant muscle strain. Capture myopathy may occur immediately or up to four weeks after capture. Great care therefore always needs to be taken when chasing wild animals to avoid over-exertion, stress, fear, unnecessary disturbance, excessive handling and resultant shock.

I had read somewhere that the condition could be reversed in zebra by the intravenous infusion of sodium bicarbonate. Giving an intravenous infusion to a rhino was not something in my current repertoire, so I prayed that the animal was not as bad as my overwrought imagination made it out to be.

Ezekial was a careful driver, which was just as well as the track was pitted with huge holes brimful of muddy water and ruts whose hidden depths had the dependant parts of the Toyota in intimate contact with whatever lay therein. Hard contact with a rock was not to be entertained.

'The road is not usually like this,' said Ezekial, 'but it has rained heavily for the past three days. Any more rain and it will be impassable and then we'll be in big trouble with the animals up here. The Animal Actors are not so used to these primitive conditions!'

He laughed.

After twenty minutes of slithering and sliding we emerged into a grassy clearing. A lorry was parked next to some tents adjacent to a couple of wired enclosures.

'The rhino's in there,' said Ezekial, 'in the back of the lorry.'

'Right,' I said. 'Let's have a look at her.'

I climbed up the side of the lorry until I could peer over the edge. 'Ye gods!' I exclaimed. The beast was enormous, far bigger than I had expected. It seemed to fill the entire lorry. All I could see was a huge grey wrinkled back, like a lichened rock on the bleak wastes of Rannoch Moor. Far to my left front there were two twitching trumpet-like ears and away to my right things sloped down to where I assumed there was a tail. Examination was going to entail difficulties not normally encountered with domestic animals. The rhino's gut was obviously working as there was great steaming mound on the floor of the lorry. Taking the temperature was not easy. Just getting near the tail involved athletics I had not thought myself capable of. By climbing part way down the inside of the lorry I was able to grab the tail. The rhino did not appreciate this and showed its displeasure by voiding several more kilos of excrement and lashing its tail from side to side and jigging violently up and down. I grabbed the tail and it was like seizing an angry anaconda. Finally, with my arm besmeared with copious amounts of ordure I shoved the thermometer into the rectum and held on like grim death for the required minute. I did not know the normal temperature of a rhino, but the reading was neither excessively high or low. At 38 degrees Celsius I deemed it to be within normal limits.

I clambered along the inside of the lorry towards the front end to try to check heart and respiration. Now I could see the rhino's head and its square lip, indicating that it was a white rhino, the more placid variety. At least I hoped so, as by now the sedative had well and truly worn off. Holding on, gibbon-like, with one hand to the side of the lorry, I leant down, stethoscope dangling from my ears and listened to the sounds emanating from the massive chest. After straining my tympana for what seemed like ages I decided, without much foundation, that all was well in that department and gingerly moved a little lower to check the heart. By stretching my arm to its uttermost limit I managed to get the bell of the stethoscope to just behind the rhino's left elbow, hoping the creature would stay still long enough for me to hear something. Just as I heard the first lub-dup of its mighty ticker the rhino suddenly lurched sideways, pinning me painfully to the side of the truck. Just as suddenly it lurched the other way. With my own heart lub-dupping in fast forward I tried again. Another go like that and I would be pressed meat, an unpleasant brand of corned beef, smeared against the woodwork. This time I was in luck. All I needed was one minute. Aha! A steady 35 thumps per 60 seconds. Would that my own heart beat so strong and true! Mine felt like the fluttering of a petrified caged sparrow.

I swarmed back up the chassis and down to join Ezekial and a small knot of members of the film crew, who had gathered in the hope of seeing me being terminally squashed.

'Is Dolly going to be all right?' an anxious nasal voice inquired. I turned to face a beaky, bespectacled American. He was wearing a khaki waistcoat, bulging with innumerable pockets from which protruded pens, pencils, sunglasses, pipes, note pads, cigars, maps, and other unidentifiable paraphernalia.

'Dolly?'

'Yes, the rhino.'

'Ah, yes. I think so. I'm going to give her a large, massive in fact, dose of corticosteroid and an antibiotic and that, together with rest and a descent to a lower altitude, should do the trick.' There was no way I was going to be able to give her i/v sodium bicarbonate. That way would lead to the death the Indian devotees of Juggernaut aspired to and which I had no wish to emulate.

From my bag I selected my longest and strongest needles, impressive four inch jobs, and attached them to my very largest syringes, which I filled to the brim with hydrocortisone and penicillin and streptomycin. I leaned over the side of the lorry and smacked the first needle into and through the horny hide. It sank in to the hilt. Dolly seemed not to object. I injected the lot and returned to earth.

I spoke to the multi-pocketed American, who seemed to be the camp manager. 'She should be OK, but get her downhill, before it rains and before the road is impassable.'

'Yes sir! I'll get onto that right away. The truck's ready to roll. Thank you, sir!'

By the time Ezekial had driven me back to the airstrip the first few spots of rain were beginning to appear on the windscreen.

Jim's jaws were still in steady state munching mode. He removed his wad of gum, inspected it carefully and popped it back into his mouth. 'Wall,' he drawled, 'did ya see her?'

'Yes,' I replied, 'she was huge and grey and wrinkled but she should be OK.'

'No, I mean, did you see Sheena? She just flew out. She's been doing a nude shoot up at a waterfall on the moorlands. You just missed her.'

Chapter Twenty

In the Lions' Den

On 26 February 1984, our first-born, Rona, slipped into the world. Despite her substantial eight and a half pounds, her entrance was uncomplicated. Berna might not have wholly agreed with a female friend, experienced in such matters, who told her – 'There's nothing to it my dear, it's just like having a massive crap,' – but she took it in her stride.

—✳—

Ol Pejeta Ranch was the sort of place which would have appealed to the likes of Ernest Hemingway and Robert Ruark. Vast plains, dotted with flat-topped acacias stretched away to the foothills of Mt. Kenya, upon whose topmost towers glaciers and snowfields sparkled incongruously in the tropical sun. Herds of soft-eyed antelope grazed those pristine plains, nibbling the short herbage in the company of knots of fat, handsome zebra and genuflecting families of alert, watchful warthog. Stately giraffe snacked on the thorny treetops, groups of elephant drifted effortlessly through the bush. In the thickets lurked the glowering black buffalo. Prides of tawny lion roared nightly, leopard dragged their prey into tree forks and hyena whooped and cackled at the moon. If the doughty pair of Nimrods felt cheated at being unable to gun down any of the above, due to Kenya's ban on hunting, they could take consolation that they could slake their mighty thirsts at a strategically-sited lodge, a five star hostelry privately owned by a Middle Eastern family, whose catholic tastes did not eschew alcohol. Here they could indulge appetites, honed by hard days and nights in the bush, by feasting on all the best that money could provide. Succulent viands and mouth-watering dishes were available in abundant supply to satisfy the inner man. And that was not all. Young ladies would be on hand to supply solace to the weary would-be hunters. In the gargantuan dining room, suspended by ropes above the vast, gleaming, mahogany table, hung, strangely, a dugout canoe. This was the 'fruit basket' containing the dessert. Once the suitably subservient waiters had cleared away the main course, the signal would be given to lower the canoe, which was filled to the gunwales with exotic fruits of every conceivable variety. There were mangos, paw paws, pineapples, melons, oranges, avocados, grapefruit. Truly a mouth-watering selection. Soft-footed flunkeys turned ratchets and the canoe slowly and gently came to rest upon the table's gleaming surface. Guests, entranced by this novel presentation of nature's bounty, leaned forward eagerly to select the fruits of their choice. Surprise and gratification lay in store. The canoe held fruits other than those plucked from the bough or delved from the earth. From below the eye catching cornucopia appeared pairs of graceful bare arms, followed by other parts of unclad anatomy, obviously female.

The appetite of the almost-exclusively male guests underwent a sudden spurt. Mangoes were munched, oranges were peeled and grapefruit sucked in a wolfish frenzy as the guests endeavoured to clear the decks of uneaten fruit. Juice from tangerines and strawberries dribbled from chins more used to the dribble of the juice of the barley. As the inanimate cargo was cleared away so the very animate cargo was revealed in the form of three well-formed, receptive maidens, naked as the day they were born, rising Venus-like from the bilges. Our mighty hunters would have been delighted.

—*—

I was often called to Ol Pejeta, despite its distance from Nakuru. The manager, John Poulton, had formerly farmed on his own account on the breezy Molo uplands. Now he was master of almost all that he surveyed, with a free hand to manage as he saw fit. His Arabian masters usually had other fish to fry and were seldom there, jumbo-jetting in from time to time as a respite from their various mysterious international activities to rest and recuperate and enjoy dessert with their friends. Sadly, I did not have the opportunity to observe the lowering of the canoe, but I was invited into the big house, with Berna, to treat a young cheetah with rickets. We were ushered into the library whose walls were covered with what seemed like thousands of books. There, charming young Arab gentlemen supplied us with small cups of thick sweet coffee while the cheetah nibbled our ears, over the back of the sofa. A stuffed leopard head glared at us from the top of a bookcase. Elephant tusks and incongruous rhino feet lined the walls. Berna went off to check out the facilities and returned goggle-eyed to report *sotto voce* on gold-plated taps, an Olympic-sized bath and a bed fit for Henry the Eighth and all six queens simultaneously. As we left, we passed through the dining room, past the great gleaming table and beneath the notorious canoe. I glanced wistfully upwards at it, hanging there innocently from the ceiling, awaiting its next orgy.

My main patients at Ol Pejeta were horses, cattle, dogs and wildlife.

The owners liked lions. So much so that any lion trapped for killing cattle on the ranch was not shot but released into a large fenced enclosure in the centre of the ranch. The female of the species being more cunning than the male, the enclosure contained fifteen large male lions and a mere five lionesses.

With fifteen males competing for five females there was a fair amount of squabbling and when things got out of hand I would be called in to doctor those who came off worst. I would arrive in my Peugeot 504 saloon and transfer to a ranch Toyota Land Cruiser pickup, together with my loaded Cap Chur pistol. The lions associated the Toyota with the arrival of meat. The first time I was driven into the huge lion-infested enclosure I was staggered to see that in the back of the open pickup were three Africans clad in denim overalls bearing the family crest of the owners, a falcon with what looked like a writhing snake, pinioned in its talons. The three were all carrying brooms. Brooms? What were they carrying brooms for? As we drove into the enclosure the lions made a concerted rush for the back of the Toyota, from which lunch or dinner was usually dispensed. As there was neither on this occasion, the three in the back of the pickup fended off the ravening horde with their brooms. Why no lion did not leap aboard and grab one tasty broom-handler was beyond me. Meanwhile, safe in the cab, I was able to identify my distracted subject and fire a projectile drug-loaded syringe into his or her backside. Once the drug started to take effect, the other lions would be lured into a separate enclosure, leaving their soporific companion behind. I would jump out, top up the anaesthetic and get to work.

In mid-1984 I received a call from the ranch to say that one of the lionesses had what looked like a tumour growing from her upper lip and that it was interfering with her eating. As this was not an emergency it was decided to go on a Sunday, when things were a little less busy, and I would take Berna, and Rona, now 4 months old, along with me.

We drove to the ranch via Rumuruti, turned sharp right at the first dukas, passed the tree-lined entrance to the Rumuruti Club, crossed the River Easo Narok and rattled up a rocky hill and onto the black cotton plains which stretched all the way to the foot of the great mountain. Rona was ensconced, like a miniature Turkish pasha, in a home-made bed on the back seat.

Rain was around. It had poured the night before and sections of the road were slick with mud. Black cotton soil dries out quickly in the sun and as it was now mid-morning I knew we would have little trouble on the outward journey. Things might be different on the way back. Already threatening cu-nimbs were developing on the distant horizon. The road was smooth and empty and we made good progress. We crossed the Pesi River and still had another 40 miles to cover. The lack of traffic on this road could be disconcerting. You knew that if you broke down no one would come along for hours. Then you might wonder *why* there were no other vehicles using the road. Was there a washed-away bridge ahead? Were there bandits lying in wait, which everyone but you knew about? The road rose over another rise and snaked away in front, far ahead over yet another tree-dotted rise. And another. After a while you drove on autopilot, hardly noticing where you were or what side of the road you were on or what you had passed. 'Look out!' Berna shouted. An eland leapt over the fence on the right, onto the road in front of the car and up the other bank, scattering stones and gravel. I slowed down.

The bush fell back and a few minutes later we drove into the ranch. It was late morning. In the back of the car Rona was stirring. At the ranch-house John Poulton was waiting. 'Come in for a cold drink and then we'll go to the lions.' The ranch was huge and I knew that it would take us at least another twenty minutes to get to the scene of the action. We were both thirsty and so was Rona. We sat on the sofa, surrounded by panting labradors and eager, salivating dachshunds. Leopard skins hung on the walls and lion skins covered the floor. An elephant's foot held a selection of walking sticks. A baboon skull adorned the sideboard. Surrounded by all this dead tissue we all drank deeply as John gave us more details about the lioness. 'She's four years old. She's got this 'thing' hanging from her upper right lip and when she eats it gets in the way of her canine teeth and as a result it's getting a bit mangled. Time it was off.'

'Right, we'll have a look at it. I've brought all my darting kit and surgical tools, so we're ready for anything.' I gave a token laugh.

'OK, then, if you're ready, let's go. You know where they are. There's a new chap in charge of the lions. He's a Goan, name of Fernandes.'

As we drove down the rocky track towards the lion enclosure a group of Red Hussar monkeys were gambolling around a termite mound. These ground-dwelling monkeys are peculiar to this area, and are generally uncommon elsewhere in Kenya. We reached the exterior gate to the group of enclosures. Berna hopped out to open it. Out of the corner of my eye I saw something large and tawny trotting alongside, and *outside,* the fence. 'Get back in!' I shouted as a large lion came loping towards us. Berna got in, fast.

John Poulton drove up beside us and stopped. 'Sorry, chaps, forgot to tell you about that. That lion has a habit of getting out and killing cattle. If I had my way I'd shoot the brute, but the owners won't have it.' What about people being killed? I wondered. I noticed that when John got out of *his* car he was carrying a heavy rifle. OK, then.

Inside this gate were two more gates, double bolted. A Toyota Land Cruiser, crewed by broom brandishing lion men stood waiting outside the last gate. The driver got out of the cab and came over to shake hands. He was a dark, stocky fellow with grizzled wiry hair and a thin moustache. 'Hi' he said. 'I'm Fernandes. Thanks for coming. The lioness is getting a bit fed up with this thing interfering with her feeding. We've moved all the male lions into the next enclosure, leaving her and the other four lionesses in this enclosure here. Once she has been darted and goes down we can shift the others out.'

'Right.'

I took my Cap Chur pistol out of its case, slipped in a fresh CO_2 cylinder and prepared the projectile syringe – the 'dart'. I looked at the lioness. She looked at me. I reckoned she was about 110 kg. So, 1000mg ketamine followed by 80mg xylazine. The only trouble was that the volume of ketamine was large, amounting to ten ml, as the only available local source came in 100mg/ml vials. I assembled the syringe, filled it with the ketamine, screwed on a 4cm barbed needle and slipped it into the barrel of the pistol.

'OK, compadre,' I said to Fernandes, 'let's go!' I got into the passenger side of the cab, John unlocked the gate and we drove into the enclosure. He then locked it behind us. The lads in the back readied their brooms. The five lionesses perked up on our entry. Was this breakfast, lunch or dinner? After a bit of circling and general weaving I cocked the pistol and slipped on the safety catch. Finally we were in position with the patient's hind leg presenting an easy target. I slipped off the safety, aimed and pressed the trigger. Bull's eye.

As soon as the syringe struck the lioness's leg one of the other lionesses rushed in and, despite the fact that the dart was barbed, removed it with her teeth. Impressive. The four undarted lionesses then played with the metal syringe, grabbing it with their teeth, throwing it into the air and generally worrying it to death. That's the end of that hyper-expensive syringe, I thought, as another set of two inch long canines bit down on the metal.

After eight minutes, the darted lioness was, to all intents and purposes, down and out. The other four lionesses were herded out and into the adjacent enclosure holding the fourteen males by driving them in front of the Toyota. I wondered what had happened to the escapee. Probably lunching on prime Boran steak. I had hoped to see the broom boys in action here but they remained safely and wimpishly in the back of the truck, from whose front I now descended, to give the recumbent patient her injection of the sedative xylazine to complete the anaesthetic dose. Within a few minutes she was peacefully asleep, ready for the scalpel.

I gave the thumbs-up sign to Berna, waiting outside the gate. John opened the lock and in she came with Rona, whom she laid under a thorn tree, next to the lioness. All nice and cosy. A bit like one of those saccharine Victorian paintings of the lion lying down with the lamb. Or vice versa. I was now able to examine the growth more closely. It was impressively large in view of its position on the lip – 4.5cm long by 3.5cm wide by 2cm deep and with a base about half of these measurements. I laid out my instruments on a clean towel, shaved the adjacent skin and got to work. Things went smoothly. The grass was soft under my knees, I was in cool shade, there wasn't too much bleeding and the few spouters were easily clamped and tied off. Berna handed me instruments as I needed them and in no time the growth had been excised and I was ready to close up. As I began to appose the subcutaneous tissue I glanced up. I felt watched. A long row of maned heads was staring fixedly at me through the wire separating us from the adjacent enclosure. 'What was I doing to their sister?' they seemed to be thinking. But one lion in particular was not pleased. He glared with ferocious menace at me and then rushed at the overhanging fence. He got three quarters of the way up before falling back down. He tried again and failed to get any higher.

'What are his chances of getting over?' I asked Fernandes, as I bent to stitch the skin with interrupted stitches of strong catgut.

'Not a hope,' he replied. 'He wouldn't be able to get over the overhang.'

'Well, that's a relief,' I said. 'He would make short work of young Rona here! Then he would start on us!' Now the lion was rushing to and fro along the wire, snarling and grunting. 'I've put in catgut stitches,' I said to Fernandes, 'so there won't be any need to re-anaesthetise her to remove non-absorbable ones.' The angry lion made one more attempt on the wire, before slinking off to sulk and mutter in a corner. 'Right, I'll give her some penicillin and streptomycin and then we'll make her comfortable and wait until she wakes up. May take an hour or so. I'll send the growth to the lab for identification.'

Leaving the patient snoring gently beneath her thorn tree we carried my stuff back to the car. Berna had discovered that the milk that she had brought for Rona had curdled in the sun. Rona was displeased.

'You'll probably get some at the big house,' said Fernandes. 'The boss would like to have you there for lunch. I'll keep an eye on the lioness until you get back. And, sorry, but I'm afraid I wasn't being entirely truthful about that angry lion.'

'What do you mean?' said Berna.

'Well, I came here yesterday to check out this enclosure to see if it would be suitable for you. I had just shot a Tommy for the lions next door and had a hind leg in my hand when I came into this empty enclosure. All of a sudden that lion in there scrambled up the wire, hauled itself over the overhang and dropped down in here and went for me. Lucky for me I had that leg of Tommy in my hand. I chucked it at the lion, who grabbed and I legged it out of here.' There was a long silence, broken only by the chirrup of birds and the buzz of cicadas. Fernandes looked distinctly uncomfortable. The tension was broken by a strident yell from Rona.

'Well,' said Berna, 'no good crying over spilt milk. Now we'd better go and find some. Just don't do that ever again, OK?'

'No ma'am, sorry ma'am.'

We drove to the big house, neither of us venturing to voice our thoughts of what might have been, had that lion got over the fence. At the house we asked our Arab hosts whether they had any milk or baby formula.

'Oh yes, we have milk and also we have a special milk formula which we are feeding to a baby zebra. It loves it. Why don't you try that?' We did and Rona also loved it and gobbled it down. Lunch was a sumptuous affair, European courses with tasteful Eastern undertones.

Nothing was spared to assuage our appetites. We had prawn cocktails, cream of mushroom soup, rack of lamb, crème brûlée, French wines, coffee and chocolates, all served with pleasing deference by squadrons of attentive waiters. Our hosts were perfect ambassadors of Arab hospitality and we were glad to be able to benefit in small measure from the proceeds of their ventures, dubious though they might be. Rumours of gun-running and the shipping of arms to doubtful recipients had been heard. Berna had another glass of wine, Bordeaux, white, chilled. I nibbled another Belgian chocolate.

I glanced at my watch. Time to check on the patient and get on the road. Thanking our smiling hosts we scooped up Rona and drove back to the lions' den. The lioness was sitting up and taking a bleary interest in her surroundings. Three and a half hours had elapsed since I had inserted the last suture.

A forelock-tugging Fernandes bade us farewell.

'You'd best get going,' he said. 'It looks like rain and the road is black cotton soil all the way to Rumuruti.'

As we drove away, the first spots of rain pattered on the windscreen and the first clatterings of the dreaded black cotton soil being thrown up under the car smote our ears. Within seconds what had been a firm, dry, dusty highway was now a fiendishly slippery Cresta Run. The main thing was not to stop. Keep going at all costs. Preferably in a reasonably high gear – third was usually best. To slow down meant a terminal slide into the ditch, from which extrication was impossible without the help of a tractor. Once stationary, even four wheel drive vehicles were helpless in black cotton soil. We were still on the ranch. The road ran straight and narrow, black and treacly, slightly up hill, with a fence on our right. I bent over the steering wheel, keeping the vehicle straight and in the middle of the track, keeping the speed up, watching the surface, scrutinising the adjacent ditches, trying not to make any sudden changes of direction.

'Elephant on the road!' announced Berna, in a calm matter of fact voice. I looked up. 'Shit!' A small group of jumbos was milling about on the road, a couple of hundred yards to our front, slipping and sliding in the mud, held up by the wire fence. One was a cow with a small calf, which she was trying to push through the wire. Unable to slow down for fear of slipping permanently into the ditch, we closed the gap with what seemed like alarming speed. But, as in one of those sweaty nightmares where your sluggish limbs are totally incapable of movement while you are being charged by a slobbering, sabre-toothed tiger, so conversely time seemed to slow down as we drew nearer and nearer, unable to prevent imminent obliteration. The elephants had now turned in our direction, ears all spread like enormous sails, trunks raised, shaking their heads from side to side, trumpeting and making short rushes towards us. Just when a disproportionate collision seemed inevitable, the elephants turned as one, and, screaming with rage, tails raised, scrambled up the bank. Surrounding the baby, they propelled it through the fence. It stumbled to its knees, regained its feet, and, protected by the covering bulk of its mother's enormous belly, moved off smartly with the rest of the group and vanished into the bush.

There was no time for sighs of relief or reaching for the smelling salts. The road was as slippery as ever and by the time we reached the Nanyuki/Rumuruti road we were beginning to wonder where we might spend the night. On the back seat Rona, gorged with zebra formula, slumbered on, oblivious to the trials facing her parents. It was still raining. Perversely we were rather glad that it was. Black cotton soil is marginally more negotiable while rain drops are breaking up the surface than when it has had time to settle. At least, that's what we had been told by the ubiquitous local experts. The road was wider now, allowing more room to manoeuvre. As there was no traffic one could drive on the left, on the right or down the middle, according to preference and the surface. We pelted on, great waves of muddy water cascading onto the roadside. Forward visibility lessened as the windscreen received its quota of the mire. It was getting dark. The mud-encrusted headlights shone dimly on the ruts and stretches of water-filled potholes. Animal eyes reflected in the flickering beams stared ominously at us as we slithered past. Broadside skids elicited yelps of irritation from the back seat. The road seemed to go on for ever. Finally we re-crossed the Pesi and as we bumped down the hill towards the bridge over the Easo Narok and onto *terra firma* it stopped raining.

It was 9pm.

The relief of being back on tarmac was immense, but now I found that I was barely able to turn the steering wheel. Up till now the inequalities of the dirt road had quite minimised such effete niceties. I stopped the car and eased myself out. Ah, the taken-for-granted benison of smooth, solid tar. Tarmacadam. Who *was* Macadam? The fellow should have been knighted. Raised to the peerage. Perhaps he was.

'What's the problem?' asked Berna.

'Steering wheel won't turn,' I replied. 'Do you have a torch?' She did. Our recent experience after an evening reception hosted by the Queen and Prince Philip at a large hotel in Nairobi remained vividly etched in our minds. Berna was eight months pregnant with Rona at the time. On the way back to Nakuru we had a puncture, on the escarpment. We had no torch. But Berna, ever resourceful, had a candle. Even so, changing a wheel in a gale force wind, in the dark, with only a flickering stub of a candle for illumination, is not to be recommended.

I peered under the car, shining the torch on what looked like several hundredweights of coagulated black cotton soil, adhering glue-like to the lower entities of the vehicle. Using a tyre lever I prised away as much as I could. Great gobbets of the stuff fell onto the road. Finally we set off on what we fervently hoped was the last leg. Things were better, but far from perfect. The wheels, unbalanced by the remaining limpet-like clods, transmitted their judderings to the steering wheel. By the time we reached Nakuru at half past ten my arms felt as though they had been partially disjointed.

The following morning I took the car to a garage where a high pressure hose removed another hundredweight of goo.

The lab report on the growth removed from the lioness revealed it to be 'an infected cyst-adenoma, well encapsulated and not malignant'. It did not recur.

Chapter Twenty One

'TROUBLED THE DEEP WATERS'

Peter Gichane, our new house boy and Njoroge's successor, had so far given us little cause for complaint. True, he had scoured the precious wedding silver with wire wool until its shining surface was like pre-Roman pewter, true, he had, during our absence, used well-nigh irreplaceable text books as firm surfaces upon which to lay his writing paper, thereby permanently imprinting their smooth covers with his deathless prose, true, he had atomised the bwana's priceless Rowland Ward beer mug, a present from grateful clients, but these peccadilloes were as nothing compared to his main defect. This was his gender.

Now that Rona was resident on the premises, we decided that we would prefer to have a house *girl*, rather than a house *boy*, pottering about the place, rearranging the cobwebs, shifting the dust and burning the toast. When we broached the news to Peter he was mortified that he was to be replaced by a *woman*. But he was in luck. Berna had chatted up the secretary of the Rift Valley Sports Club, that hoary imperial bastion, beached amid the post-colonial chaos of present-day Nakuru, and secured Peter a job as a trainee waiter. The secretary was a mildewed Ancient Briton, noted for his cantankerousness, self importance and impressive nose, which resembled the bill of a dyspeptic toucan. Narcotised by a soothing measure of Irish charm, he visibly wilted, until Berna had him wound inextricably round her little finger. Peter donned his bow tie and joined the waiting ranks, up which he rose as the years went by, serving the soup and dishing out the chicken and chips to the members with an aplomb and flourish he had never exhibited when in our employ.

Concurrent with the arrival of the new woman, we moved house to a larger establishment at Lanet, some seven kilometres from Nakuru. Moving was not difficult. Our possessions were scant and the new house, which we rented, was fully furnished. There was a large garden, full of birds and trees, we had water and electricity, friendly neighbours and the landlady was almost civil. Our cup was full.

The main road was less than one hundred yards from the house and beyond that the main railway line to Kisumu and Uganda. We made haste to block all apertures through which the rumble of traffic and rattle of trains might penetrate to interfere with our well-earned sleep. We need not have bothered. After a few nights, the Flying Scotsman could have whistled past our window and we wouldn't have heard it.

The new housekeeper was called Esther Wangari. Within a short time we called her something else. She had an alarming propensity to break everything she touched – crockery, glassware, cups, jugs, chairs, stools, ornaments, pictures, the list was endless. These innocent inanimate objects always 'fell', or 'broke' as though endowed with an irresistible suicidal urge to dash themselves to death. 'Kikombe lianguka.' (The cup fell.) 'Sahani lipasuka.' (The plate broke.) Long before the mythical Weapons of Mass Destruction dreamed up by Messrs Bush and Blair, we had a real live one living amongst us.

When she came, Esther, although she had given birth to three children sired by various fathers, was slim, fine featured and good looking. In our employ this happy state of affairs did not last long. Almost before our eyes she ballooned, fore, aft and sideways. How this was achieved was a mystery to us as we never saw her put food to her lips and our own supplies seemed not to diminish. But she was scrupulously honest, was fond of children, loved Rona, and so she stayed and stayed.

With the arrival of Rona, Berna gave up her teaching job at Blackthorn. When she was there she got around on a motorbike, a Yamaha trail, on which she travelled around the country, to the coast and even as far north as Maralal on the edge of the Northern Frontier District. After the death of a teacher friend in a motorbike accident, mown down at night by a speeding lorry, we decided that four wheels had to be safer, so Berna graduated, if that's the correct word, to a Mini Moke, a vehicle whose chassis was so close to the ground that one's buttocks felt level with the tarmac. With no door and with canvas sides and roof, this underpowered runabout was like a tea tray on wheels and was dwarfed by everything else on the road. It was overtaken by cyclists and fast walking pedestrians, could not be parked anywhere in town for fear of anything moveable therein being nicked, including the whole vehicle, and afforded the wretched driver zero protection when it rained. The Mini Moke did not remain long in the Cran stable, before it was replaced by a Mini Minor. This at least had a hard roof, and a boot, if little else. Instrumentation was almost nil, and the interior was stark, with metal where most cars had plastic or fabric. On a hot day you could have fried an egg on the dashboard.

I was doing so much mileage that I was changing cars twice, sometimes three times a year. We decided that it would make more sense to have two Peugeots. I would drive the work one, Berna would have the other, and when mine needed a service we would have Berna's one to fall back on. Without a tear we bade farewell to the Mini.

Our water supply came from a large stone tank, sited on a convenient incline behind the various houses in the compound. The tank was topped up via a pipe entering just below its rim. Twice weekly a designated employee checked the water level and if it was low, opened a valve and topped up the tank, a tried and tested method which seemed to work well.

During our first months at our new house, the water was clear and wholesome, as though sourced from some joyous mountain spring. It sprang gushing from the taps. Eminently suitable for bathing, making tea or coffee or adding to one's whisky, we rejoiced in this abundant supply.

In our previous dwelling the water came in unpredictable fits and starts, belching out of the taps at one moment, dwindling to a trickle at the next, followed by a flatulent bellow as a bolus of trapped air vented its painful imprisoned frustration. On one occasion Berna and I went to the Motor Club on the Solai road to view a nature film, prophetically entitled *And the Rains Came*. It was one of those sugary documentary biopics where the clouds rush madly across the sky and plants sprout to unbelievable maturity within seconds. On our return at midnight we found water pouring down the walls and through the ceiling. Investigation revealed that the tank in the attic had split. A night-long battle ensued, utilizing Rona's portable plastic baby bath, a hosepipe and a bucket, in a losing fight to prevent our belongings being washed out of the house. Every five minutes I sucked on the hosepipe in order to drain Rona's overflowing bath. After several hours of non-stop sucking my cheeks were almost fused together.

Came the dawn we had to engage outside assistance to render the house habitable. We recruited a pair of 'fundis', local experts of which Kenya has a seemingly inexhaustible supply. One declared that his métier was pipes, and that since he was weaned from his mother's milk he had dealt with nothing else. The other pronounced himself to be a qualified welder of unique skill and experience. For seven days they wreaked havoc and destruction. After three attempts at repair, the tank was still leaking, and twice they had put their feet through the ceiling. In an effort to stem the leak they put tar into the tank. The consequence was that the tank continued to leak and now we had tar coming through the taps and into our bath. Both experts appeared to be deeply under the influence of drink, drugs or both. By this time, at the end of our joint tether, we asked the pair to leave. They refused and became truculent, demanding outrageous emoluments. We called the police who arrived on foot. The pair protested their innocence and expertise, pointing bony fingers at us and in slurred Swahili hinting that we were a pair of reactionary racist skinflints. For once the police were on our side. The fundis were bundled into the back of our car and we drove the short distance to the police station. The police marched their now manacled captives inside and all vanished behind a door bearing a grubby and sinister sign – 'Interrogation Room'.

To the sounds of muffled shouts, yells and muted thumping, we left.

On the eighth day another fundi repaired the tank and finally brought a measure of sanity into our lives.

At Lanet we revelled in our watery bounty. Our bath was one of those massive Victorian affairs, seemingly designed for conjugal bathing. Complying with what seemed almost an imperial edict, armpit deep in the steaming tub, we nightly sipped our gins and tonic, before engaging in unbidden underwater exercises.

Then almost without our noticing it, there came a subtle change. It was barely perceptible at first, a *je ne sais quoi* alteration in colour and flavour. The formerly crystal clear water took on a slightly jaundiced tinge. Nothing was very obvious to the casual observer. There was a slightly musky, not entirely unpleasant, aroma, rising with the steam, as though an unusual and rather rare purchase of bath salts has been added to the incoming tide. The nightly ritual took on almost Turkish overtones, what with the clouds of steam drifting over the exotically coloured water, the strange, all-enveloping, exhalation, redolent of subtle Eastern joss sticks, and the flickering candlelight in which we were wont to conduct our ablutions. Harsh electric light was so unflattering to the person and bad for the eyes.

The water did taste ever-so-slightly odd, but as we rarely drank it neat found no reason to go grumbling to the landlady, who would have sent us away with a flea in our ear – 'When I was young we drew water from the well and were grateful for it. What do you want – gold-plated taps?' So we continued to make tea and soup with it, add it to whisky, and wash in it, and came to no harm.

Unbeknown to us, the employee whose task it was to check on the water level in the big stone tank, whence the water flowed, had gone on leave for a month. It seemed that, during his absence, there had been a lapse of attention to detail in that no one had been appointed to do his job.

One day, about a week before the waterman's return from his vacation, a casual labourer was assigned to trim the grass around the tank as it was growing long and unkempt. Using a slasher, a long-handled cutter with a convenient bend at the working end, he set to work.

Pausing in his exertions, he leant against the wall of the tank, wiping the honest sweat from his beaded brow. He glanced down into the depths and was surprised to see that the tank was little more than a quarter full. He looked again. There was something more. What was *that* protruding from the water? What was that white thing, which looked like a hand, with bits like white seaweed hanging off the fingers? He peered again, screwing up his eyes. The sun was strong. My God, it was a human hand! One finger was crooked, as though beckoning to the watcher – 'Come, come and join me.'

He whirled and ran, shouting. Nearby workers stared. He babbled out his news. They looked at him and then walked across to the tank, but slowly and fearfully, not wanting to see what their colleague had seen. They peered reluctantly over the rim. They saw what he had seen. They hissed with disbelief and disgust. 'Go, Mwangi,' they said, 'go and tell the Mzungu what you have seen.'

Mwangi went to the old woman, our landlady. She told him that he had been drinking and to go away. Mwangi protested his innocence and went to speak to the landlady's son, Kevin. Kevin came and looked into the tank and phoned the police.

When the police came, they ordered that the tank be drained. An exterior valve was opened and slowly the water level dropped. The pipe kept on getting blocked by something. What that something was we didn't care to think about. As the water trickled out, things were exposed which made us wish we hadn't drunk it and bathed in it with such gay and careless abandon. For there, at the bottom of the tank, now revealed in hideous mid-day clarity, was a body, bloated and coming apart at the seams. It was that of an African woman, that much was evident. The body, now chalk-white from long immersion in our putative bathwater, was bound with wire and weighted down with rocks. Whoever she was, she had obviously not just tripped on the edge and fallen in, or gone for a dip without armbands. How long she had been there was anyone's guess, but judging from the appearance of the corpse, coupled with the curious case of our changing tap water, at least a month.

The policemen gaped with undisguised repugnance. 'Wah! Who will remove this body? It is too crumbly. And, wah, it is a woman. This is a job for a woman. We must have a woman officer for this task.'

The police left, leaving the exposed body to bake in the noon-day sun.

After a couple of hours they returned with a reluctant policewoman. She stared at the body, now covered with a mass of flies, turned away and retched into the grass.

The police, men and woman, went into a huddle, piled into their Land Rover pickup, and drove away. The body continued to melt in the afternoon heat.

About an hour later the Land Rover returned, its back now filled with a gang of individuals, whose vacant expressions and sagging jaws suggested that they had no idea where they were going or what they were expected to do.

Across the road and on the other side of the railway line was the so-called Free Area, a noisome collection of shacks, tatterdemalion shops, open patches of withered grass grazed by sheep, goats, cattle and donkeys, hawkers' booths, cardboard churches, and illegal drinking dens, the whole transected by rutted lanes, ankle deep in mud during the rains and ankle deep in dust when it was dry. It was to these drinking dens that the police now made their way. The favoured tipple in these dens was changaa, a lethal home-made brew which yearly left hundreds dead, blind or brain damaged. Fermented in 44-gallon drums, it was cheap, alcoholic to the point of toxicity and guaranteed to blot out the drinker's cruel world, often permanently.

What the police wanted were patrons who were still at least partially *compos mentis*. Those who were legless, speechless or horizontal and unable to respond to the word of command would be of no use for what they had in mind. They would be rejected in the forthcoming selection process. Little did they know how lucky they were.

The drinking parlours were not advertised by welcoming signs or slogans. Here there was no *Red Lion*, *White Hart*, or *Cheshire Cheese*. Instead their presence was usually indicated by a prone individual lying comatose in the nearest ditch. Stopping beside one such figure couchant, the police battered open the door of the nearest structure and forced their way in, surprising a group of bleary eyed drinkers, who stared at them with wild surmise. 'Right, outside! The lot of you!' the cops bellowed. Those who could walk, including a number of women, staggered to the exit, blinking as they emerged into the sunlight. They were lined up in a swaying, ragged row. 'Now,' said the chief policeman, an inspector, 'you have a simple choice. You can either be charged with drinking illegal liquor, a serious custodial offence, in which case you will be taken to the cells immediately, there to spend the next six months in jail, or,' – he paused – 'you can come with us to carry out a small, but vital, governmental task. After that you will be free to go.'

The inspector was immediately overwhelmed by a show of hands. To a man, and woman, they volunteered for the unknown. Anything was better than chokey.

These, then, were the luckless crew in the back of the police Land Rover as it rattled up the hill on its way back to the tank and its deceased inhabitant. They were speedily shocked into sobriety when they saw what they had let themselves in for.

Eventually the proprietor of a roadside kiosk, a humble seller of second-hand clothes, whose stance was about 200 yards from our house, was charged with the murder of his wife. He pleaded guilty. Her nagging had got on his nerves, he said. But he did not reveal how he had managed to get her body, bound with wire and weighted with rocks, into the tank. He vanished into the prison system, taking his secret with him.

On reflection the failure to appoint someone to do the job of the absent waterman did us a signal service. If the water level had not dropped as it did, then the body at the bottom of the tank would have remained there, quietly disintegrating, the murderer would have remained at large, and we would have been left with our strangely-scented and curiously coloured bathwater.

Chapter Twenty Two

RABIES

Now that I was a Married Man with a wife and daughter, and Berna was a Married Woman with a husband and daughter, with the strong possibility of more offspring in the pipeline, so to speak, this was not the time to rest on our laurels. Looming school fees, rising prices, a weakening shilling, political instability, general insecurity, corruption, dangerous roads, disease, iniquitous taxation, a rapacious police force, doubtful medical facilities – was Kenya really the best place to bring up a family? Sensible people would have considered all of these deficiencies, weighed them up, booked their airline tickets and settled for a steady, safe, unexciting, well-paid job in Bognor or Surbiton, with a house in the suburbs and a fat pension at the end of it all.

Not being sensible and being both preoccupied with work and daily battling against the ever-increasing odds, we carried on. Each day seemed to bring forth a fresh challenge. If we had been able to harvest and market our joint output of adrenalin we would have been able to retire in comfort.

While Berna planned the setting up of a home school for local children, looked after Rona and tried to prevent house girl Esther from demolishing the house and its fittings, I attempted, seemingly vainly, to stem the rising tide of animal disease and to cope with the diurnal and nocturnal flood of emergencies and accidents.

'Barina Jerseys visit stitch mare, staked in abdomen and chest – omentum prolapsed'

'Brendon – horse torn by barbed wire on chest'

'Mrs Wedd – op. pup, chop bone lodged in stomach – open up and remove'

'Madrugada – steer with rabies – staggering, drooling, aggressive, straining, anorexic'

'To Eldoret – bleed 176 cattle'

'Technology Farm – heifer stuck down hole for one week – eating well but severely bruised and blind in one eye'

'Lowling Farm – night visit foal mare – embryotomy – two hours – mare violent, foal upside down, head/nape position – good recovery'

On a regular basis students would come to 'see practice'. They came from the UK, Kenya, Australia, New Zealand and the US. Most found the experience fulfilling but exhausting. Some found it just too much. One young local magnifico, clad in tweed jacket and tie, quit after just one morning. Others discovered the lure of the game parks and the beckoning Coast to be overwhelming. I couldn't really blame them. I would have done the same myself if I could. The young women, on the whole, had more resilience than the men, and English girls from the northern universities fared best of all.

—*—

The outbreak of rabies, which had begun in the Rift Valley in 1981, and continued until the early '90s, also affected much of Eastern Africa. It now reached epidemic proportions. Almost every day I saw a new case – in dogs and cats, cattle, sheep, donkeys and horses.

—*—

'Dr Crane?' the rising intonation was unmistakably Asian. 'This is Dr Wirdee here. I am the Provincial Surgeon.' The voice was smooth and confident. 'Look, my five month old German Shepherd pup has a bit of a problem. I am thinking he has foreign body lodged in throat.' I glanced at my watch. Ten pm. 'I sedated him with oral valium and conducted manual exploration of throat and pharynx with negative results. The ingested object I think may be in the upper oesophageal area. I would like you to examine him.'

'Right,' I replied. 'Has he been vaccinated?'

'No.'

'Did you wear gloves during your examination?'

'Yes.'

I breathed a sigh of relief.

I drove to the surgery and awaited the arrival of the surgeon.

When the good doctor, suave and suited, arrived with his dog, I was astonished that he had managed to conduct any examination at all. The animal was in a state of manic aggression, barking and snarling. Its eyeballs were jerking from side to side in a violent uncoordinated fashion. It was unable to stand. Whether the ingested valium had any bearing on this I was unable to determine, and I was not prepared to handle the dog to find out.

'Well,' I said, 'I'm glad to see that you are still wearing gloves, doctor. Because your pup almost certainly has rabies.'

'Yes, I thought it might be that,' he replied with easy arrogance, but I noticed that, under his dark skin, he blanched. But losing face was not in his book.

'Well,' I said, 'I'll have to keep your pup here. I'm afraid he will die in the next few days, and in the meantime, until we get a lab diagnosis, you will have to get yourself and all in-contacts vaccinated. I'm sure you know the form.'

'Yes, fortunately I can get the vaccine at cost. It's pretty expensive.'

'Yes, but not as expensive as a life lost, whoever's life that might be.'

He gave me a funny look, but I well knew that some people would rush off to buy vaccine for themselves, while conveniently forgetting to obtain vaccine for their workers, who were in much closer contact with their animals than themselves.

When I spoke to people who needed to be vaccinated and who complained about the cost of the vaccine, I would ask them – 'How much are you worth? Surely you're worth more than the cost of the vaccine?' And in every case they agreed and found the money. But few were keen to help others. They would rather cut corners and hope for the best, by which time it might be too late.

Dr Virdee – that was his correct name – put his puppy into a kennel and departed.

The wretched puppy deteriorated rapidly and progressively over the following three days. It yelped, it snapped, it bit at the bars of its kennel, its tongue lolled out of its mouth, it was unable to eat or drink. Towards the end it lay paralysed, whining feebly, eyes twitching. Three days after presentation the puppy died, as I expected.

I removed its head and sent it to the Veterinary Research Laboratory at Kabete, on the outskirts of Nairobi. As foreseen the brain was positive for rabies on the direct fluorescent antibody test. I conveyed this news to Dr Virdee, expressing the hope that all in-contacts had been traced and vaccinated and that, with the confirmation of the case, all concerned would now go on to receive a full course of injections. He assured me that that they would be taken care of. I hoped so.

These were the lucky ones.

One day an elderly African lady came to my surgery. She had heard, correctly, that I kept vials of human rabies vaccine in my fridge. I knew that, on Sundays or in the evening, getting vaccine to people who had been bitten by a rabid animal was a major priority. Chemists were closed and few doctors or clinics seemed to stock vaccine. So I, the vet, kept an emergency supply.

The lady came from Mau Narok, about 25 miles from Nakuru, on the high western edge of the Rift Valley. Three weeks previously she had been hoeing in her shamba with her husband when a rabid dog had suddenly appeared. Without warning the dog rushed at the pair, bent over, weeding their crop of young maize. The dog leapt at the husband, tearing open his cheek. As he staggered back the dog attacked the woman, biting her hand in the web between her thumb and forefinger. Hearing their shouting and the snarling of the dog, neighbours came running. They cornered the dog and beat it to death.

The bitten pair were taken to the local health clinic. There the wounds were cleaned and dressed. Injections of penicillin and tetanus toxoid were given, but no rabies vaccine.

Fifteen days later the husband developed the dread symptoms of rabies. Six days later he died.

Now his wife, realising that she might share the same horrifying fate as her husband came to me for help. I gave her the vaccine, wrote detailed instructions concerning injection intervals and where the vaccine should be given – in the upper arm and not, repeat not, in the buttock. She took the vaccine to a doctor I recommended and survived.

Sadly people continued to be bitten and continued to die across East Africa. The local papers told the dismal tale – '37 Karamajong die of rabies in Uganda,' 'Sixteen people have died of rabies in Kisumu District in the last few months,' 'Dar es Salaam, Wednesday – Rabies kills 12 – at least 12 people have died of rabies and 49 are critically ill in the northern Kilimanjaro region of Tanzania,' the official Tanzania news agency said today. 'There is no anti-rabies vaccine and no bullets to shoot stray dogs, cat and squirrels,' the agency quoted Regional Medical Officer E. E.

Kiwelu as saying – 'In fact, the sick are at home dying quietly, or some of them are already dead,' he said, adding that he had asked the government to order the army to shoot stray dogs. The news agency reported that '61 dogs in Kilimanjaro region have recently been found to have rabies,' 'T-9 dogs strike – the fierce rabid dogs known as T-9 have struck at Miathene sub-location of Kianjai Location, Meru district. One bit the right arm of a woman and injured her husband's leg. The dog also killed a cow and a dog.'

Day after day I was called out to yet another cow, horse or sheep which was reported to be behaving oddly. Soon I became expert at diagnosing rabies in the various species. Cattle tended to bellow hoarsely and continuously, strain as though they were constipated and drool copious volumes of saliva. Thinking that the animal had a foreign body lodged in its throat, people would carry out a manual exploratory examination of the mouth and pharynx, with potentially fatal results. Sometimes cattle and sheep were aggressive, chasing people and other cattle, smashing their way through fences and hedges, sometimes they stood quietly, staring blankly into the distance. Close observation might reveal some almost unapparent abnormality such as yawning, a slight twitching of the lip, a weakness of a leg. Docile sheep might charge a person on sight. Rabid horses were always an alarming sight and often highly dangerous. Because of their frequently irrational changes in behaviour close examination was not recommended. One moment they might be quietly contemplating the mysteries of the equine universe, the next rushing at you with snapping, foaming jaws. A distant scrutiny, even using binoculars, was recommended.

One day, after I had pregnancy-tested a batch of Friesian cattle belonging to Bruce Nightingale on his farm near Njoro, he asked me if I would look at one of his mares. 'She looks constipated to me. Not eating. Could be an impaction. You might need to give her a good dose of liquid paraffin. I've got some if you need it. But I'm not a vet, so over to you.' People were always telling me that they weren't vets. The inference was that, despite their lack of official recognition, they really did know as much, if not more, than the average vet, but because they didn't possess paper qualifications they weren't able to exercise their invaluable and unique hidden knowledge.

The mare was standing quietly in a small makeshift crush, one side of which was the wall of a stable. As I walked by the mare, en route to her rear, she bared her teeth and attempted to bite me. I looked questioningly at Bruce. 'Always does that with strangers. She's an absolute lamb with me and the syce. Must be your smell!' He laughed. As I soaped my arm prior to inserting it into the mare's rectum, I noticed that she was taking the weight off her feet by leaning against the stable wall. I recalled with frightful clarity my near-terminal encounter with the rabid pony at Blackthorn School. I pushed my gloved arm into the mare and she strained against me. Was that a normal reaction? Could be. But the rectal contents were normal. As was the temperature. Mmm. I returned to her head. On her upper lip was a small healing wound. I pointed this out to Bruce. 'Probably cut it on one of those water troughs. We saw 40-gallon drums in half. Just the job.'

'Right, can we let her out and see what she does.'

The mare trotted off in sprightly fashion to rejoin a group of horses in the lower half of the paddock. As I watched her she suddenly swerved and rushed at one horse and attempted to bite it. That horse took to its heels. The mare then attacked another horse and then another.

I turned to Bruce. 'She's probably got rabies. We need to get the other horses out of the field and if possible get her into this stable. Once that's done, no one must go near her and I'll come back in the morning.' He nodded.

During the night the mare collapsed and in the morning was found lying on her side.

Her legs were thrashing as though she was in a full gallop. Although she was unable to sit or stand she was in all-out attack mode. Anything or anybody near her head provoked an immediate baring of her teeth and a desperate lunge towards the object of her aggression.

'Got to put her down, Bruce.' He nodded. 'My best mare.' They always are.

With a modicum of care I gave her a jugular injection of a German cardiotoxic drug called T61. Using a gun was out of the question. The brain was needed for diagnostic purposes and I didn't want rabid brain tissue scattered over me or the grass.

'I've been thinking,' said Bruce as I straightened up. 'About a month ago, when I went to open her stable, first thing in the morning, a dog – a stray – rushed out and vanished. It must have bitten her on the lip. You know how curious horses are, always sniffing and nosing at anything unusual. Lucky I wasn't bitten as well.'

'Well,' I said. 'Keep your fingers crossed that it hasn't bitten any others.'

Donning shoulder-length gloves, I removed the mare's head, and, with expected difficulty, we transported it to the lab in Nairobi. Back came the anticipated result – positive for rabies.

The crossed fingers were of no avail. Two more horses developed rabies and died.

Bruce was far from being alone. On his farm on the lip of Menengai Crater, Captain Hugh Barclay had the misfortune to lose two Friesian cows and the same number of horses to rabies. One horse with a high-stepping gait involving its hind legs, generalised twitching and abrasions on its lower lip, ended up stuck in a ditch all night, where it died. On Mike Skinner's farm at Molo a rabid horse rushed around a paddock, attacking other horses and cattle. It also died during the night.

But it was dogs which were most frequently affected and which evoked most fear among the public. Horror stories were rampant. On the Galana Ranch in Coast Province a friend's servant was bitten by a dog. Taken to hospital he was only given tetanus antitoxin. Five weeks later he died of rabies. In Western Province a rabid boy attacked and bit other patients in hospital. Near Nanyuki at the foot of Mt. Kenya a trap set to catch hyenas caught instead a rabid man. A child attacked by a rabid dog at Lanet, near where we lived, had his ears torn off. A rabid dog at Prairie Estate bit four children, before being killed. Being shorter and smaller than adults, children are more likely to be bitten on sensitive areas such as the face or neck which, being closer to the brain and rich in blood and nerves, is much more likely to be fatal. The virus travels along nerve trunks en route to the central nervous system. If you are bitten on your big toe it may take months for the virus to get to your CNS and there is time to get a post-exposure course of vaccine. But a bite on the face is a matter of extreme emergency.

I was on the front line. Having been vaccinated on numerous occasions I assumed I was immune. But there was always the lurking thought that perhaps I might be the unlucky one who failed to respond.

Vincent Luis of Njoro brought in a dog which had bitten a man on his toe. I confined it in one of my kennels where it almost tore the door off its hinges. When it died I dispatched its head to the lab. Positive for rabies.

Jane Walls was driving into Nakuru. She had her Jack Russell terrier with her in the car, when it had a fit, lasting a mere minute. So she brought it to the surgery. I suggested that I keep the small creature for observation. By that evening it was in a state of terminal frenzy, snarling and attacking the wire of the kennel door with all the strength that it possessed. In the morning there was a heap of dislodged and broken bloodstained teeth lying in front of the kennel door and the terrier was lying panting and moaning on the wooden floor. Donning gloves I administered a humane injection to terminate its sufferings. Once again all in-contacts had to be vaccinated and once again we had a positive result.

My rotund Italian/Pakistani receptionist had departed. She had taken the plunge and had gone to try her hand in Italy, the land of her father and which she was visiting for the first time. I wished her well. In her place came Mandy Gore, a sharp featured, sharper tongued virago. In her first week in my employ she brought into the surgery one morning a puppy which she had found lying beside the road. 'It looked so sad and sweet, lying there all alone,' she declared. 'I just couldn't leave it.' I rolled my eyes in despair. 'I'll just put it in one of the kennels and take it home tonight.' She never did take it home, that night, or any other. I went to look at it in the late afternoon. The puppy was standing staring fixedly into the corner of the kennel. Its lips were retracted and it was growling softly. When it heard me it turned round and approached, wagging its tail in a friendly fashion.

'Mandy,' I said. 'I want the puppy to stay here overnight. I don't want you to take it home.'

'Why on earth not,' she retorted indignantly. 'My daughter was so looking forward to seeing it.'

'I'll give it some meat and milk and check it in the morning. It'll be OK.' I knew that it wasn't OK and next morning when I went to examine it the puppy was flat on its side, bent over backwards with its head almost touching its tail, in the classic position of opisthotonos, unable to rise and attempting to bite anything within reach. So, once again all possible in-contacts had to be vaccinated, in this case at my expense. Now that the puppy was obviously rabid, Mandy disowned it. Mandy was bad enough at the best of times. I didn't want her to be rabid as well.

Although many affected dogs were subject to outbursts of furious madness, which is the form most people consider to be typical of the disease, in fact most cases took the 'dumb' form, in which depression and localised and general paralysis were the main features. The one feature the two forms had in common was the eyes. They were invariably affected, usually with a fixed, glaring expression. I could tell if a dog had rabies just by looking at its eyes.

Although death was almost certain, it was not entirely so and out of hundreds of cases I saw one puppy and one cow showing classic symptoms of rabies, which did not die. The situation was further complicated by the presence of unknown carrier animals and the existence of rabies-related viruses such as Mokola and Duvenhage.

—*—

Elderly bachelors Tom and Pat Dixon lived in a run-down house off Nakuru's main street. Here they resided in spectacular squalor. In the late '50s, with their widowed sister May, they had arrived from India, where they had all been born. It was downhill after that.

May took up residence in the Stag's Head Hotel on the main street, where she specialised in feeding a monstrous regiment of cats. Tom and Pat moved into their own considerably more basic quarters.

From a privileged world of tiger bagging while perched in a howdah on the back of an elephant, diplomatic balls in Simla, punkah wallahs keeping them cool during the hot season to being drawn around Dehli by rickshaw, it was a steady decline to virtual poor white status. They were Anglo/Irish with all the easy charm of that race. All three were good looking and generous with what they had. Both Tom and Pat had been with the Ministry of Works in India and when they were 'Indianised' they came to Kenya to take up similar employment.

Now retired, they divided their time between golf and their huge collection of nondescript dogs, 25 in all. These lived within the large enclosed compound surrounding their house. As the dogs all had access to the house, conditions therein are best imagined rather than described. The house had no carpets on the floors, no curtains on the windows, filthy walls where the dogs rubbed against them and junk everywhere. The kitchen was a blackened noisome cell. If there had ever been a garden it had long ago been destroyed by the ceaseless, destructive activities of the canine horde.

Overseeing the mob was foolish, grinning Minyao, a gentle African of extraordinary forbearance, who, together with his adolescent son, did his best to keep some semblance of order in the pack. He also doubled as cook and general factotum. Lucky were Tom and Pat that their long residence in the sub-continent had rendered them immune to the most virulent of life-threatening gastro-intestinal diseases. Otherwise they would have been carried off long since.

One day Tom arrived at the surgery door in his battered blue Cortina, a vehicle, even then, harking back to a bygone age. In the back, seated on a layer of sacks, were nine-year-old Misty, a large brown bitch, and Minyao.

'Hello, Hugh,' said Tom. 'I've brought Misty to see you. She can't get up. Eats all right. Drinks all right. Just can't stand.'

Misty was overweight but that did not explain her inability to get to her feet.

Five months previously I had visited Tom and Pat to vaccinate all their dogs with rabies vaccine. As all were running free, all had to be individually caught. It was a canine rodeo. Misty was the one exception. She could not be caught. Extremely nervous and eager to bite, it proved impossible to catch her. But as the compound was completely and securely enclosed, the possibility of unauthorised entry by animal or man was deemed to be impossible.

Now she was quiet and tranquil. 'Right, Tom,' I said. 'We'd better keep her here and watch her. I'll keep you informed.'

Tom patted Misty's head and drove off in a backwash of exhaust fumes.

For three days Misty sat in her kennel, eating her head off. Apart from not being able to stand, she appeared to be quite normal. On the fourth day she was found dead without having shown any improvement or deterioration. Her brain proved to be positive for rabies. What had introduced the infection was never discovered, as nothing larger than a rat could have got into the Dixon's compound.

This was not the first intrusion of the dread disease into the Dixon family.

In India, May's husband was an inspector of police, a very senior position. The circumstances are unclear, but one day he came into contact with a rabid dog. Appropriate action was taken but he became convinced that he had been infected and would die a terrible death. He brooded more and more until he could take no more. While on leave in Britain he shot himself.

—*—

Mike Sugden, whose foal had so dramatically severed its jugular, was having a well-deserved post-prandial gin one afternoon, when his peace was rudely disturbed by a fearful commotion in his kitchen.

'Can't yoo boogers leave a man in quiet after 'is loonch?' he bellowed. The racket continued, now accompanied by barking and screaming.

'Fookin' 'ell!'Mike groaned, heaving his bulk out his armchair, 'no peace for the righteous!' and staggered towards the kitchen.

He opened the door and came across a scene from Bedlam. His four dogs – a large ridgeback, two terriers and a lurcher, were backed into a corner. All were bleeding from various wounds and all were in a state of obvious terror, barking hysterically. Perched on top of the kitchen table, holding a baby and cowering against the wall, was the servant girl. Both were bedaubed with blood. Facing them was a cat, its fur standing up on end, hissing and snarling and in full attack mode. The cat heard the door open and in a flash turned and launched itself at Mike's throat. Mike was faster and slammed the door. He heard its claws scrabbling against the door.

'Booger that,' he thought.

Grunting, he limped to his bedroom, where, beneath his four poster, he kept his shotgun. This was no time for Dead Eye Dick stuff with the revolver which he habitually wore in a holster beneath his left armpit.

By the time he had returned to the kitchen the hubbub had subsided.

He cautiously opened the door. 'Where's it gone?' he asked the quivering girl.

'Li toka. Nafikiri lienda karibu nyumba ya farasi.' (It ran out. I think it went towards the stables.)

Mike hobbled out of the house, bellowing for Arap Sang, his head syce. Lop-eared Sang came running. 'Did you see that blooody cat?' panted Mike.

'Ndiyo, bwana, it went into that stable, huko – over there.' He pointed with his chin – towards the stallion stable.

'Fook!' said Mike. He could hear the stallion whinnying and the sound of hooves crashing against the stable wall. As they reached the stable door the cat rushed out, took a passing lunge at Arap Sang, and darted into the adjacent stable, which, by happy chance, was empty. Mike cocked both barrels. 'Right, Sang, when I say so, swing open the door, and stand well back.' Sang did as instructed. As the cat came for Mike he let fire with both barrels. There was an almighty boom. Mike was a crack shot and the cat never knew what hit it. There was just enough of it left to confirm the diagnosis.

Peter Macharia, a nine-year-old schoolboy, was on his way home. Peter lived with his mother and sister in a two room shack on the outskirts of Njoro. Peter's tie was loosened, his shirt tails hung over his shorts, school was over and he was looking forward to a good meal of ugali and sukuma wiki (maize porridge and spinach).

He kicked a stone along the road and whistled.

Suddenly he screamed. A cat had leapt onto his head and was biting his ears. Peter ran, with his feline attacker still clinging to his shoulders. People stared, horrified at the sight of the boy, face streaming with blood and with the demented creature perched on his head. A man came cycling in the opposite direction. He had been to fetch water and had several full debes strapped to his bike. He stopped and with instinctive intuition, seized a full debe and threw it full in Peter's face. The cat leapt to the ground and disappeared.

Peter was taken to Nakuru where he was treated and given a course of anti-rabies vaccine by Iranian Dr Malakooti. He recovered, but never got over his phobia of cats.

—*—

Berna and I had three dogs. They were all cross cairn terriers – small, dark, hairy jobs – rejoicing in the names Dudu, Yuppie and Haggis. They had free rein in our large garden, outside of which they never ventured.

One Sunday a strange yellow dog came staggering down the hill towards our gate. It yelped intermittently as it approached. Our three dogs gave immediate tongue but they hung back. They seemed to fear the stranger. I rushed to close the gate. The dog continued on its way and vanished.

A week later we received a peremptory summons from the local chief. A child had been bitten by a dog and the mother claimed that the dog in question was one of ours.

The summons was delivered by a uniformed flunkey. I invited him in, showed him our three terriers and proffered their up-to-date vaccination certificates. The man studied them and then cautiously approached our dogs, who sat looking at him.

The chief's office was on the other side of the railway line, about 200 yards away, so we walked there, Berna and I, with the messenger.

The office was dark and dingy. We were ushered in. The chief was sitting, head bowed, behind a cluttered desk. He did not look up, but motioned for us to sit on a couple of metal chairs, lined up against the indescribably filthy wall. A headscarfed woman and a child were sitting against the opposite wall. Our accusers. The child had a grimy bandage wrapped around his left leg, below the knee.

The room did nothing to raise the spirits. A naked bulb hung from its flex from the middle of the ceiling. The window curtains, instead of being drawn aside, were tied in knots, the glass so covered in dirt as to be virtually opaque. A large bluebottle blundered through the stale air, finally crash-landing into an impressive spider's web, where it struggled and buzzed, before falling silent. I could see scatterings of rat droppings on the binders of the mouldering files stacked ceiling high in the corner. The feelers of a giant cockroach appeared from beneath a cupboard, followed a few seconds later by their owner. He ventured a few paces, before retreating to safety.

We waited in an oppressive silence. The trapped bluebottle gave a terminal buzz.

For about ten minutes the chief did nothing but study whatever was on the desk in front of him. Finally he spoke.

'So, I am informed that your dog attacked and bit this child. What have you to say?'

He stared at us. It was not a friendly stare.

I remembered the yellow dog. 'Please ask this child to tell us the colour of the dog which bit him.' The mother shifted in her seat and muttered something to her son. Too late. 'It was yellow,' he said.

'Now,' I said, 'ask your messenger the colour of our dogs.' He did.

The chief was not pleased. He turned on the woman and shouted at her. 'What do you think you are doing? Wasting our time! Accusing this mzungu when you knew you were lying! Wewe ni mjinga! (You are a fool!) Toka! Toka!' (Get out!)

'Labda iko mbwa ingine,' (perhaps there's another dog), she hissed.

'Open your mouth again and I'll have you arrested!' the chief shouted.

I raised a finger. 'The dog which bit this child was almost certainly rabid. Now, despite this woman making these despicable false allegations I am prepared to give her human vaccine at cost price. Otherwise this child may die. Tell her to come to my surgery to collect the vaccine and then she can take the child to a doctor to be injected.'

The chief spoke to the woman. She looked sullen and shifty. She had missed her chance to milk the mzungu.

I repeated my message. 'This child may die. He *must* get vaccinated. I have the vaccine in my fridge. I don't give a shit about *her* but the child is in mortal danger.'

Berna and I left.

The woman never appeared.

Later we heard that five weeks after our interrogation the child contracted rabies, and died.

Three months after the death of this child, *another* of this woman's children was bitten by another rabid dog. The mother had learned her bitter lesson. This child was vaccinated and survived.

—✳—

Another child stood in my surgery looking at a kennelled Labrador. A locked door had been opened and the child had slipped in unnoticed. She was nibbling a piece of bread. She walked across to the Labrador. 'Hello, doggie,' she said. 'How are you? Are you hungry? You look hungry. Here, have some of my bread.' She offered the bread to the dog, which sniffed at it, but refused to eat it. Saliva from the dog's mouth drooled onto the bread.

The child's mother called the child and both left to go to the nearby butchery to buy some lamb chops. When they returned the mother asked me what I thought was wrong with the dog.

'Looks like rabies to me,' I said.

'Whaaat! Sophie, what did you do with that bread?'

'Well the doggie didn't want it, so I ate it.'

'Whaaat!'

Earlier that week Jack Upperton, a master at Haverford House prep school at Gilgil had phoned me. Jack was a bit of a shock-headed Peter, with a great mop of electrified hair frizzed out style. He sported a Pancho Villa Mexican moustache and wore a gold ring in one ear. But Jack's credentials were impeccable. Of gentle birth, he spoke like an aristocrat and had attended the very best of public schools. He taught maths.

Jack needed some advice. 'Terribly sorry to trouble you, Hugh, old chap, but Lucy, my black lab has disappeared. Vanished. Problem is, she gave birth to five pups three weeks ago. They are still suckling but now they have no mother to suckle. So how do I feed the orphans?'

I gave Jack the requisite advice and turned to more immediate matters. There was a full blown riot in the street outside the surgery and a pounding mob fleeing a phalanx of armed police was trying to force its way into my premises. They succeeded.

Thirty six hours later Jack was on the blower again. 'Apologies once more, Hugh. Lucy has returned. But she's not right. Got this strange look.

Can't eat because her tongue is swollen and sticking out and she seems unable to close her mouth.'

'Jack,' I said, 'this could be rabies. Isolate her and the pups. Don't go near her head. Then get her into a crate or something and bring her in.'

'But,' said Jack, 'she was vaccinated 12 months ago.'

'Really?' I replied. I could not recall having given Lucy any injections. 'Yes, Darcy did it.'

'Darcy?' I replied.

'Yes, he got the vaccine from a government vet and stabbed it in. Seemed like a good idea at the time. Cost virtually nothing.' Meaning, I thought, compared to what I might have charged. Well, now it's going to cost a fair whack.

Eligible bachelor Darcy Macalister was a charming and persuasive pseudo-Scot who farmed an inherited spread of prime land at Olongai in the Rift Valley. Like many wealthy people he was careful both with his own money and, more importantly, that of others. Educated at Harrow and Cambridge, he had not a trace of Scottish accent. Although his forebears and current relations owned extensive tracts of the Highlands, most followed Samuel Johnson's observation and took the high road which led them to England and the colonies.

Whether the vaccine given to Lucy was improperly stored or administered, or whether Lucy had failed to respond in a normal manner was now academic. The manure had hit the fan.

Lucy duly arrived at my surgery and soon after there followed the chance encounter between her and the concerned child, who was our very own second-born, Sophie. Hence the vocalised horror of her mother, who knew the form. Sophie underwent a full course of vaccination and was none the worse for her voluntary ingestion of Lucy's saliva.

Meanwhile, back at Haverford House there was more than a mite of concern when my presumptive diagnosis was relayed to the head. Half of the pupils and not a few of the teachers had played with friendly Lucy and her pups prior to her disappearance and return. As rabid animals may for a few days prior to the development of symptoms discharge infective saliva, the concern was justified. The panic bell was rung loud and clear across the land.

Poor Lucy went downhill rapidly, accompanied by all the usual horrid symptoms. She barked uncontrollably, she salivated profusely, she was unable to eat or drink, became totally paralysed and died two and half days after admission.

Meanwhile her pups, other innocent victims, were destroyed.

Taking the usual precautions I removed Lucy's head and sent it to the lab, where it proved positive.

The school took the sensible and only possible line. All pupils and staff were given a full course of five vaccinations. The cost was considerable, but was passed on to the parents, who being who they were, could well afford it.

Chapter Twenty Three

FIRE AND BRIMSTONE

Why do unpleasing events always seem to occur in threes? Has any scientist, eminent or otherwise, come up with an explanation for this intriguing phenomenon? There is a PhD waiting out there for someone with initiative and an inquiring mind to solve this ongoing riddle, one which has troubled generations of luckless sufferers.

A week after the Haverford House misfortune, Berna and I were in a dental surgery in Nairobi. We had made an appointment for Rona to see an orthodontist in order to correct some minor dental malocclusion. As we waited for Rona to vacate the horizontal chair, the receptionist's phone rang.

The girl handed me the phone. 'It's for you.' I raised my eyebrows. I took the receiver. 'Hello?'

'Moses here from the surgery.' Well done on tracking me down, I thought. Mobiles were still about 20 years into the future.

'Yes, Moses, what's the problem?' There must be one. Otherwise he wouldn't be phoning me.

'It's the safe.'

'What about it?'

'It's been stolen!'

'What!?' The safe was bolted to the wall and weighed a ton. 'How?'

'Well, I heard that twelve men came in through the roof, prised it off the wall, broke open the back door, loaded it onto a handcart and took it away down towards the lake.'

This took the proverbial biscuit. I had had my surgical bag stolen on one occasion from my car, to be found later, buried in a maize patch. I spent hours in court over that one, until the accused was sentenced. Then I had had the back window of my Peugeot removed one night while I slept in order to extract a camera which I had carelessly left on the back seat.

Berna had had her car tape deck nicked and had her spare tyre whipped.

Now we were moving into a more professional league.

The safe had been found by some children, abandoned at daybreak on a patch of waste ground. The back had been cut open, presumably by an acetylene welding torch, and the cash, about 30,000/-, taken. This must have taken hours of unremitting toil as the safe was several inches thick. Fortunately the thieves had failed to gain entrance into a separate compartment containing valuable insurance documents, spare keys and identity cards.

Discovered, overtaken by daylight, or exhausted by hours of cutting and bashing, they had abandoned their task and had decamped.

—*—

Strapped into my Sopwith Camel I had just crossed the Hun lines.

The wind whistled musically in the struts of my trusty plane. I peered over the edge of the open cockpit. Far below I could see the trenches and dugouts of the square-headed enemy, where I imagined them to be drinking schnapps and munching sauerkraut, prior to launching an attack on our gallant Tommies.

Suddenly, above the roar of my engine, I heard the chattering of machine gun fire, and saw the sudden appearance of bullet holes in the fragile fabric of my wings.

I was under attack!

Glancing behind me I saw the dreaded outline of a blood red triplane.

The Red Baron was on my tail!

I put the Camel into a near vertical dive. Eyes driven into the back of my skull, I howled earthwards. Another burst of machine gun fire told me that my pursuer was right behind me. I pulled up the nose, and, hauling back on the joystick with all my strength, shot up vertically in an effort to gain height and advantage over my opponent. Before I could stall, I whipped the plane onto its back, barrel rolled right side up and searched the sky for sign of the baron.

The sky was empty.

A staccato series of violent hammer blows to my back and a shrill ringing in my ears, told me I had been hit. Smoke was pouring from the engine, one wing was in tatters and a curling tongue of flame licked hungrily at my flying boots. I was going down – fast. I could see the upturned faces of the square-heads staring up at me. They were getting closer and closer as I plunged towards them. I could see them raising their rifles. Bullets started to whizz past my ears. It was only a matter of time before one found its mark. Despite the icy wind whipping past my ears I was drenched in fear-fuelled sweat. Any moment now and I would be just another statistic, a charred and atomised relic, a dark stain on the wrong side of the frontline. A round struck my left shoulder, then the right. I could no longer grasp the controls. My arms hung limply. The end was now. More ringing in my ears.

'Hugh! Hugh! Wake up! Wake up! The phone!'

Berna was shaking my shoulder. 'Whaaa.. whaaa..?' The phone was on my side of the bed. I lunged for it, knocked it to the floor and scrabbled for the receiver, found it and, 'Yes?' Must be a mare stuck foaling, or a cow calving, what else would make someone phone at this time? What time is it anyway? I found the switch for the bedside light – 4am for Pete's sake!

'Jambo, bwana, wewe ni daktari?' said a gravelly African voice. (Is that the daktari?)

'Ndiyo,' I croaked. (Yes)

'Mimi askari ya duka karibu na wewe.' (I'm the guard of the shop next to your surgery.) Now that I was partially awake I recognised the voice. It was that of the Boran night askari who supposedly guarded the premises adjacent to mine. He was an affable, piratical rogue, hailing from Garba Tulla, a God-forsaken, fly-blown collection of hovels clustered beside the corrugated highway which connected Isiolo to Wajir, in Kenya's Northern Frontier District.

'Iko tabu gani?' (What's the problem?) I asked.

'Iko moto kubwa,' came the reply, 'kwisha kula duka ingine, na sasa karibu kula yako. Kuja upesi! (There's a big fire. It's already finished eating other shops and now it's about to eat yours. Come quickly!)

We threw on some clothes, checked that Rona and Sophie were asleep, alerted house girl Esther and left at high speed. As we turned onto the main road, some seven kilometres from Nakuru and the threatened surgery, we could clearly see the orange glow of a massive fire in the town. Huge clouds of smoke were boiling upwards into the clear night sky. We broke all previous speed records as we howled along the deserted road. Tearing along Kenyatta Avenue, the town's main street, we screeched into Club Lane. Enormous flames were belching out of the buildings next to the surgery. Flames were leaping up the surgery wall to a height 50 feet above the roof. A horrid crackling filled the air. A sudden crash and the roof of the next door building collapsed. A mob of goggling onlookers milled in street party fashion in the lane, obviously looking forward to the pleasing prospect of the fiery demise of my own building. A pair of slack-jawed policemen mingled happily with the crowd.

We drove round the corner and parked in the club forecourt. For a minute we sat in stunned silence, trying in vain to take stock of what looked like a hopeless situation.

The glare of the flames lit up the car park with a lurid yellow light. Great gouts of orange flame leapt skywards. A huge burst of red sparks shot up into the night sky. Berna and I just sat and stared. At any moment we expected the surgery to go up like a Roman candle.

'Right, we'd better go and have a closer look. Join the mob. Be in at the kill.'

'Bring your keys,' said Berna. I stared at her. 'Right then, let's go.'

We ran back round the corner. As we did so there was a great whoosh! and another vital organ of the building next door collapsed. The crowd gave a throaty roar of approval.

The surgery still stood intact, a miniature, plebian version of St. Paul's during the blitz. But the end could not be long in coming. As we stood gaping amidst the sweaty rabble, an inspector of police approached us.

'A fire engine is on the way coming. Open the door, get your stuff out. There may be just time before the fire takes hold.'

Berna and I looked at each other. Then we elbowed the mob aside and rushed at the door. The door had two locks, top and bottom. They had to be opened together before the door could be also opened. In my frenzy I was able to open one lock but not the other. As I fiddled frantically with the keys, a huge dark blue shadow loomed up at my elbow.

'Stand aside, my flend,' said the figure, which was that of a constable about seven feet tall and three wide, 'we know how to blake down doors.'

And with that he raised his oak-tree sized right leg, foot encased in a massive hobnailed boot, and, with one mighty kick the door was open. To my amazement the lights still worked. Inside everything looked surreally normal. If it were not for the oven-like heat, the roar of the flames busily consuming my neighbour's building and the chanting and stamping of the impi battalion in the street outside, it might have been business as usual.

'Hello, Tarquin, old fruit, sorry I'm late. Bit of a conflagration next door, what? So you think Fupi's got tick fever again eh? Well bring him in and pop him on the table.'

The door to the consulting room suffered the same fate as that opening onto Club Lane. Once again the flatfoot's size 14 sabots rendered the locks null and void. As I staggered within perspiration burst from every pore. The heat was terrific. The walls were shaking and quivering. At any moment I expected them to collapse. In a spasm of deranged curiosity I touched the exterior wall and gave a sharp yelp. It was red hot.

The giant gendarme barked an order and the waiting legions surged through the open doors. Phones were ripped from the walls, tables were dragged into the street, cabinets and cupboards splintered as they were sundered from their moorings, kennels, chairs, files, weighing scales, steriliser, dehorning shears, instruments by the hundred, drugs, reference books, filing cabinets, all ended up in a monstrous pile in the street, guarded by Berna and an ineffectual brace of constables. The chaos was total.

Just as the surgery was emptied, the fire engine arrived, and proceeded to hose down the threatened surgery wall and the now-incinerated adjacent building. The surgery contents, having narrowly escaped the threat of fire, were now in danger of being destroyed by water as the drainless street slowly filled from side to side with surplus fire engine H2O. As rapidly as we could we piled everything onto the tables. Club Lane had no street lights, so it was difficult to be sure everything was safe and sound. Furtive pickpocket-like figures flitted to and fro in the darkness. Across the street the doused fire hissed and crackled.

Dawn was slow in coming and when it did, the scene was one of depressing devastation. Saturated files, legless chairs, mounds of instruments, a cabinet with its glass shelf smashed, the legs of tables standing in ankle deep water. It was inconceivable that nothing had been stolen, that everything was intact. And there came the galling thought that, had we not taken everything out, as the inspector had advised, everything would still be lying safe and snug inside the surgery, rather than outside, looking as though it had been trampled on by a herd of elephants. If that fire engine had arrived just a few minutes earlier.....

But with the coming of daylight came timely assistance in the shape of valued friends. Berna had been on the club telephone. Nessie and Martin Evans drove in from Rongai to help shift our stuff. As did the Gilanis. Patti Neylan loaned us her pickup. Moses cycled in early, arriving at 7am. Speed was now vital. Tens of thousands of people were now surging along the street, intent on looking and pillaging. Soon we would be overwhelmed, outnumbered, outmanned and outwomanned. Seven premises had been gutted so there were no pickings to be had there. We were a soft target. Frantically we piled as much as we could onto the pickup. Hands were grabbing things. A child scampered down the street with a pair of towels streaming out behind him. A woman grabbed a bucket. A man reached out to take a pair of gumboots off the back of the pickup. I bellowed at him. He backed off, looking aggrieved. It was time to go.

At the house we took stock. A lot of stuff was missing. Our helpers had helped themselves to over 80,000/- worth of equipment. We were insured, but replacing some items would be difficult. I returned to the surgery and, with the staff, spent the whole day cleaning up the mess, repairing doors, replacing locks and trying to treat patients amid the debris. Next door the remains of the gutted building still smouldered. Glue-sniffing kids were dragging away what they could find – sheets of corrugated iron, half burnt planks, window frames. We ferried buckets of water and poured them onto the smoking mounds of red-hot ash and cinders. A phone call to try to obtain the help of the private presidential fire brigade went unheeded. It was Saturday afternoon now, and for hour after hour Berna and I lugged buckets round the corner and sloshed them onto the embers. We seemed to be getting nowhere. It was like trying to extinguish an erupting Mt. Etna by pissing into the crater.

When we returned at 3am on Sunday morning to monitor the situation we were met by a fiery bed of crimson coals. Plumes of acrid smoke drifted across the street. Also drifting across the street as we surveyed a scene which would have dismayed even the most fearless of Fijian firewalkers came three members of the paramilitary General Service Unit. Red bereted and arrogant, armed with automatic weapons, their burnished boots glinting in the firelight, they were not friendly.

'Wat are you doing here at three o'clock in the morning? Do you know that we could arrest you for loitering?'

At 3am Berna was not in the mood for light conversation. 'That's my husband's surgery there and at any minute it is liable to go up in flames, while all *you* can do is polish your boots and sit there warming your bottoms!'

This did not go down well with the men in uniform, especially coming from a woman.

They hissed like angry cobras and bristled like circling wolves.

'Madam, we are here to protect property from looters and thieves, of which there are many. If the fire looks like spreading we will at once inform the Nakuru fire brigade, who will swing into action.'

We both laughed.

'Swing into action? If they come as quickly as they did yesterday morning,' I said, 'there'll be nothing left for them to swing into! That's why we're here.'

They moved closer, intimidating and threatening. One of them, a huge, bullnecked, glowering individual with the build and demeanour of an all-in wrestler, held out a meaty palm.

'Nipa sisi kitu kidogo!' (Give us a little samthing!)

Dumbfounded, we stared at them – big, strapping, gun-toting men, togged up in their smart, clean uniforms. We presumed they were adequately paid. Yet here they were, demanding money, almost at the point of a gun, from those who, via their taxes, were contributing towards their salaries.

They moved closer still.

I rummaged in my pocket, finding nothing but loose change. Forty five shillings and ten cents..

Giving the Idi Amin look-alike my brightest smile, I poured the coins into his cupped palm, which awaited my contribution like a collection basket proffered by a vicar's flunkey to a reluctant parishioner.

The coins vanished as though dropped into a dark well.

The fingers of his other hand gave a peremptory snap and he rubbed his thumb and forefinger together. 'Ingine!' the giant demanded. (More!)

'Hakuna ingine! (There is no more!) I shouted in sudden rage. 'I've just had 80,000/- stolen from my surgery last night and there is no more! Hakuna! Sikia?' (None, do you understand?)

'And if you ask for any more, we'll report you to your commanding officer,' barked Berna.

'Madam,' the ogre replied, 'I *am* the commanding officer! You may go!'

We spent what was left of the night pouring buckets of water onto the threatening embers, and vocalising our contempt for the so-called Guardians of the Law in particular, and random, light-fingered opportunists in general.

—*—

After this sort of thing, getting away to climb a remote mountain was actively therapeutic. Thrashing one's way through dense thickets of flesh-tearing thorns or crawling up some beetling crag was positively relaxing compared to the daily stresses of life at the sharp end.

On certain very clear, rain-washed days, when I was engaged in winkling out a long-dead foetus from a near-dead cow, mare or heifer, or suturing an unappreciative stallion, I would lift my eyes to the heavens in search of succour and enlightenment and espy, far to the north-west, at the furthest edge of vision, a sharply topped purple mountain. This was Tiati, a noble peak in the land of the pastoral and warlike East Pokot. On most days it lay hidden, screened from rude public view by the ever-present heat haze and plumes of ochreous dust rising from the surrounding thorn covered plains. Mysterious and rarely climbed, it beckoned the dormant climber, even more so when he was on his long suffering knees, praying that both he and his patient be soon delivered from their current predicament.

Stanley Whittle was my climbing partner on this occasion. Berna was encumbered with the cares of motherhood. Besides, the Shompole episode was still clearly etched in her memory and she was not keen to repeat the experience. Stan was a fine fellow, reliable, efficient, possessing an equable temperament – and a Toyota pickup. He did, however, have two distinct disadvantages as far as I was concerned. He was tall, very tall, about six foot six, with legs which appeared to sprout from somewhere near his armpits. He was also about fifteen years my junior. I could see that I was going to have to run to keep up with him.

Stan lived with his wife Tabitha at Njoro, some twelve miles from Nakuru. Rising betimes, I crept out of the house. As I did so I advised Berna with the optimism of ignorance that I would be back by teatime on the morrow.

By 6.30 we were on the road, heading due north towards Lake Baringo and Tiati. The road was now carpeted with an indeterminate layer of bitumen, sufficient to allow us to move at hitherto unattained speeds through the bush. This was just as well, because once abeam of the lake, some 60 miles from Njoro, the tarmac ended with brutal finality. One moment we were zipping along, a song on our lips, hair ruffled and uplifted by a refreshing breeze, the next labouring from rut to rut and from boulder to boulder, with the first unwelcome trickles of sweat beading our dusty brows. Normally I would have vented my opinion regarding the surface of the road in plain unvarnished Anglo-Saxon prose. Stan, before his union with the fair Tabby, would have done the same, rending the air with four-lettered vim, letting off pent-up steam, lessening tension and extending his allotted earthly span. Now all that was part of his wicked past. Under the new matriarchal regime, to stub one's toe and let out an oath was verboten. To ingest so much as a dry rusk without having given due thanks to one's Maker was almost worthy of transportation. Alcohol was taboo and all flamboyance and frivolity in dress or behaviour were severely sanctioned. Stan was a changed man. I had hoped that once freed, albeit temporarily, from his matrimonial bonds, he might have unwound, torn open his hair shirt and sunk a Tusker as soon as he was out of sight of the happy home. But Tabby's talons had sunk deep into his vitals. Her iron grip held him fast by his quivering gonads and I could see that he was doomed. So I stayed my pent up verbal flow, bowing my head and giving thanks to my Maker that my own Beloved was a free-living giver and taker, with no conjugal hang-ups. And charming and attractive and damned good looking, all those things which Tabby wasn't.

Past the derelict shacks of Loruk we rattled. In the spindly shade old men lay asleep, stretched out as though they had just died, necks propped on their head rests. No one seemed to be awake or to notice our passing. After another hour or so of more Toyota bashing we were in the southern vicinity of Nginyang, the nerve centre of East Pokot, another dispiriting collection of humpies and iron-roofed lean-tos, teetering on the edge of the Burususwa river. As we approached the ragged outskirts a lone figure sprang into the road and waved us down. This turned out to be the chief of the area. When we told him we were on our way to climb Tiati he looked grave. 'Ah my flends, you have a hard task ahead of you. The mountain is fa, very fa, there is no water, the road is very bad, the people there do not like strangers, especially they do not like the wazungu, the sun is too fierce, the bush is full of wild animals.' I looked at him. 'What is your name?' I asked.

'Jeremiah – Jeremiah Koskei,' he replied. We dropped Jeremiah off at the bridge which spanned the river. The bridge had been partially washed away in recent floods. Debris in the form of branches and tree trunks hung 20 feet above the river bed.

A picturesque knot of Pokot women, obsidian-eyed, clad in skins, mounds of red beads encircling their necks, dark features expressionless, watched silently as we drove past and onto the road to the Kito Pass and Tiati. Now the road was uphill all the way, and the chief was right – it was very bad. As on the road to Nginyang, we saw no other vehicles. A breakdown therefore was not advisable. We crossed innumerable luggas. Some were soft and sandy. Others were obstacle courses of rocks and cunningly concealed tank traps. To the accompaniment of a worrying crescendo of bangs and rattles we crashed our way to the other side. The edges of these luggas were sometimes sheer, so that time had to be spent finding a way down to the dry river bed. Going full tilt was to be avoided. The prospect of being embedded, even temporarily, in the bedrock of East Pokot did not appeal.

The Pokot are a fiercely independent people, indifferent to, if not actively intolerant of strangers, strongly traditional, conservative, and hostile towards their tribal neighbours, the Turkana to the north and Samburu to the east. They are not a demonstrative lot. They don't wave cheerily to passing Wazungu as do the extrovert Samburu. They tend to stare in a rather disconcerting way, fingering their arrows and spears, making you wonder just what would happen if you did break down. On the other side of the Kito Pass, at a place called Kollowa, there was a monument beside the road, dedicated to the memory of a handful of brave British officers and askari, who had died during an uprising by the Suk, as the Pokot were then called. One Elijah Masinde led an anti-colonial sect, called Dina ya Msambwa, which met its nemesis at Kollowa. There was no mention on the monument of the scores of brave Pokot who had also died at Kollowa. As the bloody confrontation took place in 1950, well within the memory of some of the local inhabitants of the area through which we were now passing, it was perhaps little wonder we were not greeted with open arms.

After what seemed like hours of dedicated inhumanity to the internal combustion engine we reached the summit of the pass, which turned out to be long and flat and not the dramatic Khyberesque defile I had imagined. Our rather scanty preparations had informed us that there were two missions in the area. On the left, as seemed appropriate, there was a Protestant Africa Inland Church set up, while further on, on the other side of the pass and on the right, as was fitting, was the opposition, in the form of a Catholic redoubt. We tried the Protestants first as they were closer. The only intelligible occupant was a lone American. He was sitting on the steps of the main complex staring moodily into the surrounding bush. We clattered up and ground to a halt, covering him in a light patina of dust. He unfolded himself and stood up and it was like watching a giraffe get to its feet. He was immensely tall, six foot eight easily. He had enormous feet, spindly legs and a tiny, pointed head. Disfiguring his upper lip was a small gingery Hitlerian moustache. Judging by the delighted grin which spread across his cherubic features we were the first palefaces he had seen in many a long day.

'Waall, lookee here, ain't you a sight for sore eyes,' he drawled as we switched off the overheated engine. I was pretty sure that neither Stan nor I had thought of ourselves in that regard. A generator thumped somewhere behind the building.

'Hi! The name's Dorsett, Chuck Dorsett.' He stuck out a large fleshy hand.

'Cain Ah get you fellas some iced tea?' he asked.

Iced *tea*! For the past couple of hours I had been dreaming of ice cold beer and here was this chap offering us chilled tea! Politely I declined and asked him if he could give us any info about the route up Tiati.

'Waall now. Let me think.' He thought for a long time. 'Yup, Ah did a trip up that a way once with donkeys. Got pretty high up as Ah recall. 'Bout two years ago. Seems there was some sort of track, but Ah cain't rightly recall where it was. Perhaps it wasn't Tiati but some other mountain. Sorry fellas. A'm not much help to you, am Ah?' No, indeed I thought, as we took our leave.

'By the way,' I asked, 'what's the name of this place?'

'Moron,' he replied. It figured.

We pressed on to the Catholic Mission at Barpello. Here we had more luck. Two Irish sisters and an English friend of Tabitha were in residence. Compared to Chuck they were icons of efficiency and competence. In no time we had an audience with the local chief, who sent a swift runner to summon possible candidates for the post of guide and askari. After about 20 minutes two men shuffled into the chief's breeze block office. One was very tall and thin and one-eyed. The other was shorter and gazed in wonderment around the office, rather like a tourist staring open-mouthed at the wonders of the Sistine Chapel. In his hand he carried a bow and a cluster of wickedly barbed arrows. Both men wore short black shukas, tightly wrapped around the waist and ending above the knee. A few beads and leather sandals completed their wardrobe. They looked lean and mean.

The open-mouthed archer, who was to guard the vehicle from unwanted incursions during our absence on the mountain, knew no language other than his native tongue. I turned to our one-eyed friend and quizzed him in Swahili.

'Wewe unajua njia mpaka juu ya milima?' (Do you know the way to the top of the mountain?) He slowly turned his head to regard me with his one good eye.

'Ndyio, bwana, mimi najua.' (Yes, I know the way)

'Aiya, tuende,' I said. (OK, let's go.) But first the men had to get some posho (maize meal) to see them through the next 24 hours. I gave them some money and they trotted off, returning in a short time with a small bag containing the vital grain.

We thanked the chief for his help and piled back into the Toyota, the men standing in the back, and set off back up the hill. Directly opposite the road leading to where Chuck sat sipping his iced tea and listening to his generator, an almost invisible track led into the bush. As Stan turned the wheel there was an unwanted clattering from beneath the bonnet. Stan switched off and I hopped out and raised the lid. The battery had come adrift. The archer's jaw sagged as he gazed in amazement at the entrails of the Toyota, now exposed to view, and at the two palefaces as they seemingly expertly put the beast's innards back together. Eight kilometres and 45 spine-jarring minutes later we reached the abrupt termination of the track. An open, treeless, rocky clearing marked journey's end. A little further on two small streams trickled musically down the mountainside. This was to be the last water, other than that we carried on our backs, that we would see until we returned.

Knowing it would be a cold night we asked One-eye to tell the askari that he could shelter in the cab and that we would leave the door unlocked. Consciences thus satisfied we hefted our packs and, with One-eye in the van, set off. It was two in the afternoon and the sun was at the very peak of its powers. Before we had gone more than a few yards I was soaked in sweat. My rucksack weighed a ton and I half toyed with the idea of turning back and ditching my tent in the car. But already Stan and One-eye were striding ahead, eating up the ground as though they were wearing seven league boots. Panting and gasping I struggled to keep them in sight as they loped up a rocky path, entered a patch of tall bush and disappeared. By the time I reached their vanishing point I was almost hyperventilating. Then I saw them hopping from rock to rock far below me, where the path dropped down with inconsiderate steepness for several hundred feet to the head of a bush-choked valley. My thumping heart was glad to be given a break, but I knew that this was only a temporary respite and that once down we had to painfully regain the height lost. I staggered down the bouldery path. By the time I had reached the bottom I had gained my second wind and steadily caught up with my companions who were ascending a path of unique rugosity, whose surface was more rock than anything else. The gradient eased as we reached a col. Then it was down again to the head of another valley. I was wearing trainers and my toes were not in agreement with their regular impact against iron hard stone. Then it was up again to another col choked with trees and dense vegetation. One-eye, unencumbered by rucksack, camera or other impedimenta, slipped through like a dusky wraith. We, on the other hand, quickly became entangled with briars, roots, thorns and vines whose consistency rivalled that of tensile steel. Hats were torn from heads, rucksacks became immovably wedged in low-slung branches, blood was shed and cries of anguish rang through the thickets. Finally, on all fours, gasping and panting like a pair of unfit gun-dogs, we emerged into a welcome clearing.

I stood up. Here was green grass and shelter from wind. A good place to camp. Stan agreed. Even One-eye thought so and said that he would descend into the valley to spend the night in a manyatta. I looked at my watch – 5pm. We had been walking for three hours. But there was still time for another hour. One-eye agreed. Stan was not so keen. It was two to one. We pressed on, and struggled up onto a ridge, through another belt of shirt-destroying vegetation and into another clearing where there was the remains of an old manyatta.

One-eye said he would drop down to an occupied manyatta some 1500 feet below, but would be back at six in the morning. He gave a casual wave, loped off on his stick-like legs and was soon lost to sight.

We dropped our loads and made to pitch our tents. I pulled mine out of its bag and laid it out. Something pretty vital seemed to be missing. Shit! Where was the bloody ridge pole? I rooted around in my rucksack. It wasn't there. Damnation! The ridgepole, as the name suggested, held up the ridge of the tent, which otherwise would sag dramatically in the middle. It did sag, such that when I crawled into it my head and chest were in one small cavity at one end and my abdomen and legs were out of view in the other. Another problem arose when I tried to zip up the tent. Such was the instability of the tent minus its ridgepole that any attempt to zip up the door resulted in the tent collapsing. I would have to sleep with the door open, hoping that nothing carnivorous came along to nibble my extremities. To add to my discomfort a clear sky and a full moon promised a chilly night. At least I hadn't forgotten the tent pegs – that would wait for another best-forgotten trip with my long-suffering spouse.

Stan, meanwhile had smoothly set up his domed habitation, and was casting what appeared to be disdainful glances at my sharp-angled snuggery. Time now for a well-deserved meal. Out with the Gaz burner, get the matches, boil some water for tea and soup, then the baked beans, followed by an orange and a can of Tusker, ignoring Stan's disapproving look. Not having camp chairs in which to loll back and enjoy the evening, we lay in the wiry grass. Our ridge faced due north, towards Tiati's sharp summit. Shadows lengthened, light softened and swiftly the sun dropped below the western horizon.

As the sun descended so did the moon rise, until its silvery light flooded the clearing and lent some minor dignity to our squalid encampment. The old manyatta now resembled a romantic warrior outpost, while our lonely tents might have set the scene for a chapter in *King Solomon's Mines*. Mine, especially. Stan's modern dome didn't quite fit with Rider Haggard's imaginative vision.

Crickets chirped, night birds called, a jackal yelped, a hyena whooped. A distant tinkling of a cow bell far down on our left indicated where One-eye was probably enjoying home comforts.

I felt a tickling on my right thigh. I shone a torch onto my manly limb. There, marching northwards in the direction of my essentials, was a phalanx of tiny ticks – pepper ticks, so small as to resemble grains of pepper. Barely visible, and all hastening to the fertile feeding grounds. Hastily I brushed them off. Stan was likewise engaged. I should have known. An old manyatta, and its surroundings, with cattle, goats and sheep grazing nearby, would be alive with ticks.

Hoping, but not believing, that we were tick-free, we crawled into our respective tents, and composed ourselves for the night. It was only 8pm but at least I would have an early night for a change. I fell asleep almost at once, only to wake at 1am. I was freezing. With the tent door wide open a chill wind was numbing my lower limbs and creeping up my sleeping bag. I tried curling up in the foetal position, which is difficult in a sleeping bag. Finally in desperation I kicked at the pole and the tent collapsed onto my legs.

Immobilised but warm, I fell asleep.

We were up at 5.15am. In the lightening dark we ate a less than hearty breakfast and drank as much fluid as our stomachs could hold, reasoning that the more we drank the less we would have to carry on our backs, a theory since proved to be fallacious if not downright dangerous. But we at the time thought it was a Jolly Good Idea. At 6.03am, One-eye not having appeared, we set off, leaving the tents empty but still pitched –half pitched in my case.

'We'll pick them up on the way down,' I said. 'No point in carrying them all the way to the top, just to carry them down again. No one will touch them here. And it would be a good idea to leave some water here for the descent.' So saying we stashed a two litre bottle of water in a bush next to Stan's tent.

It was now just light enough to see where we were going, so we pushed our way through a patch of scrub and saw above us a narrow ridge, leading towards the still distant summit. A 45 minute struggle brought us to its crest. It was an exhilarating position. The ridge was no more that twelve inches wide, with swooping drops on both sides.

'Bloody lucky there's no wind, or we'd be soon over the edge,' I laughed. Stan nodded. I looked around me – deep gorges, narrow ravines, soaring ridges, indigo blue valleys, dark cliffs, forbidding crags vanishing into shadowy depths. The snake-like outline of a dry river bed, fringed by tall trees, could be dimly seen far to the west. On our right, as the earth wheeled on its equatorial axis, the sun rose above a ridge, flooding us with light and warmth. Far below on our left I could see a manyatta, and above it, a tiny figure climbing up in our direction. One-eye was on his way to join us. Deep in a valley on our right was another minuscule manyatta, fringed by two cultivated fields.

With Stan leading, we tightroped our way along the ridge, descended to a col, and then followed a path which led upwards, in a series of rocky switchbacks to drop down to a pocket-sized platform, where there was a miniature manyatta and a small herd of cattle, quietly chewing the cud, attended by a young boy. As we greeted him, we saw One-eye, seated on a rock, smoking a cigarette – waiting for us. He looked as though he had been there for some time. With a sigh of relief we also sat down. Not for the first time I marvelled at these mountain men. Pencil thin, with legs like blackened twigs, they romped up near vertical slopes, chattering away at sixteen to the dozen, puffing on a fag, never getting out of breath, sandals or flip flops on their horny feet, rarely drinking or eating and remaining invariably cheerful and relaxed. Without their help and their knowledge of the mountain paths, ascents of Africa's remoter mountains by outsiders would be nearly impossible.

The presence of people living on and around Kenya's mountains, grazing their cattle, sheep and goats on their slopes, fetching water from their streams and springs, setting honey hives in their trees and collecting medicinal plants from their forests, is part of their unique attraction. In other parts of the world, mountains, although often beautiful and containing rare species of animal, bird and plant, are often devoid of human habitation and therefore, to my mind, somewhat sterile. In the mountains of Kenya the unexpected encounter with a spear- or rifle-toting tribesman, a waving child with his flock of goats, a smiling woman carrying calabashes of water, lightened the upward or downward toil and made one feel privileged to be there. After all, this was where they lived. To them this was home.

This tiny manyatta was perched high on the mountain to escape the predations of the Ngoroko, hit-and-run Turkana bandits who roamed the wilderness to the north of Tiati. The Pokot and Turkana do not see eye to eye. Although superficially physically similar, they speak different languages and follow different customs. Raiding and stealing each other's livestock are age-old traditions, with frequent killing of members of the opposing tribe.

We rose and shouldered our packs, grateful for the cool breeze fluttering the tops of the thickets through which we now forced our way. A brilliantly coloured sunbird flitted in front of us. A small striped mouse darted across the path, which at this point was blessedly horizontal. This respite did not last for long and soon we were toiling up yet another rocky hogback. But now the summit was looming closer, a stony knob surmounting a small but annoyingly steep forest. Down into the trees, deep loam underfoot, thickets of nettles, cool shade, slog up, pack digging into the shoulders, feet slipping on soft unstable earth and then out into the sunshine, a final gasping scrabble and there were Stan and One-eye on the top. I glanced at my watch – 9.03 – exactly three hours from our campsite. Holding my breath and trying to appear nonchalant and supremely fit I sauntered casually onto the summit. And stood and gaped. This was a view to die for. A great sweep of rugged country, jagged peaks, distant blue escarpments, to the north-east the sere amber wastes of the baking Suguta Valley, to the south-east a glimpse of the waters of Lake Baringo, westward to the Marakwet Escarpment, eastwards to the rising hills of Samburu and to the south the long line of the Tugen Hills.

We sat and ate our stale sandwiches, sipped our warm water and drank in the view. A pair of black dots in the sky dropped down towards us – fan-tailed ravens, friendly sociable birds, they swooped and hovered, croaking conspiratorially, before landing on a nearby rock. They hopped closer. I tossed them a sandwich. They pecked at it with gusto, watching us with their beady, probing eyes. One-eye regarded me disapprovingly.

A large male baboon barked from a nearby crag, voicing his annoyance at our presence. He swarmed onto its summit, staring at us. He was in a furious temper, shaking his head from side to side and rushing backwards and forwards, barking. One-eye stood up and laughed at him. The baboon was beside himself with rage, jumping up and down, baring his massive canines. Stan looked concerned. 'Perhaps it's time to go,' he said.

'I've only just arrived,' I said, 'need to recharge the batteries. It's a long way down.' That's the trouble with climbing with super-fit people with legs like stilts. They power ahead, eating up the miles, have their rest, and, just as you pant up, soaked in perspiration, wheezing like a chap with terminal emphysema and gasping for a drink, they rise leisurely to their Niked feet, toss their sacks onto their perfectly muscled shoulders as though they were filled with thistledown and glide off, leaving you bent over, wondering if you're going to have a heart attack.

About a thousand feet below us a pair of black and white eagles glided effortlessly through crystal clear space. Verreaux's eagles, noble birds of remote cliffs and lonely crags. I envied their ease and grace, knowing that in the space of minutes they could cover a distance which was going to take me hours of sweated toil.

The ravens had gone, their ham sandwich pecked to the last crumb. It was time to get going. Two and a half hours later I tottered into camp. Due to the undulating nature of the ridge a considerable part of the descent seemed to be as much uphill as downhill, which did not please my aching limbs. Stan and One-eye seemed to make light work of these antisocial physical features, romping along far ahead and were ready to move off as I staggered through the final bushes, thoughts on the cached water supply. Dropping my pack I went to the bush where we had left the two litre bottle of water. It was gone!

Gone! I had been looking forward to a good long drink for the past hour, imagining the flow of cool H20 over my desiccated tonsils and now all I had was rising bile. Had some passing herdsman found it and taken it? We had seen no game larger than a mouse so animal intervention was unlikely. Four hours to the car and our water was down to what we had in our packs. Great! I had a litre and a half left. Stan had a litre. One-eye appeared not to drink at all, which was just as well as we would have little to spare. I also had an orange and an apple. Already my mouth felt dry and rancid.

We packed our tents, shoved them into our packs and set off. In no time Stan and old One-eye had vanished from my ken. My toes had taken a major bashing on the rocks on the way up and were now taking even more on the way down as the forces of gravity exerted their toll. I crippled along like a lame Quasimodo, hobbling from rock to rock and lurching blindly through the thickets which barred our way. Blood was shed. Words were spoken. While limping across a stretch of bare rock I glanced down and saw carved into the rock was a double row of holes for playing bau – that fiendishly difficult backgammon-like game played all over East Africa. And in another was a trough for watering livestock. Both looked ancient, but there was no time to pause and examine these exciting phenomena. It was ever onwards and downwards to the waiting vehicle, over the rocks and through the bush.

The sun was now at its zenith. Shade was almost non-existent. My shirt was soaked with sweat and my hat hung limply over my streaming brow. My eyes stung with my personal salt, which attracted a loyal squadron of eager flies, who stubbornly resisted my frantic rebuffs and followed me for miles. What they fed on when I wasn't intruding into their personal space defeated me. The area was bereft of human and animal activity. It always amazed me that in areas seemingly totally devoid of mammalian life, you just had to pause for a moment to scratch your ear or spend a few quiet seconds voiding your straining bladder and you were almost immediately visited by legions of flies, all keen social bonders, willing and able to go to almost any lengths to make your personal acquaintance.

I tumbled on down the path. My battered toes dislodged a loose boulder. A large pale yellow scorpion scuttled out. My sudden adrenalin-fuelled leap surprised a somnolent lizard which with a flick of its tail vanished into a crevice. I was catching up with the others. Were they flagging? Was the tortoise catching up with the hares? There was a long green twig athwart my route. As I raised my dusty foot to surmount this minor obstacle it moved and slithered into a nearby thicket. A hornbill perched in a thorn tree gave a raucous cackle. My rate of descent increased. I passed Dick and One-eye, squatting panting in the minimal shade of a spindly acacia. They rose and followed. I had my third wind. But the path seemed to go on forever. Rocks, dust, thorns, unstable boulders, low branches, gullies, cactus, spiny plants, and always above us the sun, beating down with ferocious intensity. Where was the bloody vehicle? We plodded on, automatons, lurching speechless through the dry bush. Now we were so tired and dehydrated that when one of us slipped or barked his shins we did not have enough oral spit to vocalise our discontent. We just staggered on, mute and glassy eyed.

After about four hours of this seemingly endless march we met the second of the two streams we had crossed after leaving the car the previous afternoon. Good Lord, was it only yesterday? It felt like a week ago. Heaving sighs of relief we dumped our packs and drank deeply at the fountain, caring not whether men or baboons had shat in it upstream. We poured water over our heads and washed the blood from our legs and arms, lifted our loads and pressed on, knowing that our footwork was almost done.

There was the Toyota, at last, seemingly intact, with the askari and another man sitting beside it. We approached and bade both good morrow. The askari seemed somewhat out of sorts, as though he was a bit liverish or was suffering from a hangover. Any problems while we were away on the hill? He looked a bit sheepish and didn't answer. The other man spoke up. He was a herdsman and had been looking for a lost goat when he came across the parked Toyota. The time was noon and the sun was at its zenith. It was as hot as Hades. Seeing no sign of life, he approached the vehicle. He noticed that the windows were closed and all steamed up. He tried to peer inside but was unable to see through the grey opacity. As he stood there, pondering, a clawed hand appeared and raked a window, leaving long finger marks on the glass. He leapt back in alarm. The hand appeared again. The herdsman fitted an arrow to his bow and came near and put his eye to the five-fingered porthole. Another eye, bulging and bloodshot, peered back at him. Once again the herdsman did a backward skip. He heard a hoarse cry and a banging. There was someone inside trying to get out. He tried the door handle. It opened easily and out tumbled the askari, at his last gasp, chest heaving, grey-faced, hyperthermic, speechless and with his tongue lolling from his slackening jaws.

The herdsman dragged him into the shade of a nearby tree, ran for water from the stream, bathed the man's steaming forehead and forced a few drops between his teeth. Slowly he recovered his senses and told his story.

This had been his first time inside a vehicle. He regarded the interior with trepidation, like entering a leopard's cave. But as darkness approached and the temperature dropped he had decided to take shelter inside the cab, as we had suggested. It was getting cold and there might be hyenas around. There was a handle and the door opened easily enough, but once inside with the door slammed shut he no idea how to get out or how to open the windows. All was well until the morning when the sun rose and with it the temperature inside the cab. Very soon it was like an oven, then a pressure cooker and then a microwave. The poor chap was almost fried alive. If the herdsman had not come along when he did we might well have found a charred corpse inside the cab.

We paid off our men – thirty shillings and a water container to One-eye and the same to the parboiled askari. They were more than content. We drove back along the rocky track to the road, where they disembarked. They set off home with a song on their lips and a spring in their step. I hoped that their voices were lifted in praise of the generous if somewhat demented bwanas come to climb their mountain, but I feared that they were comparing notes on our various deficiencies.

Another three hours of dedicated vehicle destruction saw us back at Baringo and onto the blessings conferred by tarmacadam. The relief to be free of the incessant lurching and jolting and crashing into potholes was immense. If we had not been so late we would have gone down on our bloodied knees and kissed the stuff. But it was now 6.30pm, the shades of equatorial night were fast approaching and it was rather past the teatime deadline I had so blithely given to my ever lovin' as I tiptoed into the misty dawn the day before.

Back at base the alarm bells were ringing. Rescue parties were being assembled. Berna had taken me at my word and had phoned Tabby and together they had set out on the road to Baringo in an attempt to locate the missing duo. They had also phoned friends. Suspecting that something of the sort might have taken place we made a fruitless effort to contact them from Marigat, a best-forgotten township at the southern end of the lake. Driving like a hurricane force wind we tore back along the road to Nakuru, flashing our lights at every vehicle we met.

Finally, at the village of Kampi-ya-Moto, the Hot Camp, 25 kilometres from Nakuru, we met them. Berna was driving the practice Peugeot. Tabby's relief was mingled with a measure of self-satisfied matriarchal rancour and I could see that Stan was going to get it in the neck, if not in other parts of his anatomy, when he got home. As they drove away in Stan's Toyota I could see Tabby's jaws clattering like castanets as she vented her pent-up spleen. Stan was hunched over the steering wheel, a mute, suffering St. Sebastian, pierced by Tabby's verbal shafts.

Berna drove us slowly home. 'I was beginning to get a tiny bit worried there. Look at the time! Eight pm! *You* said you'd be back by teatime! Teatime!'

'Sorry about that, my darling. Took a tiny bit longer than expected. It won't happen again.' Berna snorted.

'How are the girls?'

'Fast asleep. Esther is looking after them.'

A soft winged owl drifted in the car's headlights. A spotted genet darted across the road. A full moon flooded the land with a soft yellow light.

Back at home I drew off my battered trainers and surveyed my battered toes. Several of the nails were blackened and rather the worse for wear. Berna regarded them with distaste. 'Well, if you will go off rambling across the country you've got to accept the consequences. Isn't that so, my love? I just hope they don't sully the sheets, that's all. Esther has just changed them.'

As I quaffed an essential cold beer, Berna gave a yelp. 'What's *that* crawling up your leg?' *That* was a tick, one of several.

'Well, you're certainly not getting into the same bed as me until you've got rid of your revolting parasites! I'm running a bath and filling it with the tick dawa we use to wash the dogs.'

Later, smelling less like a rose of Araby than a vat of disinfectant, but at least tick-free, I composed myself for sleep. Thankful to be in the conjugal bunk and not on the hard, cold couch, I wondered where Stan was spending the night. Within minutes I was fast asleep. It took rather longer for my mortified toenails to fall off and re-grow. But it was worth it.

Chapter Twenty Four

BACONHEAD AND FRIENDS

It was half past eight in the evening and there was someone at the gate, blowing their car horn. 'Baaa! Baaa! Baaa!' it went. 'There's someone at the gate, my poppet,' said Berna, rather unnecessarily, as big, and getting bigger, Esther arrived with the pudding, her *specialité de la maison*, rhubarb crumble.

'All right! *All right*. I'm coming!' I muttered as I marched down the drive, skirting the pepper tree in which a colony of unfriendly bees had made their home. 'Baaa! Baaa!' Whoever it was hadn't turned their headlights off. Gestapo-like beams blinded me as I fumbled to unlock the gate.

'Who is it?' I asked.

'It's me,' shrilled a female voice.

'Who's me?' I reasonably inquired.

'It's Cara, and I have an emergency. Do hurry up! It's a matter of life and death.'

Cara was Cara Bloom, a personable, if emotional, young woman.

'Cara!' I said. 'What's the matter?'

Cara was still invisible in the darkness. I heard a sob. 'It's Mr Baconhead!'

'Mr Baconhead?' I echoed.

'Yes, he's been mauled by my dogs. You must help him!'

'Come in! Come in!' I said, no wiser at to the identity of Mr Baconhead.

Cara drove up to the house. I followed on foot, again skirting the bee-infested pepper tree.

By the time I reached the house, Cara was inside, cradling a cardboard box to her shapely bosom. Berna was on her feet, pudding forgotten. Rona was agog with interest. Sophie peered down from her high chair. Esther had her ear to the kitchen door.

'Right,' I said. 'Let's see the patient.'

Cara opened the box to reveal a rather bedraggled rooster squatting within. I could see why he was so called, as his impressive comb was just like a rasher of streaky bacon.

'He was just going to bed when my horrid dogs grabbed him and if I hadn't been there they would have eaten him. It was terrible.' A tear trickled slowly down her ivory cheek. Gently she lifted him out. Mr Baconhead was in a mess. One eye was closed. There was a rent in his chest, another down one leg and a gash in his left wing. But the worst damage was to his vent. Things were sticking out which shouldn't have been sticking out.

Cara suddenly placed Mr Baconhead on the dining table next to Rona's pudding bowl and raised a hand to her snowy forehead. 'Can I use your loo? I feel a bit faint.' Mr Baconhead looked around him and, encouraged by Rona, had a few pecks at the rhubarb crumble.

Berna whispered, 'Just put it out of its misery!' But then Cara was back.

'Hugh! You must save poor old Baconhead! You will, won't you? Please!'

Cara nuzzled Baconhead's comb. I glanced regretfully at my bowl of cooling crumble. 'Right,' I said, 'let's take him to the surgery and see what we can do.' Berna rolled her eyes. Rona looked pleased. Sophie had polished off her pudding and to make the point plain, had placed her bowl on top of her head. The kitchen door creaked as Esther shifted her weight and her ear.

'Can I come and help, Dad?' asked Rona. Berna rolled her eyes again.

In the surgery I inspected the damage more carefully. A section of gut was protruding from Baconhead's rear end. By upending him this was persuaded to return to its proper position. Then it was a case of carefully suturing everything back in place. It was as well Rona had volunteered her services as after the first few stitches Cara had to sit down and mop her alabaster forehead. After about an hour of dedicated avian cosmetic repair Mr Baconhead was ready to be returned to the personable bosom of his family. I gave the appropriate guarded prognosis, citing shock, sepsis, internal adhesions and wound breakdown. Cara would have none of it. 'You're going to be fine, Mr Baconhead, now that Hugh – and Rona' – Rona beamed – 'have put you together.' And he was.

Cara was a lovely person, young, friendly, very good looking, easy to talk to, but in moments of crisis hysteria took over and normal communication went out of the window. So after the Baconhead Affair I hoped that there would be a decent respite, banking on the false assumption that lightning does not strike twice in the same place.

Some two weeks later, we were sitting down to the evening repast, when the phone rang.

I raised the receiver to my ear. At first all I could hear was gasping and panting. I was about to put the phone down and return to the table, on the assumption that someone was playing the fool, when a shrill cry almost burst my right ear drum.

'Hugh, is that you? Are you there? Can you hear me? It's my puppy. She's dying! She's choking! She swallowed a bone and now it's stuck in her throat. She can't breathe! Oh my God! I'm coming in right now!'

Before I had time to reply the phone went dead.

Cara lived at Rongai, 35 kilometres from Nakuru. We lived 7 kilometres from the surgery. Berna and I drove to the surgery as fast as we could, to find Cara already there. How she had achieved this feat we had no opportunity to discover. Cara's car was parked in the middle of the road outside the surgery, doors open, engine running, lights blazing. Cara was pacing up and down. In her hands was a limp puppy. Cara was hysterical.

'Do something!' she sobbed. 'She's dying! Can't you look at her under the headlights? Look, there's the bone stuck in her throat.'

I took the puppy from Cara and quickly examined it. It appeared to have stopped breathing. Then it gave a convulsive gasp. I gave the pup to Berna and opened the surgery.

'Cara,' I said, 'I'm going to sedate the puppy to see if relaxation will move this bone. If not...' Cara began hyperventilating again.

'Perhaps,' I thought, 'I should zap her as well! In her state she would hardly feel the needle!' I weighed the pup and carefully gave the computed dose into the small hind leg.

'Now,' I thought, 'this will either push it over the edge or...' Cara was sitting down, tear-stained face in her hands, whimpering quietly. Berna made comforting noises. I watched the pup like a hawk. Its mucous membranes were still a horrid purple colour and its breathing came in unpredictable fits and starts. I palpated the lump in the throat. A mistake. The breathing stopped. Quickly I compressed the chest and with a rasp it came back to life.

Slowly the pup relaxed, the breathing steadied and slowed, the tongue and conjunctiva were now a healthy pink. But the bone was still there in the lower gullet, telling me that we were not out of the woods yet.

'Cara,' I said. 'I propose that we take the puppy home so that we can monitor it throughout the night. There's a good chance that the bone may shift while the puppy is sleeping.'

'Let me come as well! I can sleep on the floor beside her. Please! I'll be no trouble!'

I was firm on this one. With Cara in the house we weren't going to get a wink of sleep. She would be pacing the boards all night long, badgering us with questions and knocking on our door and giving us a minute by minute bulletin on every aspect of the puppy's progress – or otherwise.

'You go home and get a good night's sleep, Cara,' I said. 'Leave this to me and Berna. There's nothing more for you to do. And don't worry. We'll do everything that's necessary and we'll phone you in the morning.'

'She will be all right, won't she?' she asked.

'I'm sure of it,' I replied, not feeling very sure at all.

'Well, then if you're sure, absolutely sure, then I'll go home. You don't mind if I give you a ring now and again?'

'No indeed, any time. Drive carefully. You're in no hurry now.'

Cara bent and kissed the sleeping puppy and departed. Berna rolled her eyes. There was a lot of eye rolling where Cara was concerned.

Back at home we laid the puppy on a blanket on the floor beside the bed, checked that it was breathing normally, hopped between the covers and switched the light out. Five minutes later the phone rang. It was Cara.

'Hello, Hugh, how is the puppy? I'm so worried.'

I switched on the light and bent down to check the patient. All seemed satisfactory and I conveyed this to Cara, and switched off the light. Fifteen minutes later the phone rang again. It was Cara again.

'Sorry, Hugh, I just couldn't sleep. How is the little darling?'

On with the light, check the patient and report back, flop back and turn out the light. Fifteen minutes later it happened again, and again.

'My God,' groaned Berna, 'it might have been better if we'd let her come and sleep here with the puppy.'

To say that the night was disturbed is a gross understatement. Finally at about 4am the calls stopped. We assumed that Cara had finally fallen asleep. Shattered, we also fell asleep.

The alarm went off at 6.30. With difficulty I opened my eyes, and focused on the puppy's blanket. The puppy was no longer there. It was busy defecating in a corner, concentrating grimly on its chosen task. I staggered across and checked its throat. The bone was gone. Shifted into the stomach, the chances were that it would now be slowly digested and/ or excreted. Which it was. And Cara was grateful – and quiet – for a while.

Chapter Twenty Five

GUSSIE

John and Amanda Perrett, formerly of Mogotio, now lived on Ol Maisor Ranch, an hour's journey north of Rumuruti, on the Laikipia Plateau. Here they ran camel safaris, reared angora goats, and catered for adventurous, not to say, foolhardy, tourists. It was no good telling anyone that the ranch was so many kilometres from Rumuruti. That meant nothing without some idea of the state of the road, which was generally awful. Just outside Rumuruti was an insignificant rivulet. If this was in flood, your journey might end before it had even begun. In the rains, a lorry slewed across the road might hold you up for hours.

The ranch was owned by Amanda's father, Jasper Evans. Japper, as he was generally known, had his fair share of eccentricities, and this trait was handed down in full measure to daughter and son-in-law.

John and Amanda lived in a self-built house on a euphorbia-covered bluff overlooking the Rumuruti/Maralal road. The steep bouldery climb up to the house made the road one had just left seem like a tarmac highway and the rocks which littered the final section resembled a storm driven sea suddenly frozen by an Arctic blizzard. Onward progress was abruptly terminated at the gateway to the Perrett demesne by a flinty barricade of thigh-high granite. The house was hidden by dark jungly thickets, through which snaked what in other circumstances might be called a drive, but which in the case of the Perretts was more of an obstacle course. A crate full of empty beer bottles, a pile of discarded bottles of Terramcyin, an old Land Rover drive shaft, heaps of mouldering camel and cattle bones, a dog kennel, a leopard trap, chicken houses, and as you negotiated your stumbling way, packs of various canines rushed forth to investigate and obstruct your approach. At the back door various domestics would be engaged in activities of a furtive and unknown nature. The house was not built on a horizontal plane, but on various interesting levels, finally ending at the cliff edge overlooking the road. Here was the guest wing, which consisted of a thatched rondavel and a bathroom. The latter was open plan. Very open. A rocky ledge contained the usual items, such as wash basin, shower, toilet seat and so on, set into the stony wall of the cliff. An overhanging tree provided a degree of cover, but otherwise all was exposed to the elements, to the birds of the air, scuttling hyraxes, lizards, the occasional snake and to any passing peeping Tom on the road below. Apart from a few strategically-sited thickets of thorny vegetation, nothing separated the unclad user of the ablutions or the desperate sitter perched precariously on the throne from the penetrating gaze of the sharp-eyed strollers below. Such being the case, occupancy of the facilities was usually short and hurried. When anxious guests queried John about the lack of outer wall he laughed –'the road down there is so rough that no one looks up. They're all staring at the ground trying to avoid the rocks!' We hoped so.

The interior of the house was a chaos of dogs, cats, ancient mildewed magazines, bottles full and empty, jars of pickle, dusty pictures, photos so faded that it was impossible to determine their subject matter, chairs and sofas upturned to prevent the canine horde from lying on them, a child's tricycle, a lion's skull with the former owner's faded skin spread over the floor, piles of old newspapers, innards of combustion engines.

In one door leading into the main room was what appeared at first glance to be a cat flap. It was in fact a pig flap. One day the Perretts brought me a piglet, which had been badly burnt. I treated it and it recovered. The piglet was so grateful it attached itself to the Perretts and became one of the family, trotting in and out of the house through the pig flap. Some months after the piglet had been presented, I was on the ranch and came into the house to examine one of the ubiquitous dogs. As I bent to my task I was interrupted in my examination by the most horrendous porcine squealing. Turning around I saw a large snout trying to force its way through a now ridiculously small aperture.

'Yes,' said John, 'Porky's grown up but he doesn't know it. He can't come in now and we're running out of bacon so problem solved! We'll all be happy – well he won't be quite so happy, but he's had a good time, and all good things must come to an end!'

John was lean, almost cadaverous, favoured long 'empire builder' shorts, baggy shirts and was invariably shod in sock-less plimsolls. Amanda ran a knitting enterprise, turning out fashionably heavy sweaters emblazoned with images of camels padding across the wearer's chest. These sold well to participants of the Perrett safaris, more as a symbol of survival than as a fashion accessory – the camel saddles were excruciatingly uncomfortable. In cool weather both John and Amanda clad themselves in these shapeless, knee-length garments.

Both had a highly developed, sardonic sense of humour, were laid back to the point of horizontality and were fazed by nothing. In situations where others would be reduced to panic-stricken jelly the Perretts were the very embodiment of the wartime maxim 'keep calm and carry on'. Vehicle breakdowns, stock theft, camels killed by lions, attacks by bandits, they took them all in their daily stride.

From time to time the Perrett household would be home to four-legged creatures other than dogs, cats and piglets. One of these was Gussie, a fully-grown female cheetah, who had the run of the house. Why this lovely animal was called Gussie, rather than a noble feline name like Sheba, Athena or Sappho I never discovered. At least it was better than Spots.

One Friday evening as I was endeavouring to close up the surgery, an earlier attempt having been thwarted by the late arrival of a dog suffering from tick fever, compounded by a long-standing hookworm infestation, the phone rang. It was John.

'Hi Hugh,' he said, 'we seem to have a bit of a problem with Gussie.'

'Oh yes,' I said, 'what sort of problem?'

'She seems to have broken a hind leg.'

'How did she do that?' I asked, visualising the cheetah streaking across the open plains after her legitimate prey and being bowled over by a hartebeest or being kicked by a zebra.

'She was doing the wall of death round the lounge and slipped. Looks high up, swollen, and she can't put it to the ground. It's her left hind.'

I tried to imagine the cheetah in full flight around the Perrett lounge and found it difficult. The very word lounge suggests discreet order, soft lighting, carefully arranged comfortable seating, soothing music playing gently somewhere in the background. Perhaps even flowers, chocolates and wine. The Perrett lounge was more like a commando assault course.

'Right,' I said, brain working overtime. 'Right then, can you bring her in?' I had pinned dogs' and cats' broken legs but never a cheetah's. What about anaesthesia? Still, I had knocked out a few lions so the principle must be roughly the same. Better check Harthoorn's *Chemical Capture of Animals* though, to be on the safe side.

'We can bundle her into the car and be with you late tomorrow morning, if that's OK with you,' replied John.

The Perrett car was a small, battered, low-slung Datsun saloon. How it negotiated the monstrous irregularities of the Rumuruti/ Maralal road was one of life's ongoing mysteries. Most of its interior was normally crammed full of containers of cattle dip, cow hides, sheep skins, groceries, various dogs, spare tyres, machine parts, a battered and apparently much-used child's potty and innumerable miscellaneous, unidentifiable oddments. Where they were going to put a fully-grown cheetah was beyond me.

That evening I boned up on the little information I could glean from my textbooks.

I decided that the well-tried xylazine/ketamine combo was the anaesthetic to go for. And fortunately I had a good selection of large intramedullary pins on hand.

Late morning turned into early Saturday afternoon. I let the staff, including Moses, go. But I had my faithful back-up crew in the form of Berna, Rona and Sophie, all keen and eager to rub noses with a real live cheetah.

I prepared the instruments which I knew would be necessary.

The street outside the surgery was thronged with people, hawkers shouting their wares, passers-by, shoppers, beggars, loafers, street kids, shoe shine boys, all seemingly bawling in unison. The noise was deafening. At 1.30 precisely the Perrett conveyance turned the corner and, negotiating the crowds, came to a stop in front of the surgery. I could see that the back of the car had been cleared of its customary debris and there, lying on a cushion of blankets, reclined Gussie. I was not the only one to see her. A rubber-necking vagrant, perhaps hoping to improve his lot by relieving the Perretts of anything portable left lying on the back seat, peered in and immediately leapt back. 'Chui!' he roared, 'chui! Iko chui ndani ya gari!!' (Leopard! Leopard! There's a leopard in the car!) At once there was a rush, a tsunami of humanity surrounding the car, goggling and gawking at poor Gussie. There is a limit to even a placid cheetah's patience. Gussie gave a growl and lunged at the window where one seemingly demented adolescent was beating on the glass. With a uniform scream the crowd surged backwards. Now was our chance. We opened the door and quickly carried Gussie inside the surgery. She bore this indignity with equanimity, I was glad to observe. With a neap tide of uninvited, vocalising humanity at my heels I closed the door with all possible speed.

Getting her onto the scales proved to be impossible. I estimated her weight to be approximately 50-60kg. She was big. The upper part of her left hind leg was badly swollen. The femur must be broken. I did not have an X-ray machine and getting her to a local facility was out of the question. Quite apart from the difficulty of manhandling her onto an X-ray table, it was quite likely that we would have a riot on our hands as soon as we went out of the door.

Gussie stood quietly, a stunning creature, with John and Amanda beside her, but I knew that as soon as I injected her she would react, possibly violently.

'OK, folks,' I said, 'I'm going to give her a sedative first, wait for ten minutes and then give her the anaesthetic. Fortunately the volume of the sedative is about a quarter of that of the anaesthetic. Just hold on. I don't want her leaping for my jugular!'

'What about *our* jugulars?' said John.

'Well,' I replied, 'there are two of you and she can't get both of you, and besides *I've* got to remain intact in order to do the op.'

'Well, that's OK then,' said John, 'off you go.'

Berna and the girls stood by as I filled the syringe. I had to be quick. John held Gussie round the neck as I smacked the needle into her good hind leg and emptied the syringe into the muscle. Gussie gave an outraged snarl and leapt forwards but it was too late. The deed was done.

Ten minutes later she was sufficiently drowsy for me to inject the larger volume of the anaesthetic ketamine without restraint. Very soon she was out for the count. We heaved her onto the table.

'Right,' said John, 'we'll leave you to it. Got things to do, like having a beer or two in the Men's Bar!' Amanda gave him a look. They left.

I manipulated the leg. I hoped it *was* a fracture. Getting in there and finding it wasn't, would be a bit embarrassing. I also hoped that the break was a clean one, not one of those splintered jobs, with shattered overriding shards all over the place, the bone split up the middle and no place to insert a pin or place a plate. A vet's nightmare. I could feel crepitus, the sensation when raw bone ends grind together. I knew all about that, having had my own femur broken when a cow kicked me, not long after I arrived in Africa. Distinctly unpleasant. I was glad that Gussie was unconscious.

'Is it broken, Dad?' asked Rona.

'Yup, so get me a razor blade and I'll shave the leg.' I lathered the area over the femur and shaved a wide area, from the pelvis to the stifle.

'Hey, look,' piped Sophie, 'her skin's spotted just like her fur!' So it was.

I draped and disinfected the surgical site, Berna brought the tray of instruments and I made a long incision through the skin over the line of the femur. A few arteries spouted dramatically. Rona whistled. I clamped them off and her whistling stopped. Now it was a matter of delving between the muscles without cutting through them. Cutting the muscles results in a sea of blood totally obscuring everything, quite apart from putting the animal at risk. Using scissors I carefully pushed the blunt points between two muscle groups, making an opening large enough to insert my finger. I pushed it in, forcing it between the muscles. There was a rush of dark clotted blood. Rona whistled again. Sophie's nose was perilously near the incision. Berna was more restrained.

'Right,' I said, 'I can feel the fracture and thank goodness, it appears to be simple.'

'Simple?' said Rona, 'it doesn't look simple to me!'

'It just means it isn't smashed to hell and gone,' I replied. 'It doesn't mean the job's easy!'

Carefully I separated the muscles, until I could feel both ends of the fractured bone. The break was clean, thank goodness, and was in the middle of the femur with minimal overriding of about an inch. I pushed my finger under the lower end of the upper fragment and, not without difficulty, levered it upwards, and clamped bone-holding forceps onto it. Not easy.

'Right, Berna my love,' I said, 'can you give me the biggest intramedullary pin.' She did and I inserted the sharp point into the marrow cavity of the bone.

'Now, bring the chuck and fit it onto your end.'

The chuck was a T-shaped instrument which was screwed onto the opposite end of the pin. Grasping the bone-holding forceps in my left hand, with my right I forced the pin up the marrow cavity. It fitted snugly, I was glad to see. A loose pin results in poor healing. The pin reached the end of the marrow cavity. Now was the hard bit, shoving the stainless steel pin through the dense bone and out through the skin. The pin would then be withdrawn, the two broken ends of the bone brought together and the pin pushed back down into the marrow cavity of the lower fragment. Easy. Except sometimes it isn't.

By the time I had pushed the pin through the upper fragment the perspiration was beading my honest brow.

'Gosh, Dad,' said Sophie, 'that's hard work, eh?'

'I'll say,' I replied. I removed the chuck and transferred it to the top end, pulled the pin out until the lower end was just flush with the fracture site and handed the instrument to Berna to hold.

Now comes the tricky bit – lifting the lower end of the broken femur, levering it upwards and downwards and aligning both fragments just so and pushing the pin down from the upper into the lower half of the bone. More perspiration, grunting, heaving, the odd expletive, until – 'Right, Berna, start pushing the pin now. Twist it a bit, that's it.' Once in the lower fragment, it was just a matter of screwing and forcing the pin down until it was well seated in solid bone, having measured the length of the pin against the length of the femur.

'Right, that's it. Now we just stitch up and cut off the bit of the pin that's sticking out at the top end and Bob's yer uncle!'

Rona and Sophie laughed. Neither was fazed by the cutting and the blood. I stitched the long wound and cut the pin flush with the skin with a hacksaw. A solid steel pin takes a lot of sawing to get through. A couple of stitches to close the small hole and we were done.

Gussie was still out cold, but breathing quietly and steadily. I gave her a covering shot of antibiotic and we lifted her onto a blanket to recover.

Four hours after I had given her the anaesthetic she was trying to get up. The same anaesthetic combination given to a dog or cat lasts for less than an hour.

There was a knocking on the surgery door.

'That'll be the Perretts,' said Berna. And it was.

'Hi John, hi Amanda, all done, stitches out in a fortnight, pin out in about two months and fingers crossed! Keep her quiet. No more wall of death nonsense!'

'Will they drive back now?' asked Rona, 'It's six o'clock and they'll be driving in the dark.'

'No problems,' said John, 'any baddies will run a mile when they see Gussie!'

In the street outside, the original mob had got tired of waiting for us to emerge. Now we had to get Gussie into the car before the new crowd became aware what was happening. Just as we got her into the back of the car the cry went up, but it was too late. The Perretts sped away into the gathering darkness.

Two months later, beside the road to Nyeri, in an abandoned

quarry, I sedated Gussie and removed the pin. She was walking well, and went from strength to strength. For the next couple of years she lived on the ranch, fleet and active, hunting the odd dik dik and gazelle, spending nights with the Perretts.

Then she took to killing sheep and goats on nearby farms owned by local Africans. She was unafraid of people so when a tribesman, armed with a spear, approached her, she did not immediately flee as wild cheetah would have done. He killed her.

Chapter Twenty Six

LUMPS AND BUMPS

On the penultimate day of the year 1988, at 9.55am precisely, Kim Ross Cran emerged into the light of day, weighing in at 9lb, and completing our trio of delectable daughters. Her arrival had been medically predicted for Boxing Day, my own birthday. Berna's mother and sister had come from Birmingham to lend a helping hand in the birthing process, but were due to return to Blighty on the 2nd January. Boxing Day came and went. Something had to be done to speed things up. Anxious to avoid the discomfort of a threatened induction Berna took her sister, aged parent and full-term foetus on a roller coaster, self-driven, infant-expelling ride around Lake Nakuru Park. Barely able to fit behind the steering wheel, she roared along the rutted tracks at forbidden speeds, leaping over hidden humps, crashing over boulders and rattling over car-destroying corrugations. This manic exercise almost wrote off the car, and had a traumatic effect on all four occupants, including Kim, who decided that further uterine residence was contraindicated, emerging forthwith, without protest, the following morning.

Meanwhile, something else was emerging from the foetid shores of the Majani Mingi swamp, to the north of Nakuru.

A few miles to the south of the swamp, on their farm, Jo and Janet Mills bred racehorses and milked a herd of Jersey cattle. Whenever Jo phoned I knew there was trouble afoot, be it a mare unable to give birth, a yearling with colic, a gelding which had run into wire, or a cow with a prolapsed uterus. Jo did not phone over trivialities. So when I heard Jo on the blower at 0730 hours one Monday morning my heart sank as I waited for the worst.

'Hugh,' Jo said, without preamble, 'we have a couple of cows here with lumps and they don't look happy. Can you come out?' My heart rose. This was a darn sight better than a large bowel impaction or a skittish filly with a tear down the inside of a hind leg.

As I drove down the Mogotio road I wondered what this might be. On my right lay the lip of Menengai crater, fringed by fields of wheat and maize. A ground squirrel darted across the dusty track. A black-headed heron lifted itself out of a roadside thicket. A man on his one-gear bicycle toiled up the hill, standing on the pedals, perspiration on his brow.

Driving into the farmyard, I saw Jo standing looking at two cows. I drew up and stopped. Jo was one of those people who are invariably cheerful, no matter what the circumstances. His best stallion might have just broken his leg, his prime milking cow might have died of bloat, but Jo would greet you with a beaming smile and say, 'Hugh, how *are* you?' Which is what he said now. His gap teeth gleamed in the sunshine, his battered, sweat-stained hat sat squarely on his crinkly grey hair, thin sunburned legs poked out of his short shorts.

'I'm fine,' I replied, 'but those cows are not. How long have they been ill?'

'A couple of days, maybe more. Stopped eating, then started to salivate. Looked like three day sickness, but they've got worse, not better as they normally do with three day.'

Both animals were dejected, their coats were standing on end, saliva drooled from their muzzles, their eyes were inflamed and they were panting. But the most immediately obvious symptom was the lumps. There were dozens of them, scattered over the animals' skins – on the head, the neck, their legs – round, firm lumps about an inch to two inches in diameter. Both cows had roaring temperatures. I felt their lymph nodes in front of the shoulder. They were massively enlarged. I felt the lumps. Firm and sited within the skin.

I stood looking at the animals and thinking. I had never seen this before, but I knew what it was. 'Jo,' I said, 'this is Lumpy Skin Disease.' A pair of hadada ibis flew overhead, their harsh calls echoing in the still air. A dove cooed relentlessly and monotonously in a thorn tree.

'Right,' said Jo, 'and what is it? I've heard the name but never seen it.'

'Neither have I, but I'm certain this is what it is. A viral disease of cattle, similar to sheep and goat pox, carried by blood-sucking insects, with no treatment and sometimes heavy mortality.'

'Great!' said Jo, 'just great! And what about prevention?'

'Well, there is a vaccine but it's too late for vaccination in your case, I'm afraid, and as it's spread by flying insects there's not much you can do about that either.'

'Sounds like shauri ya Mungu to me,' said Jo, as we had a cup of coffee in the farm office.

'In the lap of the African gods – again! Par for the course!' he laughed.

Over the next few days more animals were affected. Some were covered with hundreds of lumps. Some had a grossly swollen leg with hugely enlarged lymph nodes. A few pregnant animals aborted. In some cases the skin overlying the lumps began to slough, leaving large, open suppurating wounds. In others apparent healing was followed weeks later by the separation of a central core. This plug would eventually fall out and the resulting hole would slowly heal, but the hide was damaged and the animal's value diminished. Milk yield declined and fertility slumped.

From the original focus of infection around the swamp the disease slowly spread southwards, carried by affected carrier animals and their attendant insects. The disease had not been seen in the province for many years and as a result vaccination with the locally produced sheep/goat pox vaccine had been neglected. As a result the entire cattle population was susceptible and the epidemic spread far and wide. Thousands of animals were infected. Farmers who vaccinated their cattle when they were incubating the disease blamed the vaccine for infecting their animals.

By the time the epidemic petered out it had reached as far south as Morogoro in central Tanzania.

—*—

In southern Kenya a crocodile-infested river flows through a dry and hostile land before entering the Indian Ocean. To the north of the river a vast tract of territory had been demarcated as an enormous ranch. It was so large that one had to wonder what had happened to the original inhabitants who at one time must have lived there.

Here another strange and unpleasant cattle disease had reared its ugly head. The general manager, a strong-minded individual, generally known as the Commandant, a consequence of the forceful imposition of his iron will on his cowering subordinates, asked me to examine the affected herds and give my opinion on the situation. I accepted with alacrity. I had heard that the area was a positive hotbed of tropical ailments, a veritable pathologists' paradise. Here were diseases which most vets would give their eye teeth to see. Trypanosomiasis, anaplasmosis, redwater, botulisim, heartwater – even that rare malady besnoitiosis was rumoured to be rife. And now there was an outbreak of the almost mythical bovine farcy among the herds. I couldn't wait to get there.

In order to ferry us to the field of endeavour the Commandant arranged to meet us at a grass airstrip on the shores of Lake Elementaita. As we drove up, a gleaming flying machine shot over our heads, landed, turned and taxied towards us. This was no two-seater, fabric-covered string bag. Compared to what I was used to, this was luxury indeed. The Commandant was at the controls, the very picture of aeronautical efficiency. Beside him sat Ingrid, his vivacious honey-blonde wife and in the rear perched their young daughter. But there was room for all of us and we piled in – Berna, Rona, Sophie, Kim and myself, plus our luggage. Introductions were curt. I had heard that the Commandant had a very possessive nature. Socializing was verboten. We were there to work, not to fraternise, engage in idle or frivolous banter and certainly not to ogle.

The plane rose over the lake. Drifts of pale pink flamingos scattered in panic as we roared overhead. A spiral of circling pelicans coiled upwards over the far shore, rising with the warming air. Behind the pelicans lay Delamere's Nose, a singular volcanic feature, which from certain angles did bear a certain resemblance to the late Lord's prominent profile. We gained height and set course for the distant ranch, passing the Aberdare range on our left and then Nairobi on our right, before flying over the brown, coastward-descending land of the Kamba people and the sere wilderness of Tsavo National Park.

My own flying career was almost over. I had gained my private pilot's licence in December 1976 and had flown light aircraft for ten years. But with the arrival of our three little darlings and the looming prospect of hideously expensive school fees, flying for pleasure had to end. I learned to fly in a Cessna 172 and then graduated to a Piper Super Cub, a fabric-covered, tail wheel, two-seater plane, in which I had a half share. This was a marvellous machine. With its narrow fuselage and broad wings it would leap off the ground in a ridiculously short take-off run, which was shorter that its landing run, a singular advantage in the case of a forced landing. It had a very basic instrument panel, had two seats one behind the other, and was flown by means of a long joy stick between the knees, as opposed to a yoke in most conventional aircraft. Having a tail wheel meant that in order to get the machine airborne the tail had to be raised by pushing the stick forwards to gain enough ground speed before pulling back to lift the plane off the ground.

The Super Cub did not have the usual doors found in most aeroplanes. Instead the side window on the right of the plane folded up while a wedge-shaped section of the fuselage folded down. Double-jointed hips were a distinct asset when it came to entering the machine. But the wonderful thing was that you could fly the Super Cub with the side of the plane open to the elements. Flying at hundreds or thousands of feet above the earth at 90 miles an hour with the door and window wide open sounds pretty chilly. Not so. The Cub's exhaust pipe emerges from the engine and is directed towards the right. The result was a delicious blast of warm air flowing past the open side of the plane.

Being able to fly the Cub with the door and window open had distinct advantages as I discovered when taking part in an air rally which involved a bomb-dropping competition. The 'bombs' were brown paper bags full of flour which burst in a pleasing manner when they hit the ground. My bomb aimer sat in the seat behind me and we swept over the target at what other competitors regarded as an unfairly low altitude. My one-man crew stuck his head out and dropped his bomb right on target. Unfortunately he was wearing a pair of impressively large horn rimmed spectacles at the time and these were instantly torn from his nose by the slipstream and never seen again.

I used the Cub to fly to clients in various far-flung spots, such as Laikipia, Naivasha, Baringo, Sotik, and Mau Narok. But as the costs of maintenance rose ever higher my co-owner and I decided to try to recoup our outgoings by putting the plane out for hire. This proved to be a fatal mistake. A professional hunter, one John Alexander, made a basic error of judgement at Naro Moru airstrip near Nanyuki, hit the boundary fence, overturned and destroyed the plane, but not himself. I felt as though I had lost a dear friend or a close relative. The passing of Five Yankee Alpha Hotel Sierra was observed with the reverence and regret accorded to military heroes and doughty explorers who fell in the course of duty.

Following the demise of the Cub, I went back to flying the Aero Club's 172, with Berna as frequent co-pilot and navigator. We flew to Ferguson's Gulf on the western shores of Lake Rudolf to fish and visit crocodile-infested Central Island, we flew to Lake Baringo, Nanyuki and many other places. Then the plane was sold and I hired, from a friend, his Cessna 182, a larger, faster, but more expensive, machine, which I flew for another year, before the light of financial reality finally dawned.

But I loved the sensation of flight, the isolation from the earth-bound world, the feeling of personal control and, for a while at least, the getting away from the constant problems of the practice. And it beat driving hands down. I loved the roar as the engine burst into life and the swift vanishing of the propeller into a diaphanous whirling circle, the rocking of the wings in the slipstream, the lift as the plane left the ground, the satisfaction of a smooth landing as the wheels brushed the grass, the smell of hot oil and the cracking of the engine as it cooled down.

We were nearing our destination and descending. We could see the river, lined by green trees, oiling its way towards the distant ocean. Beside the river were buildings and the long brown smudge of an airstrip. The Commandant spoke into the mike, reduced power and lowered the flaps. As we lost height the plane lurched and bucked in the columns of hot air rising from the land below. A dark shadow plummeted vertically in front of the windscreen. A violent wrench on the controls and we narrowly avoided the falling vulture. Yelps of alarm from the infants in the rear seat. More power as we approached the threshold of the runway. A solid thump and we were down.

We taxied to the end of the runway and stopped opposite some buildings. The Commandant switched off the engine, got out, grabbed a briefcase and marched off without saying a word. Berna and I looked at each other. An African with a club foot limped up to the plane and helped us to hump our things to a house overlooking the river. Like many Africans with disabilities he was friendly and cheerful, chaffing the children until they giggled and laughed.

It was hot, crickets sang in the dry, burnt grass, a few birds chirruped lifelessly in the spindly trees and the air felt thick and stifling. Lizards scuttled below stones. We settled into our rooms and, while the girls amused themselves, stood on the verandah looking at the river. The dark water slid by between tall mud banks without a murmur or ripple. A kingfisher, a flash of cobalt blue, shot upstream. What was that sullen splash? A crocodile? A monitor lizard? The sun, a blood red orb, sank below the riverine trees and suddenly it was dark, a moist, warm, clammy dark. Mosquitoes began to whine. A servant called and we went in for dinner.

We found the Commandant already seated at the table and halfway through the first course. While we seated ourselves he continued to devote himself to his personal platter, steadily working his way across the plate until it shone in the lamplight. With lowered eyes pudding was demolished in the same remorseless fashion, at which point he stood up and, without uttering a syllable, vacated the room. Berna and I raised joint eyebrows.

With his departure the atmosphere palpably lightened. Ingrid proved to have a wicked sense of humour and the children were in top form, excited by their surroundings.

Beneath the mosquito net that night I boned up on Bovine Farcy. The generator had coughed its last asthmatic cough and I studied the printed page by the fast-fading light of my torch. Beside me Berna snored gently, enlivening the tropical night with a light, musical alto. Outside the net the maddening song of clouds of frustrated mosquitoes filled the night. The river was silent. Now and again a night bird squawked and once I heard the grunt of a distant lion.

Bovine Farcy, I read, was a bacterial disease, caused by an organism called Nocardia farcinica, transmitted by infection of skin wounds, and that ticks and lice might also be involved. It was also able to survive in the soil. The main symptoms were the appearance of firm, painless subcutaneous nodules, which showed no tendency to rupture, and which might persist for months or years. The nodules contained a thick, creamy, yellowish or greyish yellow pus and ultimately they spread internally. There was no effective treatment and control was by treating all wounds promptly, reducing the tick population and, most importantly, by the isolation and slaughter of all infected cattle.

It sounded all quite straight-forward. I yawned. I had heard mention of another disease called Besnoitiosis lurking somewhere in the backwoods of the ranch. I read on, eyes drooping. It would never do to confess ignorance, having come all this way. Having absorbed the gist I could keep my eyes open no longer. My book slipped from my fingers and I slept.

I was up next morning with the birds and tiptoed to the dining area. I intended to demonstrate my impatience to get down to brass tacks by being there all hot and eager for the fray, before the Commandant had even got out of bed. To my chagrin I found him already at the breakfast table, head bent over a bowl of porridge. He looked up, gave a grunt and resumed his attack on Scotia's national dish.

As I got to work on my own bowl, he briefed me on the situation on the ranch.

The outbreak had started a year ago, to date about a thousand animals had been affected, 50% severely, and all attempts at treatment had been ineffectual. They had tried streptomycin, sodium iodide and potassium iodide, all to no avail. It was thought that the disease had been brought in with cattle from the Tana River area to the north, where it was endemic. The game seemed not to be affected.

I inquired about tick control, knowing from my nocturnal reading that ticks could play a part in transmission of the disease. Because the ranch was so big – one and a half million acres – dipping was only possible during the dry season when the cattle were brought in to be near sources of water. When the rains came they were then dispersed over the vastness of the ranch. 'And,' said the Commandant, 'there is a risk of loss of immunity to anaplas and redwater if we dip too regularly.'

I nodded. He was right. Give him his due, he knew his onions. The humped Boran cattle are relatively resistant to these tick-borne diseases and calves possess an innate resistance enhanced by maternal antibodies. By allowing calves to become infected, a state of co-infectious immunity is created, associated with the persistence of the organism in the peripheral blood. This immunity may last for years. With too efficient tick control there would be no exposure to infected ticks, no immunity and as a result a herd wide open to infection by these potentially fatal diseases. But now we had another disease situation in which ticks were potentially involved, with the likelihood of not being able to do anything about it.

I finished my porridge, drank my tea and stood up. 'Anything else I should know about?' I asked.

'Well, we've got tryps along the river and luggas but we've put out tsetse fly traps to try and deal with that. And we get heartwater in the sheep.' This was another much-feared tick-borne disease, one which could wreak havoc in susceptible flocks and herds and which was transmitted by the bont tick, Amblyomma. This was the same tick, I knew, which was suspected of being involved in the transmission of Bovine Farcy. 'Oh, and we don't feed any minerals so we get a bit of Botulism. We get Foot and Mouth on a regular basis and the odd outbreak of pleuropneumonia from time to time and we've got some Besnoitiosis I'd like you to look at.'

'Right,' I said, 'I think that's probably enough to be going on with for the moment.' The Commandant gave a thin smile.

Out in the yard stood a Toyota pickup, in the back of which sat or stood a number of hard-looking Boran herdsmen. Already the sun was hot and I was glad of my hat. We drove out of the yard, heading for the distant boma, where the infected animals were waiting. The land was table flat, biscuit-brown and dry. The only glimpse of greenery was along the river and by the dry river beds. Here the indigo-blue box-like tsetse traps had been sited. The flies are attracted to such dark colours and, lured in by attractants simulating ox breath, the traps are remarkably successful in reducing tsetse fly numbers.

For an hour we drove across parched, withered plains, covered in brittle scrub. The monotony of the sparse landscape was broken by the occasional anthill and isolated flat-topped acacia, dancing crazily in the shimmering superheated air. A group of mineral-deprived cattle gnawed listlessly on a scattering of elephant bones. A trio of red-earthed warthogs dashed across the track. To our left a column of needle-horned oryx, dust clouds streaming from their galloping hooves, vanished into the haze. The track surmounted an almost imperceptible rise and there, in front of us, was the boma, full of white, humped cattle.

The truck rolled to a halt and the men in the back jumped down. Even before I got out of the dust-filled cab I could see the nodules on the affected animals. Some had only a few, but others appeared afflicted with what looked like bovine leprosy. Some had large nodules in the parotid area of the neck, others chains of lumps extending along the neck, shoulder and along the flank. In front of the shoulder the pre-scapular lymph nodes were enormously enlarged. The forelegs of some animals were grossly swollen with a mass of disfiguring lumps.

I walked through the thick dust into the boma. The cattle appeared to be in no way disturbed by their unsightly afflictions. All were in good condition and were relaxed and at ease. But it was patently obvious that no drug on earth was going to cure this disease. The Age of Miracles was past and if I was expected to produce a wonder drug the Commandant was going to be grievously disappointed. The only solution, if it could be called that, was early isolation of the affected animals and slaughter. Prevention lay in tick and fly control, keeping animals out of areas of thorny vegetation and the prompt treatment of any wounds. I put this to the Commandant, standing beside me in the boma. He remained silent, gnawing on his lip, face puce in the growing heat. The herdsmen stood watching us.

'Look,' I said, 'you've already got about a thousand infected cattle. The more that get infected the more will get infected. You've got 20,000 odd cattle on the ranch. Better to cull a thousand now than ten times that number in a year's time. Most can be sold for meat as in most cases the nodules are superficial and can be trimmed off by the butcher.'

'Right,' he replied, 'we'll see what we can do.'

'If you can dip, then dip. If you can't then try to get insecticide ear tags or pour-ons. But you have to start selective culling before the situation gets out of control.' It's probably already out of control, I thought.

'Cull all the worst cases, and maintain separate streams of potentially-infected and potentially-non-infected offspring until the disease has subsided to a low level.'

I swatted away a cloud of flies buzzing round my head. Gad, it was hot. There were more cattle outside the boma. I walked through the bush to look at them. Many had nodules on their necks, on their flanks and nearly all had swollen pre-scapular lymph nodes. All must go, I thought. Any dilly dallying, foot dragging and procrastinating would worsen an already bad situation.

I returned to the vehicle. The Commandant was already at the wheel, engine running. 'Right,' I said, 'let's see the other outbreak.' The herdsmen once more piled into the back, apparently ready to receive another covering of red dust. We drove for another hour across an interminable plain, on which the only sign of life was a pair of bat-eared foxes whose siesta in the middle of the track we rudely disturbed.

The affected cattle were standing in an apathetic group in a fenced enclosure. Compared to the outbreak of Bovine Farcy this was small beer – a mere 40 animals infected with the protozoal organism Besnoita besnoiti. But these animals were ill and had been so for a long time. They stood, heads lowered, eyes glazed, thin and weak. Their skins were thickened and wrinkled, some had diarrhoea, others had enlarged lymph nodes; some had swellings on their bellies.

I walked among them, shirt soaked in sweat, still swatting flies. It was furnace hot. I was told of the numerous drug trials to which the wretched animals had been subjected, on the spurious basis that because this was a protozoal disease it might respond to drugs used to treat other protozoal diseases such as East Coast Fever. But I knew that there were no known curative drugs and that now these animals, if they recovered, would be life-long carriers of the organism and as such a potential source of infection for other animals. Once again I advised the Commandant to cull all infected animals and to abandon further treatment. He looked at me as though I was Jeremiah re-born.

There is considerable confusion as to how this strange disease is spread. Some authorities mention the cat as the final host, but there were no cats in contact with these cattle on the ranch. Others refer to a reservoir in wild game such as kudu, impala and wildebeest, with transmission by blood-sucking insects, such as horse flies, tsetse flies and ticks. But the important thing is that as the parasites multiply in the tissues the intermediate host reacts by forming cysts packed with thousands of parasites. And so the unfortunate host becomes a life-long carrier. The only vaccine available is one made in South Africa and it is so fragile that it cannot be used outside its location of manufacture.

Apart from the buzzing of a squadron of stowaway flies, there was an ominous silence in the cab as we drove back to base. The sun was sinking over the plains, lending them a mystique and beauty lacking during the harsh light of day. The Commandant, morose, silent and uncommunicative, stared fixedly through the dusty windscreen. He put his foot to the floor.

As we leapt wildly over irregularities in the track and tore round blind corners I fumbled desperately for my non-existent seat belt. I had brought no comfort to the beleaguered guardians of the ranch. Indeed I was little more than a grim judge donning the black cap.

Once back at base my chauffeur vanished into his office. Berna and the girls came rushing out, telling me what a wonderful day they had had in the swimming pool by the river.

'And how was *your* day, Dad?' shouted Rona.

'Great,' I said, 'just great.'

Ingrid appeared. 'Ah, Hugh, you're back.' she smiled, 'As you're here would you be so kind as to look at my dogs? Nothing much, but one's a bit lame and another has a skin problem.'

'With pleasure,' I replied. At least I wouldn't have to advise that they be culled.

I followed Ingrid through the house and out to the kennels. I spent some time examining the dogs, palpating legs and scrutinising skin. Having delivered my verdict I took a step back and trod on a foot. Startled, I spun round, to find the Commandant standing behind me. He had crept in and had stood silently in the shadows watching while I checked the dogs in the company of his wife. What did he think I might do? Have her on the kennel floor?

Next morning we flew back to Lake Elementaita. Our designated pilot on this occasion was the livestock manager and the plane was, by strange chance, the same Cessna 172 in which I had trained to fly. But it was an obvious demotion. There was barely room in the cabin for us all, and were it not for the fact that the runway was at a mere 900 feet above sea level we would not have got off the ground at all. The flight, over Tsavo East, the Yatta Plateau and the parched hills of Ukambani took three hours.

I had hoped that action would have been taken on my advice. Not so. My gloomy predictions came to pass. The disease spread and the following year 9,000 cattle had to be culled.

Chapter Twenty Seven

TIME FOR A TORTOISE

It was 9pm. I had finished the day's bookwork. The girls were all in bed. Berna and I sat in the lounge and pondered on whether to have a cup of tea or a glass of Gilbey's and decided, without too much discussion, to opt for the latter. I was pouring the first tot when there was the most infernal battering on our verandah door.

'What the shoot? Who the ....?' This being Kenya one's immediate thoughts were of thugs, burglars, Mau Mau.

'It's me, Irene!' a voice shouted. Irene was our neighbour, married to Seamus, who was a farmer and pilot.

'Can I come in?' I opened the door. Irene was of South African Afrikaner descent, born in the Karoo. When she was excited she spoke in the pinched accents of her birthplace. She did so now, to such an extent she was almost unintelligible.

'It's Seamus,' she babbled, 'he's been arrested, he's in the cells and it's all the fault of those damned tortoises!' Berna and I looked at each other. What *was* she talking about?

'Sit down, Irene,' we said, 'would you like a drink?'

'I bloody well need one, but there's no time. It's all Rafael's fault! Bloody idiot! What was he thinking about? Leaving those tortoises there! Left them on Presidential land, didn't he? Very clever! And now he's gone! To Leicester or Hackney, or wherever all the Asians go when they leave here!'

'Sorry, Irene,' I said, 'we're a bit lost. Can you clarify just what's going on?'

'Right. Well, as you know, Rafael D'Mello has been working for Seamus for years and years. Anyway, he decided that it was time to settle in the Motherland, although he'd never ever been there.' Irene snorted. 'The day before he was due to fly to London, the day before,' – her voice rose to a shriek – 'he suddenly remembered that he hadn't disposed of, or found homes for, his kids' five tortoises. So, what does he do? Does he phone up Seamus, or a friend, to say – 'Would you look after these five tortoises for me until you find a home for them?' No, he puts them into the boot of his car, which is Seamus's car, a company car, jumps in and drives down the Baringo road. Does he wait until he finds an unoccupied piece of bundu? No, he stops where the road runs through Presidential property, opens the boot and offloads five large tortoises.'

'What time was this?' Berna asked.

'It was dark – about 8pm or so.'

'Carry on.'

'As Rafael was in the process of decanting the tortoises, an askari hoves out of the darkness and asks him if he can help. Rafael says no thanks, jumps back into his car and zooms off, never to be seen again. All this was about three weeks ago. The askari is curious to see what were these heavy round objects which Rafael has dumped into the Presidential field, and finds five tortoises! All with names painted on their shells, names like 'Speedy' and 'Rocky', you know the sort of thing. But, more importantly, he wrote down the number plate of the car, Seamus's car! Perhaps I'll have that drink after all.'

I poured a generous measure into a glass and waited until Irene had knocked back a substantial slug.

'Go on,' I said.

'Well, as you know tortoises do not have a good reputation in the African mind. They are associated with drought and with bad luck. So why, they might think, would anyone want to release tortoises on the land of the President, unless they meant harm? Unbeknown to us, an ad was put in the paper asking anyone seeing Seamus's car with the recorded number plate, to report it to the police!'

If this had not been so serious we might have burst out laughing. But now that the Kenyan police were involved, things began to take a more sinister turn.

'Seamus flew in this morning from the farm, to find a posse of police waiting for him. They told him that he was under arrest for releasing tortoises on Presidential land. He didn't know what the hell they were talking about. They said that his car was seen at the scene of the crime and that the askari said that a non-African had opened the boot and taken out five tortoises and so he was being charged. They took him to the Central Police Station where he was interrogated for five hours! Five hours!' The South African accent was really strong.

'Then he was taken to the police station next to the President's farm where he is in the cells! In the cells! For what?' Irene's voice rose again to soprano heights.

'You're the British rep here. You've got to come and help poor Seamus. God knows what he's going through.'

'Right, let me phone the duty officer at the High Commission in Nairobi.'

I rang the relevant number. After about ten rings I was just about to put the phone down when it was answered. Judging by the background noise: music, ribald laughter, shouting, and the clashing of glasses, it sounded as though the duty officer was attending some sort of debauch.

'Yesh? Djohn here?' John who for crying out loud!

'Are you the duty officer?' I inquired.

'Yesh, that's me.'

Well mate, I thought, pin your ears back and listen to this. I gave him chapter and verse and waited for his response. There was a short pause and he burst into laughter, adding to the din behind him.

'Are you having me on?' he asked.

'Listen chum,' I said, 'this is serious. The man's inside and we've got to get him out.' He seemed to sober up at that.

'Right, there's not much I can do at the moment. Can you go and see him, perhaps take something to prove to the cops that he's not the man who dumped the tortoises. Can you contact a lawyer, either now or first in the morning? I'll pass this on to the consular chaps first thing.' And with that he was gone, back to the party.

Lucky chap I thought.

Berna had heard all of this.

'Hey, wasn't Rafael at our wedding?' she said, 'maybe we've got a snap of him in our wedding album. If you show that to the cops it will prove that Seamus is innocent.' And off she went to search for the album, coming back a few minutes later, triumphant.

'Look, there he is.'

We looked and there was Rafael, all togged up and looking like an extra in a Bollywood movie. He was wearing a hideous pink and yellow tie, his moustache looked as though it had just been brilliantined and, judging by the inane expression on his map and the half empty tankard of beer in his right hand, this was not his first pint of the day.

'Yes,' said Irene, 'that's him all right. Looks totally smashed!'

'And looks nothing like Seamus.'

'Thank God for that!' said Irene.

I carefully removed not one, but two images of the cause of all our troubles from our album and placed them in an envelope.

'Right,' I said. 'I'll just phone Rajni Sheth, the lawyer, and we'll be on our way. First class chap. Nothing ever fazes him. I've got to go to Kericho and Koru for work in the morning so I want him to know what's going on.' Rajni fortunately was not partying and listened carefully to what I told him and said he would speak to the police in the morning.

Irene finished her drink.

'Poor Seamus won't have had a particle to eat or drink since he was arrested,' she said. 'I've got some sandwiches in the car and a flask of coffee to keep him going and I'm bringing a camp bed as well. From what I've heard the prisoners have to doss down on the stone floor. Sounds awful.'

'I'll bring a couple of light bulbs and a camp chair,' I said.

Bidding Berna farewell we set off into the night. We reached the police station at 10pm. The place seemed to be in darkness. We got out of the car and saw that there was a dim light in what passed as the reception area.

Irene's normal temperament was nothing if not volatile and I harboured apprehensions that she might queer our pitch if she lost her rag when we met the gendarmerie.

'Look, Irene,' I said, 'let me deal with this. We don't want both of you in chokey do we?'

'Very well,' she said through gritted teeth.

We entered the building. The air was dank and chill. Faded posters peeling from a formerly white wall, now a leaden grey from years of accumulated grime, advised us in imperative terms how to avoid contracting AIDS. Graphic, primitive art drawings showed what happened when you did not drive with the due care as advised by the authorities. All they lacked were a few gobbets of real blood. A rogues gallery of Wanted men and one woman stared at us from a glassed-in frame. Irene shivered.

'God, I wouldn't like to meet any of them on a dark night.'

I approached the large sloping counter. On our side bars extending from ceiling to floor prevented me from prodding the constable slumbering on the other side. His forehead lay on the pitted woodwork. I coughed. No response. I rattled the bars with my car keys. Nothing. I looked at Irene. I rapped the wall sharply with my knuckles. He stirred and looked up.

'Yes?' he mumbled. He did not look friendly.

'Good evening officer,' I said, showing him my brightest smile and my official High Commission card, 'I would like to see the European you are holding here. He is British and should not be here.'

'We will decide that,' he snapped.

'Can I see the officer in charge?'

'He is off duty.'

'But he lives here, does he not?'

'Yes, but he will not be pleased to be disturbed.'

'I understand that, but this is important.'

'Very well,' and he slid from his stool and shambled off.

The officer, Inspector Kiprono, was not overjoyed to be routed out at this late hour, but he invited me into his office to discuss the matter. I showed him the photos of the inebriated Rafael.

He laughed.

'My, he's had a few. I'm surprised he's still standing.'

'Yes, and *he's* the chap who dropped off the tortoises, not poor Seamus whom you have in your horrid dungeons.'

'They're modern cells, not dungeons, and for me this is a small matter, but my instructions have come from above. If it were up to me I would release him but I cannot, until I am told. Let me show these photos to my boss who will know what to do. Meanwhile you can see the prisoner.'

Preceded by the constable, I returned to Irene. We were led down a short corridor to the cells, of which there were only four. All were in darkness. The constable unlocked a door on the right. Above the door on the left was a sign – 'Male Lunatic Wing'. At least Seamus wasn't in there.

'Can you switch on the light?' I asked the jailer.

'No bulbs,' he grunted. In the gloom we could make out the figure of Seamus, sitting on the floor in the far corner. He leapt to his feet as we entered.

'Gosh, am I glad to see you,' he said. 'This place is like the Black Hole of Calcutta and I'm absolutely starving.'

'You poor darling,' said Irene, 'and all because of that idiot Rafael.'

While they comforted each other, trying to ignore the ferret eyes of the watching flatfoot, I returned to the car to collect the food, camp bed, stool and bulbs.

Seamus attacked the sandwiches like a starving wolf. While he sipped his coffee I explained what we had done so far.

'Don't worry,' I said, 'we'll get you out. Try to get some sleep and we'll see you tomorrow.'

The following day I was off to Kericho and Koru, a round trip of about 200 miles. On my way back to Nakuru I drove to the police station. It was 3.30 in the afternoon and Seamus was still incarcerated and getting more than a bit desperate. By this time, having driven on indifferent roads a distance equivalent to that between London and Land's End, done a full day's work, lost a large chunk of my previous night's beauty sleep and desecrated our photo album, I was getting a little testy. I suggested to the inspector, on no basis whatsoever, that a phone call to higher authority in London might be required to rectify the situation. Satisfied that he looked a trifle concerned, I left.

Back in the surgery I spent the next hour on the phone, speaking to the lawyer, the Consular Department of the High Commission and to Julie, a government official in London, who made no effort to disguise her open-mouthed incredulity.

'At least it makes a change from news of famines and civil wars,' she laughed.

During the course of these seemingly interminable phone calls there were dark mutterings about international arrest warrants, Interpol and lengthy custodial sentences. Rafael was a Wanted Man. But my prime contact was Berna, back at base camp, and adjacent to the home of the luckless Seamus.

In the late afternoon a phalanx of police had turned up. Equipped with long slender wands, ideal apparently for detecting tortoises, they had fanned out across the property and for the next hour poked and prodded the vegetation in a vain hunt for reptilian evidence with which to incriminate Seamus. They found none. But, prior to this bizarre act in the ongoing pantomime, they had been to Rafael's home to quiz the servants and neighbours, who corroborated the fact that the place had indeed been a home-from-home for tortoises and that the children had spent their waking hours in close proximity to the creatures.

At 7pm Seamus was released. But his car was impounded, he was required to report to the police weekly and he was to try to persuade Rafael to come back to face the consequences of his actions. And if Rafael did not return Seamus would be held personally responsible for the whole episode.

Meanwhile the wretched tortoises had been found and taken to Lake Nakuru Park where they were closely confined, under armed guard, and carefully watched for any sign of aberrant behaviour. Who knows, perhaps they had time-bombs secreted beneath their shells.

Ten days later the case was dropped. Rajni Sheth had nobly offered himself in place of Seamus. The car was released and Seamus was left without a stain on his escutcheon. The same could not be said of the distant Rafael.

The fate of the tortoises remained unknown, one common to many hapless prisoners in Africa.

Chapter Twenty Eight

OFF THE MENU

In February 1990 foreign minister Robert Ouko was murdered in mysterious circumstances in Western Kenya. The case, like so many others, has yet to be solved. The killing triggered off country-wide demonstrations and riots. These seemed to morph into later unrest associated with a call for democracy and a multi-party parliament – something not looked on with favour by the government in power at the time.

Nakuru, being a melting pot of tribes from all over the land, was much caught up in these disturbances. For months and even years, the town echoed to the sound of gunfire and the baying of mobs surging along the streets. The smashing of shop windows and the staccato rattle of army helicopters circling overhead was a frequent everyday background noise. We became used to the sight of lorries full of steel-helmeted police roaring along the streets, en route to quell another demo. Students would regularly go on strike and hold up the traffic, break car windows and erect barricades across roads. Columns of heavily-armed cavalry would clip-clop past the surgery. They were members of the Anti Stock Theft Unit, formerly and unfortunately called the Stock Theft Unit, until it was pointed out that their role was to counter stock theft, not to engage in it. I treated their horses and they would give me a friendly wave as they trotted past.

Stampedes past the surgery were commonplace and if I did not close the door quickly, fleeing residents would seek refuge within, until the threat had passed. Sometimes up to thirty frightened people would be packed inside. The Club across the street was not immune and shooting in the car park indicated that the authorities were in hot pursuit of anti-government elements. Several people were shot dead in these disturbances and hundreds arrested. The jails were full. The opportunity to benefit was too much for some, as looting was easy. During one sudden uproar my long-time general worker, Bernard, fled. He turned up next day, smart and dapper and clad in a new shirt and trousers.

I would come back from my rounds to find the town deserted, rocks scattered over the streets, and civilians being marched, hands in the air, police rifles pointed at their backs, towards unknown destinations.

But life had to go on.

I came home one afternoon to find that Berna had arranged a singing show to be performed in our living room, by a number of children, including our own. As their treble voices piped their infant numbers, a mob was busy rioting on the main road a hundred yards away and singing loudly to a different tune.

Disease and accident carried on as before. Cows had difficult calvings, bitches had to be spayed, ticks brought infection to dogs and cattle, horses ran into wire and had to be stitched, sheep got worms, legs got broken and had to be pinned or plastered, animals died and had to be autopsied.

During this period of social unrest many essential drugs became scarce. The supply dwindled, shrank and finally dried up. Dog vaccines, horse sickness vaccine, certain antibiotics such as oxytetracycline, snake bite anti-serum, drugs for treating East Coast Fever in cattle and tick fever in dogs, all became unobtainable. We were back to basics and before. Ancient remedies, lost in cobwebbed antiquity, were dragged out and, not without some misgivings, put to the test. The death rate rose, but if I had done nothing it would have been much higher.

—✳—

It was 2am and I was sleeping the sleep of the just. I had spent a good part of the day on ranches near Nanyuki, about a hundred miles from Nakuru. One in particular, El Karama, had occupied much of my time. It was owned by former white hunter Guy Grant. Guy was a splendid fellow, the very salt of the earth, kind, hospitable, friendly and interested in everything. Bearded to his bushy grey eyebrows, Guy was always clad in safari shorts and his lean teak-brown legs ended in sock-less feet thrust into sandals of such immense size that he resembled a human lily trotter. But he was not nicknamed 'Lightning' for nothing. Guy talked very slowly and with great deliberation. If he phoned me up for a chat about some animal problem, I would say, 'Hang on a moment, Guy,' while I dragged an armchair across to the phone, for I knew that I might be on the blower for all of half an hour. Things moved on El Karama in a similar stately fashion. Everything had to be done in the correct order. There must be no rush. No animal must be stressed or flustered. No voices were to be raised.

The ranch staff followed these Grantian dictates to the letter. They carried out their allotted tasks in a curiously soporific manner, almost as though they were sleep-walking. This was wonderful as long as one wasn't in a hurry, which I usually was. So I moulded myself to the system and, to my gratified surprise, it worked. Festina lente, more haste less speed, was Guy's motto and one with much to recommend it. In future, when confronted with a knotty problem, instead of rushing at it bald headed as I had done so often in the past, I would give it thought, take my time and then go for it and then still make mistakes, but in a more orderly, leisurely fashion.

There was always a lot to do – camels and colts to castrate, bitches to spay, Sahiwal cattle to examine, horses' teeth to rasp. On this occasion it was horses with contracted tendons, resulting in club feet. After anaesthetising the patients, I performed an inferior check desmotomy – severing the check ligament to relieve the tension on the deep flexor tendon. Once again much time was spent on my long-suffering knees. But it was worth it as the results, provided the horses were presented early enough, were usually highly satisfactory.

Lavinia, Guy's wife, was tall, elegant, erudite, and artistic. She was fond of dogs and cats, including the memorably-named Soft Grey Bear. She also was a dab hand when it came to the rearing of orphans of the wild. Species of rodents barely known to science were billeted in wire-mesh enclosures in the master bedroom, their quarters almost dwarfing those allotted to the lord and lady of the manor. On one occasion Lavinia took it upon herself to instruct a trio of abandoned adolescent hadada ibis in the arts of obtaining their daily crust. This they normally do by prodding the ground with their long curved bills in search of grubs, insects and the like. Young ibis are normally taught this by their parents. We arrived one day to find Lavinia crawling over what passed for a lawn, a large papier-mashe ibis head, complete with beak, attached to her own head, resolutely stabbing at the grass, and watched with what looked like avian incredulity by her three feathered pupils. But they caught on and very soon all four were hard at it, frantically blunting their beaks on the unreceptive earth.

As an addendum to my work on the ranch I had been asked to spay a bitch for Kob Johnson, who lived on a sort of enclave called Combretum on the other side of the river Easo Nyiro which formed the property's westerly boundary. Kob was a local legend. Burly and bespectacled, he lived in two rooms attached to a ruined house sited in a green meadow surrounded by bush. Kob was a master cobbler, a genius with leather, and here he made saddles, harnesses, belts, bridles and boots. He had dogs, horses and donkeys, no car and when he wanted to go somewhere he walked, through the bush, dodging elephant and buffalo, skirting lion and wild dog.

El Karama was full of game and it was always a pleasure to drive from the ranch-house across the undulating hills and valleys to Kob's retreat. Herds of impala, Thomson's gazelle and zebra, both Burchell's and the endangered Grevy's, were everywhere. Knots of needle-horned oryx galloped off as I approached. Families of stiff-tailed warthog trotted away in mock alarm as the car drew near. Buffalo glowered from dams and swamps. Reticulated giraffe ambulated in seeming slow motion among the acacias. And over all was the huge African sky, blue and dotted with white clouds which cast dappled moving shadows over an enchanted landscape.

We bumped down to the plank bridge over the river. Wheels on the planks, bridge just wide enough for the vehicle, now don't look down at the brown water foaming 20 feet below, no sides to this bridge remember, rumble slowly across and thump onto the sandy track on the other side. Then left, past the old cattle crush, splash through the stream, disturbing a dozing hammerkop, and crawl up the rocky hill to Kob's domain.

Operating facilities were minimal to non-existent. I spayed the bitch on a ramshackle table set up on the wrecked verandah of the ruin. A late afternoon breeze got up and a loose section of the corrugated iron roof flapped and banged in the wind directly above my head.

Halfway through the operation I had the feeling that I was being watched. I looked up. A small group of baboons was sitting on the grass about twenty yards away, staring intently in our direction. I lowered my eyes and continued with the operation. When I looked up again, they were gone.

—✳—

It was 2am. I was not quite full fathom five, but pretty close. Something like the tolling of a ship's bell pealed into my unconsciousness. I clawed my way on deck and grabbed the phone beside the bed.

'Hello,' I croaked.

'Hello, Hugh,' an infuriatingly cheery voice boomed in my ear. 'This is Julian here. Got a bit of a problem. Need your invaluable assistance.' *This* was Julian Fox, Anglo-Irish, without a trace of the brogue. In fact he spoke rather like *theeat*.

'Oh, yes, what's up?' I said.

'It's our young stallion. The wretched syce puts a mare in season into the stable next door to his and buggers off. The stallion tries to get at the mare, mounts the rail and has done something serious to his vitals. It's all hanging out and swollen to the size of a rugger ball. Doesn't look good.'

I bet it doesn't, I thought bleakly.

'Right,' I said, 'we'd better come and have a shufti and see what we can do. See you in a while.' Julian's place was about 25km away so it would take a good half hour or so to get there.

By this time Berna was also wide awake. 'I'm coming with you' she said. No argument there. I was glad. It always helps to have someone with you who has a vague idea what you're up to, especially when you're working in the dark. In more ways than one, I thought.

By the time we were ready to go Rona was also awake.

'What's the matter with the horse?' I explained that it sounded like a prolapse, without going into specifics.

'Can't it wait until morning?' she asked. I explained that while some things, such as wine and children, improve with age, others, and prolapses were one, definitely do not. She nodded, and trotted back to bed.

At about 3am, when most of life was at its lowest ebb, we reached the entrance to Foxy's establishment. The gate askari seemed to be included in this depressing category, and only after several stentorian blasts on the car horn did he hobble, troll-like, from his sentry box to raise the portcullis.

We drove straight to the stables, where we could see a light twinkling in the gloom.

The light was held by Julian. He was a broad, bulky chap with a mass of dark curly hair, a large nose and a jocular attitude to life. I hoped this would stand in my favour should things not go according to plan. As yet I had no plan.

'Well done, Hugh,' said Julian as I opened the car door. 'Thanks for coming. Ah, I see you've brought the memsahib. Things will be OK now!'

He gave a great booming laugh. He turned towards the stable.

'Well here's the patient. Chaka Zulu. Randy bugger, just like his namesake! Black as your boot as well! Hey, arap Sang,' he turned to a tall, thin syce standing motionless and unseen in the darkness, 'take this torch and shine it on the damage so the bwana can see what he's come to sort out!'

As yet I had not even seen the horse. The night was pitch black and so was the horse, an inky black stallion, which whinnied and shied away as the syce approached with the light.

The beam flickered across the stable. The stallion did not like it and reared, pawing wildly at the air, and as he did so I caught a glimpse of a grossly swollen penis, protruding grotesquely from his sheath.

'Right,' I said to Julian, 'I've seen enough. He's got a massive prolapse of his penis, probably traumatised as well. We'll have to knock him out and try to shove that lot back inside.'

'I'd be traumatised if that had happened to me!' said Julian. 'OK. I suppose you'll need some warm water?'

'Water, soap, towels and an extra pair of hands if possible.'

'The other syce, the bloody idiot who put the mare next door, is off and doesn't live on the premises. The house girl is away having her umpteenth baby and Samantha, my better half, is at a hen party in Nairobi.'

'Right then,' I said, 'so it's just as well Berna's here eh? Four of us should be enough. By the way, what's he like with injections?'

'Hates them! Goes ballistic when he sees a needle.'

'Great! How about a twitch then?'

'Not a hope. Up on his hind legs and tries to bite and goes for you with his forelegs.'

'Wonderful! Perhaps he hates men but likes women. Berna? Would you like to have a go?'

'Me? The only needle I've ever used is the one to stitch the holes in your shorts. I wouldn't be able to find the vein if I tried and, besides, I'm here in a humanitarian, supporting role, not as a member of a suicide mission.'

'Right. What about the syce? Perhaps the stallion is racially motivated in his likes and dislikes – hates whites but love blacks.'

'No go,' said Foxy, 'this one hates all humanity.'

'OK, looks like I've drawn the short straw. I'm going to use the finest possible needle and see if I can slip it into his jugular without him noticing it.'

'Are you joking? He'll make mincemeat out of you.'

I filled the syringe with a stallion-felling dose of Xylazine.

'When I was a schoolboy,' I said, 'and got bored during lessons, and nearly all the lessons *were* boring, I used to while away the tedium by sticking pins into the back of my hand – funny sort of thing to do but there you are – anyway I discovered that if you did it really slowly it didn't hurt at all. You could shove one in almost to the hilt and it was totally painless. Whether it was because the nerves of sensation are widely spaced or the pin was so fine and sharp I don't know. I'm going to give it a go on his nibs.'

'Why don't you breathe up his nostrils while you're at it,' laughed Foxy. All right for him. He was on the outside of the rails. All too soon I would be on the inside.

Arap Sang opened the stable door and I followed him inside. The stallion snorted in alarm but allowed the syce to put on a head collar. I turned my back on the horse. I could sense him looking at me. I waited for five minutes before turning round. I laid a hand on his flank. He shivered but did nothing.

'Now,' I said to arap Sang, 'slowly raise his head.'

He did so and I placed my fingers in the jugular furrow, raising the vein. Very slowly I pushed the point of the needle against the skin – no reaction – then through it and finally into the vein itself. Blood flowed into the syringe and slowly and carefully I injected the contents into the vein. Chaka Zulu did not move.

I turned away, wearing a small, smug smile. I smiled too soon. There was a crack like a pile driver on the back of my thigh as the stallion lashed forwards with a hind leg. I staggered and almost fell.

'You bastard!' I shouted.

'Yes, he's a mean one, all right,' said Foxy complacently from the security of his bunker.

'Are you OK, Hugh?' gasped Berna.

'Yeah, fine, fine,' I articulated between gritted teeth, 'Never better!'

I hopped out of the stable on one leg, thinking that this was taking the stiff upper lip nonsense a bit too far. But the deed was done. Two minutes later, the stallion's head was drooping to the level of his knees and he now offered no more resistance than a geriatric donkey.

We pushed him outside, where I gave him a second injection, this time of ketamine. He swayed, staggered and fell on his side with a thump.

I fished a couple of ropes out of the boot of the car and looped them around his lower legs.

'Right,' I said to my team, 'pull him onto his back. We're going to need all the gravity we can muster to get this lot back inside.'

'This lot' looked like an enormous black pudding, bulbous and protruding at all the wrong angles and bent backwards like a Spanish question mark. I mentioned this, to my mind, rather apt resemblance, to Foxy. He said nothing. But when I compared the diameter of this gruesome mass with that of the prepuce from which it had been so violently extruded my heart sank.

Foxy's light was wavering all over the place. One moment there was light, the next there was none.

'On the target please, Julian, if you don't mind!' I demanded.

'Sorry, folks, feeling a bit faint. Came over all hot and cold. I'm rather partial to black puddings and now seeing that lump there I'm off them for life.'

'Right, well there are alternatives. Try haggis. Now, have you got the warm water and soap? Lux or Imperial Leather if you don't mind, not that ghastly laundry soap. And while you're at it bring a kilo of sugar, preferably caster or icing. In the meantime I'll try to tenderise Chaka's essential member.' I could feel Julian staring at me.

Then he was gone and Berna held the torch steady and true while I poured obstetrical fluid over the prolapsed mass and proceeded to massage and knead the organ in an effort to reduce it to a returnable size. I seemed to be getting nowhere when Julian returned.

'Got the sugar,' he said. 'Icing – it's my birthday next week and Sam was going to bake me a cake. I say *was* because this is the lot and it was the last bag in the grocer's.'

'Chaka's need at the moment, Julian,' I replied 'is much greater than yours.' I cleaned off the lubricant and sprinkled a light frosting of sugar over the engorged penis. 'The sugar should draw out the trapped fluid – that's the theory anyway. I've used it on prolapsed bovine vaginas and uteri – is that the plural of uterus? – and it works.'

'Yes,' said Berna, 'I think that's correct. But I'll check in Chambers when we get home. And, for your information, the plural of vagina *can* be vaginas, but the purist would tend to use vaginae.'

'I'll remember that,' I said. 'Hey, look!' Berna held the torch closer to Chaka's swollen organ and sure enough, drops of fluid were now appearing on its surface.

'Have a look at that, chaps!' I said, addressing myself to Foxy and the supportive arap Sang. Neither seemed overly keen on a close inspection. 'We're getting somewhere!'

But as I said those words Chaka Zulu stirred, a hind leg twitched and he gave a low whinny.

'Sounds as though he still wants to get at that mare!' laughed Berna. However I was ready for this contingency and had prepared two syringes with half doses of Xylazine and Ketamine, which I had left lying on a clean towel. Quickly I rinsed my hands, grabbed the syringes and injected their contents into Chaka's jugular, deftly illuminated by Berna's spotlight.

'Right,' I said, 'back to the grindstone.' Although outside the circle of light which illuminated the scene of struggle all was pitch dark, I sensed Julian's shudder. But now we were on the home straight, the final furlong. A few more purposeful kneadings of the dough and the offending organ was decently out of sight and returned from whence it came. A purse string suture of strong monofilament nylon round the prepuce to hold everything in place, a shot of an anti-inflammatory and an antibiotic and we were done. I stood up. My leg had stiffened like a poker. During the heat of the action I had barely noticed it. Now I could barely move. I dragged myself to the car and leaned against it, waiting for Chaka to recover from his anaesthetic. Berna quickly and efficiently tidied away the crude evidence of our recent endeavours.

While we waited for Chaka to show signs of recovery, Julian produced a leather-bound hip flask of impressive proportions and proffered it to us. I took a substantial slug of the enclosed whisky which seemed to bypass my stomach, rushing directly to my cerebral cortex. I felt light-headed and very much better. Even Berna, who loathed the stuff, took a modest sip.

Chaka slumbered on. Long periods of suspended breathing were interspersed with deep inhalations. During an especially extensive period of apnoea, Julian said, 'I say, Hugh, are you sure he's still alive? I haven't seen him draw breath for about five minutes!'

'Mmm,' I replied, 'I'm afraid he's probably gone to commune with his ancestors. Perhaps I gave him too much when I topped him up!' I knew that the anaesthetic was extremely safe and that these were normal signs, and, as I spoke, Chaka swished his tail, flicked his ears and sat up.

Julian laughed. 'You bugger, Cran! Sam dotes on this stallion. If anything happens to him she'll have my guts for garters! And yours as well!'

Chaka sat quietly for another five minutes before rising smoothly to his feet.

'Right, Julian, I'll be back in four days to remove that suture. He'll be able to urinate past it in the meantime. And keep him away from the girls!'

I looked at my watch. 'Ye gods! Four thirty! Home, Scarlett, home to Tara!'

'Tomorrow's another day!'

'You mean, today's another day!'

Chapter Twenty Nine

THE STARE OF THE SCORPION

After a spate of cases like this I was more than ready for a break from the harsh realities of veterinary life on the equator. So when the Mountain Club announced that it was having a family meet to Silali, to the north of Lake Baringo, I suggested to Berna that we participate.

'Should be fun,' I said. 'There's a river for the kids to play in, shady trees to loll under, and the mountain is hardly a mountain at all. In fact it's almost horizontal. And, an added bonus, the natives are really friendly.' Berna looked sceptical, but gave the OK.

We had acquired an ancient Toyota Land Cruiser, and, being large and capacious, this was our vehicle of choice. The beast had only three gears and in the eyes of most people, usually those owning top-of-the-range five-gear air-conditioned spacemobiles, our wagon was little better that a four-wheeled single gear bicycle. It had a massive engine powered by petrol which it consumed at a prodigious rate, so much so that as one drove along one could see the fuel gauge needle dropping with every passing kilometre. The bonnet was so long that its end was almost out of sight. It was like driving a terrestrial aircraft carrier. The vehicle's only positive attribute was its powerful four wheel drive. Almost as soon as we bought it we tried to sell it, a process which took an inordinate length of time before a welcome sucker came along.

On the appointed day, under Scorpio, the eighth sign of the Zodiac, after having attended to several dogs in the surgery, we all piled aboard and set off to the rendezvous on the dirt road north of Lake Baringo. Here we met the rest of the party, who were drawn from Nairobi. There were about a dozen in total, mostly unknown to us. But among the group I was glad to see fellow masochists Paul Clarke and Graeme Watson, veterans of previous close encounters with thorn and rock. Paul was tall and lean, Graeme was a bit like an overfilled punch bag on legs. Both possessed an alarming determination to press on towards distant summits long after lesser, or more sensible, mortals, had turned back.

We continued along the rocky road to Silali, passed through the collection of shacks which constituted the best-forgotten township of Nginyang and on towards Kapedo. Kapedo, which cowered at the base of Silali, contained a mission set up by saintly Finns and a collection of humpies inhabited by a motley collection of less-than-saintly Pokot. The reason for Kapedo's existence lay in the fact that close by was the source of the Suguta River, which bubbled up in hot springs, tumbled over a waterfall and flowed northwards into the fearsomely hot Suguta Valley, there to finally expire in a waste of baking mudflats.

Just north of Kapedo was the boundary between the territory of the Pokot to the south and the Turkana to the north. They were not friends, clashes over water and grazing were common and stock theft and armed attacks kept the area in a constant state of tension.

After lunching in one of the innumerable luggas which transected the road at tiresomely inconvenient intervals we pressed on to Kapedo, where we were welcomed by an excited throng of colourfully-clad inhabitants. Kim, now aged ten months, was an object of especial interest. A young chap carrying a bow and a quiver of arrows pushed his way through the crowd.

'Na weza saidia?' he asked. 'Can I help?'

'Yes,' I said, 'we want somewhere to camp.'

'I will show you.' He climbed into the back of the Toyota. The girls goggled at his weapons and at him.

He directed us onto a rough track which led across country towards the distant river. A sudden short rainstorm laid the dust which was billowing up from our wheels. The drop in temperature was welcome. It was very hot. The sweet smell of rain falling on dry earth was pleasantly cool and refreshing. We stopped on the river bank and gazed down at the wide, shallow muddy water. I turned to our guide.

'Iko mamba?' I asked. 'Are there crocodiles?'

'Ndiyo. Iko.' 'Yes, there are.' Berna pursed her lips and raised her eyebrows.

I turned the key in the ignition. A horrid grinding sound. Had the starter jammed? I tried again. The engine caught. It was very hot.

We found a grove of trees by the river bank and pitched our tents –

Rona and Sophie in one and Berna, Kim and me in the other. The tents were not large. Luckily nor were we.

Our guide turned to us.

'I go now. Me Pokot. This Turkana land.' I thanked him and gave him a few shillings. He loped off.

The rest of the party arrived and soon there were several tents scattered under the trees. A gaggle of Turkana children turned up, clad in little or nothing. I asked them about the crocodiles.

'No problem sir. We know them very well. Your totos can bathe, and will be safe. If we see a crocodile coming we will shout 'mamba! mamba!' and then they can scramble out! They will be safe and sound!'

And so they were, that day and the next.

The children brought us fish, which we bought and cooked. Ravens appeared. We tossed them scraps. The sun descended behind Silali, which suddenly seemed rather larger than before. A trick of perspective I thought. The river gurgled musically on its way to the Suguta Valley.

At the appallingly early hour of 4.30am I struggled from my sleeping bag. I brewed some tea and breakfasted sumptuously on a bowl of weetabix. I stuffed some oranges into my rucksack, together with three litres of water. It was going to be a hot walk, but a short one. No need to burden myself with masses of surplus food. Other figures could be seen groping around in the darkness.

Berna was awake. 'When do you expect to be back?' she asked.

'In time for tea, I hope, so have the kettle on the boil!'

These pre-dawn starts are all very well, but it takes an age to do what in the bright light of day would take a fraction of the time. So it was not until 6am that everyone was ready. Eight of us squeezed into a Land Rover and were driven in considerable discomfort back to and through a sleeping Kapedo, crossed a small river of the same name and after several bumpy kilometres on the road to Nginyang arrived at our jumping off point. Our driver turned his vehicle in preparation for returning to camp and, presumably, bed. I asked him when he would be back to pick us up.

'I'll be here at four,' he said. In other words, just in time for tea.

We set off. For some reason those in charge of the expedition had not recruited a local guide to show us the way. Most of the mountains in the lands of the Pokot appear to be sacred to them so perhaps no one was willing to show the white strangers the way. On the other hand arrogance and ignorance may have got the better of people more used to the tamer conditions of the so-called First World. But threading one's way through dense East African bush without a guide can take an inordinate length of time and can result in getting irretrievably lost in unfriendly terrain.

We wound our way through a maze of black volcanic boulders beneath tall acacias and crossed the dry bed of the Nginyang River, which further downstream joined the Kapedo to become the Suguta. The trees thinned and we plodded across a bare, dusty plain towards the distant mountain. The sun was rapidly rising and shade was nowhere to be found. Far off, where the mountain met the plain, camels were browsing.

As we trudged along I asked Graeme about our objective.

'Well,' he said, 'Our Leader's plan is to walk to the crater rim – Silali's got the most enormous vertical walled crater – have lunch there and then return to the roadhead, where the vehicle will pick us up.'

'In time for tea!' I replied.

'Exactly.'

'OK, that's all very well, but what about the summit? The summit's to the north, while we're heading due east.'

'That's not on the agenda,' said Graeme.

'Well,' I said, 'it's time it bloody well was.' Paul had joined us, and it was agreed that after lunch on the crater rim we would form a splinter group and head for the summit, with anyone who cared to join us.

We reached the camels. They were being herded by a Pokot woman who made signs that she wanted water. But we had none to spare. We asked her in Swahili about the way to the crater. She stared at us, as did the expats in the group. Neither understood the language. A few spindly white cattle appeared, drifting through the bush. They also stopped and stared, wondering who these strange creatures were, invading their territory.

We found a path, steep, stony and rubbly, heading roughly in the right direction. We followed it, getting caught at frequent intervals in overhanging branches of wait-a-bit thorn. No one found this to their liking. A hard faced Pokot man carrying a spear and a polished wooden head rest came walking easily down the path, not getting caught in any thorns. He wore a tight black cloth from waist to above the knee, leather sandals and a bead necklace. An ostrich feather bobbed jauntily in his elaborate mud pack chignon. He looked at us, said nothing and passed on his way.

'Gosh,' said one of the party, 'not overfriendly was he?'

'Well,' I said, 'like Gibbon's Aethiopians, the Pokot are encompassed on all sides by their enemies. Turkana to the north, Samburu to the east,

Tugen to the south and across the Ugandan border, the Karamojong. So any stranger in this part of the world is suspect. Plus we don't have a local guide to introduce us.'

We pressed on, losing the path more often than finding it. But at 10.30 we reached the crater rim. The crater was vast, surrounded by vertical walls of rock. Far to the east we could see the hills to the north of Maralal and the stunning viewpoint of Losiolo. As soon as we sat down to eat and rest a pair of fan-tailed ravens appeared to join the feast. In my case it was less a feast than a snack. An orange and a slug of water. Others had Bakewell tarts, slices of pizza, cans of beer, slabs of chocolate, packets of crisps and in one case even a bottle of wine. I was all for gobbling and going for the summit. But decorum dictated otherwise. Also, mountaineering ethics dictate that the party should not be split until it is safe to do so.

Finally at noon we rose and retraced our steps. Canvassing the others had failed to recruit any volunteers to join us in our summit bid. We three split off to the north while the others carried on downwards to the distant road. There was no path to the summit and there was no shade either. It was fearfully hot, with not a breath of wind. We ploughed our way through a vast tract of long, fibrous grass, raising dust and clouds of disturbed insects. We struck a ridge and began to toil up it. I could feel myself dehydrating as I walked. The very ground radiated heat. The sun was vertically overhead. This was the very worst time to be indulging in this sort of nonsense. Even the lizards were seeking shade under rocks.

Graeme was lagging behind. Suddenly he stopped and vomited violently. Paul and I turned back to find Graeme sitting on a rock, looking pale and holding his head in his hands.

'Sorry, chaps, I'm totally wiped out. You carry on. I'll meet you on the way down.' Graeme was in no immediate danger, so Paul and I carried on along the ridge. Normally as one gains height on mountains the temperature drops and a breeze gets up to cool the heated climber. Not so on Silali. The air shimmered, the rocks danced crazily in the sun. I pulled my hat lower over my streaming forehead and concentrated on avoiding the next boulder.

Another 45 minutes of sweated toil and we stepped onto the top. We exchanged an ironic handshake and looked around for comfortable rocks on which to rest. There were none. I swallowed a few mouthfuls of warm water and sucked an orange. Two left. I looked around. North to the khaki-coloured wastes of the Suguta Valley, west to Tiati of fond memory, down to the just visible clump of trees around Kapedo, south to the black lava flow on the sacred mountain Paka. I looked back the way we had come. Through the juddering air there were faint signs of life. Graeme was on the move. Slowly he clawed his way up to us. Paul and I cheered him on. Finally he staggered on the summit and collapsed, gasping from the exertion. He mopped his brow and drank deep and long from his water bottle.

I looked at my watch – 2pm. Time to get moving. Graeme appeared to have recovered. We rose, shouldered our packs and chose a different ridge for the descent in the hope that it might prove less arduous than that we had just ascended. It was worse, steep, and covered in long wiry grass in which were hidden countless antisocial elements in the form of innumerable boulders. At 4pm we regained the crater path and set off towards the distant plain, still far below us. As we bashed our way through the boulder-fields, continually losing our way, Graeme had another bout of vomiting. We stopped to allow him to recover his equilibrium and then pushed on. By the time we reached the edge of the plain the shadows were lengthening and dusk was almost upon us. I glanced at my watch – 6pm. Another hour should see us at the road. As we set off on the last lap a knot of camels appeared, herded by a pair of spear-carrying Pokot. We asked them the way to the road. They pointed with their spears in the way we were going. Then they were gone.

We staggered on, dry throated, dehydrated and exhausted. By the time we reached the river bed it was completely dark.

'Got a torch, Hugh?' asked Paul.

'No, I assumed we'd be back in time for tea so I didn't pack one.'

'What about you, Graeme?' Graeme shook his head and croaked. We took this to be a negative.

'Well, neither have I,' said Paul. Still, I thought, we're only a few hundred yards from the road. Shouldn't be a problem.

I felt the rise of ascending bile and a spasm of giddiness. I turned aside and vomited into a bush. Feeling better I looked around. I might as well have done so with my eyes closed. I couldn't see a damned thing. The volcanic rocks were black and there was no moon. I could hear the others stumbling around in the darkness. Muffled curses from Paul. Gasps and groans from Graeme. Then a light appeared, barely a bowshot from where I stood. It was a vehicle on the road. We were saved! I could hear the sound of the diesel engine. The light swivelled, shone in our direction, turned, there was a grinding of gears, the light faded and the vehicle was gone.

'Who the hell was that?' said Paul, 'that didn't even stop or hoot?'

'Must have been one of the group,' I said.

'Well, why didn't the bugger stop? If he didn't see us on the road then where the hell did he think we were? Taken a short cut back to camp?'

We cussed and fumed for a few minutes and then decided to fumble our way in the total darkness towards the road. Hands outstretched I shuffled towards the spot where we had seen the vehicle's headlights. Within a minute I was painfully and inextricably entangled in a thicket of wait-a-bit. For what seemed like hours I fought to disentangle myself. Finally with shirt in tatters and streaming blood from a multitude of unseen wounds I emerged backwards, to immediately go base over apex as I tripped over a hidden log, cracking my head on a rock.

Cursing, I staggered to my feet. A few feet away in the sooty darkness I could hear Paul and Graeme cursing as they too floundered in the satanic groves like inebriated walruses, knowing not where they were going. Suddenly there was a great whoop, a moment of silence and then a whump as though a sack of cement had fallen from a building site onto the pavement far below.

'What the shoot was that?' I called. Again silence. Then a muffled voice came calling, as though from below ground. It was Graeme. He sounded almost bereft of speech.

'I've fallen into some sort of pit,' he gasped.

'Where are you?' I called. 'God knows,' he wheezed. I shuffled towards his voice and found it emerging from an inky emptiness below my feet.

'I'm down here,' he said. 'Must be part of the river bed, a waterfall or something. If we carry on like this someone, most likely me, is going to break a leg, or worse.' After an age of desperate scrabbling and what sounded to my keen veterinary mind rather like Cheyne-Stoke's respiration, Graeme emerged from his pit. He sounded rather the worse for wear. Paul emerged from outer to inner darkness and we decided that we had to call a halt to this nonsense. Our only option was to doss down until the moon rose and by its light make our way to the road.

'When does the moon rise?' I asked.

'Search me,' replied Paul.

I looked the luminous dial of my watch. 7.30pm. In the event the moon did not rise until 2.30am. Meanwhile, we lay stretched out on our individual patch of sandy earth, earth which grew harder and harder with each passing hour. Above us we could see, through the fine tracery of the acacias, the star-studded, but moonless sky. Down at ground level, among the volcanic boulders, it was as black as the pit. Conversation languished. I had sucked my last orange dry. All my water bottles were empty. Dehydration was uniform. We could barely enunciate, let alone hold a rational discourse.

As I scanned the heavens, the winking light of a high flying jet crossed the firmament. I remembered that we lay below the flight path of planes from Nairobi bound for Europe. With hideous clarity I could imagine the air-conditioned passengers lolling back in their seats, watching their movies, quaffing beakers of chilled champagne, sipping glasses of claret, nibbling on morsels of chicken breast, munching crackers and cheese, and being fawned over by well proportioned stewardesses..

With cruel regularity the aircraft passed overhead, mindless of our sufferings below. My reverie came to an abrupt end.

'Shit!' I shouted as something inserted its pincers into my backside. 'What the hell was that?' I scrambled to my feet. The something scuttled away.

'Bloody hell. Whose idea was this anyway?'

'Yours, I think,' said Paul.

'Well, *you* agreed pretty fast, with Watson there close behind.' This topic occupied us for a useful 30 minutes. The hours slowly dragged past. Finally at 2.30am the faint light of the rising moon shone down on our beds of pain. Outlines of rocks appeared, trunks of trees became visible, thorny thickets showed themselves. We rose to our feet and within ten minutes were on the road.

By the soft light of the risen moon we plodded in silence towards Kapedo. It was hot. Our mouths were so dry that we were incapable of speech. We arrived at the bridge spanning the Kapedo river, to whose bank we now tottered.

The water was stagnant and warm and there was no flow. Heaven alone knew what it contained in the way of bacteria, fungi and protozoa. We scooped it up eagerly and drank deeply.

Marginally refreshed, we pressed on.

'You realise, don't you,' said the cheerful Paul. 'that we have another five kilometres to cover *after* Kapedo? I estimate that we've walked 40km so far, so what's another five?'

'With a bit of luck we might be back in time for early morning tea!' I said.

311

By the time we reached the suburbs of Kapedo the fluids imbibed at the stream had evaporated and our mouths were like cement. We trudged past the outer humpies towards the mission.

'Hey, look,' croaked Graeme, 'isn't that the Land Rover we came in yesterday?' Sure, enough, there was a white Land Rover parked outside a stone house.

'Shall we knock?' said Paul.

'Why not,' I said, 'it's only half past three.'

We knocked, and almost immediately the door was opened by a beaming African. 'Come in! Come in! We have been expecting you!'

Really?

We filed in. The room was lit by a Tilley lantern and a couple of candles. Kapedo was far beyond the reach of such comforts as electricity. Our host was Charles Munyua, a catechist from Meru, on the north-east slopes of Mt. Kenya.

'Yes, your friends said you would be along some time, so we' – he gestured to a buxom, smiling woman hovering behind him – 'knew you would be hungry and thirsty.'

'So sit down! Sit down!'

Charles and his wife were Christian hospitality personified. They produced pots of hot tea, cool water and mountains of fresh pancakes, which we devoured to the last morsel.

'Now,' said Charles, 'here is the key to the Land Rover. Drive to your camp and rest!'

We shook hands with the splendid couple.

'Safari njema!' they called as we trundled away.

We sat in silence for a while, humbled by our experience.

It was 5.30 and still dark as we approached our camp. A nightjar fluttered up from the dust in front of our headlights. A soft winged owl drifted through the trees. A jackal, head turned in our direction, trotted into the bush and vanished.

We cut the engine and free wheeled into the sleeping camp.

Silently we opened the doors and stiffly tiptoed towards our respective tents.

Still torchless I knelt down to crawl into our waist-high two person teepee. As I fumbled with the zip, I realised that there was a basin on the ground beside the entrance. Mmm, I thought, that's pretty careless. I could easily have stumbled over that. Then, wait a mo! There was a bottle lying in the water, with, yes! an opener tied by a string to its neck.

In the now half light, I held it up, the better to scrutinise the label. Yes! Tusker! Time for a Tusker! Berna's thoughtfulness and foresight had come up trumps. She would have known that I would be gasping for a beer on my return, no matter what the hour. I snapped off the top and in two enormous gulps, drained the lot.

Berna was awake.

'So, Mr Cran,' she said, 'back in time for tea, eh? I seem to have heard that said before. A trifle late, aren't we?'

'Yes, sorry about that. We were overcome by the elements and were obliged to bivouac until the moon rose.'

'Oh, yes, and what elements were those?'

'Darkness.'

'By darkness? Do you mean to lie there like a great beached whale and tell me that three so-called experienced mountaineers went out to climb a mountain without so much as a penlight? I wouldn't even cross the road without a torch!'

'We each thought the other would be carrying one. Besides we *had* intended to be back in time in time for afternoon tea!'

'Well, in about half an hour it will be time for early morning tea!'

For 30 minutes I slept like the dead, before being roused by daylight and what seemed like a great deal of unnecessary activity and unwarranted noise. After breakfast we packed the tank and drove back along the track to the road, before trundling through Kapedo. No welcoming committee was on hand this time. The inhabitants all appeared to be still abed.

We reached home at 1.45 in the afternoon. The day, however, was not yet done. At 4pm I was in the surgery treating dogs, desperately trying to keep my eyes open.

That evening, as we were unpacking the tent on the verandah, out of its folds scuttled a large, sooty-black scorpion, sting-ended tail erect, pincers snapping in fury. We looked at the scorpion. It looked at us. 'Well,' it seemed to be saying, before vanishing into an adjacent untrimmed thicket, 'was it really all worth it?'

'You bet your spiny ass it was,' we replied, 'and what's more, we'll be back for another round.'

Also published by Merlin Unwin Books

And Miles to Go Before I Sleep Hugh Cran

A Farmer's Lot Roger Evans
Over the Farmer's Gate Roger Evans
A View from the Tractor Roger Evans
A Job for all Seasons Phyllida Barstow
My Animals and Other Family Phyllida Barstow
The Yellow Earl Douglas Sutherland
The Byerley Turk Jeremy James
Saddletramp Jeremy James
Vagabond Jeremy James
The Poacher's Handbook Ian Niall
The Way of a Countryman Ian Niall
The Naturalist's Bedside Book BB
The Countryman's Bedside Book BB
Training your Puppy Fiona Baird
Venison José Souto

www.merlinunwin.co.uk

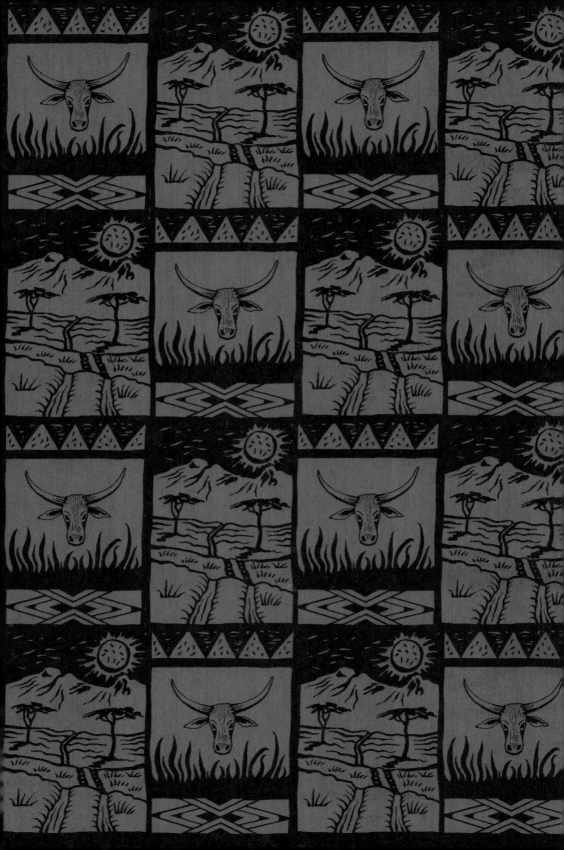